Edited by
Wayne Martin,
Oksana Suchowersky,
Katharina Kovacs Burns,
and Egon Jonsson

Parkinson Disease

Edited by Wayne Martin, Oksana Suchowersky,
Katharina Kovacs Burns, and Egon Jonsson

Parkinson Disease

A Health Policy Perspective

WILEY-VCH Verlag GmbH & Co. KGaA

The Editors

Prof. Dr. Wayne Martin
University of Alberta
Movement Disorders Program
Edmonton, Alberta T5G 0B7
Canada

Prof. Dr. Oksana Suchowersky
University of Calgary
Movement Disorders Program
Hotchkiss Brain Institute
Calgary, Alberta T2N 4N1
Canada

Dr. Katharina Kovacs Burns
University of Alberta
Health Sciences Council
Edmonton, Alberta T6G 1K8
Canada

Prof. Egon Jonsson
University of Alberta
University of Calgary
Department of Public
Health Science
Institute of Health Economics
10405 Jasper Ave
Edmonton, Alberta T5J 3N4
Canada

Series Editor

Prof. Egon Jonsson
University of Alberta
University of Calgary
Department of Public
Health Science
Institute of Health Economics
10405 Jasper Ave
Edmonton, Alberta T5J 3N4
Canada

Cover   Photo by Walter Tychnowicz/Wiresharp
Photography Edmonton, Canada

Library of Congress Card No.: applied for

British Library Cataloguing-in-Publication Data
A catalogue record for this book is available from the British Library.

Bibliographic information published by the Deutsche Nationalbibliothek
The Deutsche Nationalbibliothek lists this publication in the Deutsche Nationalbibliografie; detailed bibliographic data are available on the Internet at <http://dnb.d-nb.de>.

© 2010 WILEY-VCH Verlag GmbH & Co. KGaA, Weinheim

Composition   Toppan Best-set Premedia Limited, Hong Kong
Printing and Bookbinding   betz-druck GmbH, Darmstadt
Cover Design   Adam Design, Weinheim

Printed in the Federal Republic of Germany
Printed on acid-free paper

ISBN: 978-3-527-32779-9
ISSN: 1864-9947

Contents

Parkinson Disease – A Health Policy Perspective. Edited by Wayne Martin, Oksana Suchowersky,
Katharina Kovacs Burns, and Egon Jonsson
Copyright © 2010 WILEY-VCH Verlag GmbH & Co. KGaA, Weinheim
ISBN: 978-3-527-32779-9

Preface

Two years ago, the Institute of Health Economics (IHE) initiated a discussion about different aspects of Parkinson Disease. The aim was to identify potential gaps between findings from research and health policy and practice. Initially, the IHE invited a small group of researchers to these discussions; however, the pilot scheme quickly grew into a larger project and eventually involved 18 people representing clinical and health services research, patient associations, and persons with Parkinson Disease.

In order to make a difference for people with Parkinson Disease, this group felt that they should focus on the policy aspects of the disease, namely the organization and management of services for people with this condition.

This book is written for a broad audience – not only for health policy makers but also for anyone interested in this condition, such as people with the disease, family members and other caregivers, healthcare professionals, and community health and social services providers. It includes recommendations of what might be done at the policy level to improve the situation for people with this ailment.

Parkinson disease is a complex, chronic condition that presents challenges not only to those living with it but also to their caregivers, to their healthcare providers, to Parkinson societies, and to health policy makers. As one of many chronic diseases, it is important to not lose sight of Parkinson Disease and the associated impact and burden, particularly in view of aging populations and the projected increases in the numbers of people that will be affected by this condition.

We would like to acknowledge the contributions of all those individuals who shared their personal stories and experiences of Parkinson Disease, who contributed to the chapters and their editing, and to the IHE staff that provided administrative support, namely Wendy McIndoo, Kris Schindel, and Melissa Waltner.

Institute of Health Economics

Egon Jonsson, Paula Corabian,
and Liz Dennett

Acknowledgment

The printing of this book has been made possible by a grant from The Parkinson's Society of Alberta.

Summary and Policy Considerations

Wayne Martin, Oksana Suchowersky, Katharina Kovacs Burns and Egon Jonsson

It is estimated that six million people worldwide have Parkinson disease (PD), with about one million cases in the US [1] and 100000 in Canada [2] (although prevalence estimates vary widely from study to study [3–8]). In the Province of Alberta, there are about 7000–8000 people with the disease (see Chapter 11). Moreover, as the population continues to age this number will increase substantially.

Parkinson disease is a both chronic and progressive condition, which causes significant disability, handicap, and suffering and impairs the quality of life for the affected person and his or her family. The management of the condition may be improved in many different aspects. A major theme of this book is the need to coordinate services to more effectively utilize existing scarce expertise in the field, and to provide more coherent services from interdisciplinary and multidisciplinary teams composed of expertise in different aspects of health, social and community care for the person with PD.

There is, therefore, a need to develop a comprehensive strategy for early and accurate diagnoses and effective treatment, support and care for patients with PD. Such a strategy would require a more detailed investigation than has been presented in this book. However, it is suggested that responsible authorities establish a special committee to review the findings presented here, along with other data and facts about the situation for people with PD and other neurological diseases, and subsequently develop a proposal of how to improve the services for these patients. It is also recommended that actual or virtual centers for PD are established (where needed) that would consolidate the research, expertise and other resources in the best possible manner.

The following is a condensed overview of the common themes presented in this book.

A Structured Surveillance System for PD

Some countries and states have established registries of different diseases that are used in the planning, monitoring, and assessment of the provided services. Currently, there is no structured surveillance system or registry for PD in Canada

Parkinson Disease – A Health Policy Perspective. Edited by Wayne Martin, Oksana Suchowersky, Katharina Kovacs Burns, and Egon Jonsson
Copyright © 2010 WILEY-VCH Verlag GmbH & Co. KGaA, Weinheim
ISBN: 978-3-527-32779-9

or in its individual provinces (see Chapter 11). Moreover, a lack of information on the prevalence and incidence of the condition, particularly as the population ages and more people are diagnosed with PD, may hamper health planning, including the appropriate allocation of resources. A PD Registry and structured surveillance system are needed to more accurately and consistently track relevant data about PD, including population-based trends. This would also address the gap in epidemiological data that currently exists.

Accuracy of Diagnosis

Even with advances in clinical assessment and developments in medical technology, the accurate diagnosis of PD remains a major challenge (see Chapter 2). At present, there is no reliable technology or test that clearly distinguishes PD from other similar conditions. Currently, the diagnosis is based primarily on the patient's history and clinical examination, with examinations often carried out in a primary healthcare setting, without necessarily having access to a specialist in brain disorders. Therefore, in order to avoid underdiagnoses or misdiagnoses, it is important to coordinate the available capacity to increase timely and easy access to specialist evaluation and treatment.

Availability and Access to Needed Treatment and Services

An early diagnosis and appropriate treatment is of fundamental importance for all patients. In PD patients, this alleviates stress and anxiety regarding physical and psychological signs and symptoms (see Chapters 2 and 3). A tailor-made management approach using various therapies is critical for optimum care, while easy access to selected treatment choices may minimize any functional disability and maximize the patient's quality of life. This includes the prevention of adverse reactions to medications, and the coordination of different appropriate therapies (Chapters 3, 6, and 7). Interdisciplinary teams are critical to the success of managing PD.

As indicated in Chapters 12 and 13, it is also important to consider the needs of the caregivers, who are often spouses or family members. Indeed, PD will have a substantial impact on the health and social well-being of caregivers – an issue that has been well documented (see Chapter 13). Evidence from clinical practice makes it clear that an holistic approach to treatment and care is essential to ensure that individuals with PD are able to maintain their independent functioning capacity, and have an acceptable quality of life (Chapters 3, 12, and 13). Availability and access to different services are high priorities for people with PD. Highly sought-after services include access to specialists and movement-disorder clinics, as well as to various therapies (physiotherapy, physical, speech and occupational), counseling, support groups, home care, adult day care, respite for caregivers, and others. One serious barrier to accessing services for people with PD who live in rural communities is the fact that many of them cannot drive or do not have transportation available (see Chapters 12 and 13).

Impact on Quality of Life and Personal Cost for Persons with PD

Parkinson disease has a clear and strong negative impact on both the physical and mental aspects of the health-related quality of life, and this has been well documented in the scientific literature (see Chapters 12–15). One personal burden for those with PD and their caregivers is simply to understand and cope with the physical and mental changes and deterioration that result from PD (see Chapters 12–15).

Many people with PD have to make substantial financial sacrifices in order to maintain their quality of life. PD is common among older individuals who are close to retirement or who have retired, and who are often living on a fixed and modest income or have had to stop working at an early age. They may lose their driving privileges and independence, and have to pay out-of-pocket for some medications, nonprescriptive supplements, home renovations, medical devices, and much-needed therapies. By the same token, the caregivers' health and well-being will also be affected; they may have to stop working in order to become a full-time caregiver, or perhaps start working to supplement the household's income (see Chapters 12 and 13). Whilst the contribution of the caregivers clearly reduces the burden on the healthcare system, the extent of this has not been well researched, and neither is it recognized in healthcare policy making (Chapters 8 and 13).

As PD progresses, the severity of the condition increases such that the patient requires more access to specialists and to specialized services, care, and assistive devices (Chapter 12). This not only places greater demands on the health system but also adds to the overall cost burden of PD (see Chapter 8). Moreover, as the population continues to age and the projected rates of PD increase, the burden of costs will rise accordingly unless strategies are put in place to address these various cost-escalating factors.

Existing Research Evidence and Future Research Needs

A review of the literature published between January 2006 and October 2008 revealed 18 relevant systematic reviews and 11 practice guidelines related to PD (see Chapter 9). These selected studies reflect and confirm the findings in some of the previous chapters, and also provide health policy makers with useful evidence for their decision making. However, as they are limited in their range of topics, there is a need for more systematic reviews concerning many other aspects of PD.

The gaps in PD research, including basic research, epidemiological studies and risk factors, as well as the impact of therapeutics and therapies in clinical studies, and policy-related research, are highlighted in Chapter 10. Although both genetic and environmental influences related to the development of PD have been identified to some extent, the complex interaction between these factors remains largely unexplored. Close collaborative links between basic and clinical neuroscientists will enhance the likelihood of developing relevant new insights into the mechanisms underlying the etiology and inexorably progressive nature of PD. There is also an identified need for health services research related to PD, especially in view of the fairly good availability of research findings of the management and organization of services in other chronic disease areas (see Chapter 12). Other research gaps are noted in areas such as the burden and costs of disease and treatments (Chapter 8), and in comparing various interventions and their impact on quality of life (Chapters 3–7, 12, 13, and 15).

Specific policy considerations for Alberta are presented in Chapter 16.

References

1 Michael J. (2006) Fox Foundation for Parkinson's Research [Internet]. Parkinson 101. Available at: http://www.michaeljfox.org/living_aboutParkinsons_parkinsons101.cfm (accessed 8 May 2009).

2 Parkinson Society Canada, Health Canada (2003) *Parkinson's Disease: Social and Economic Impact*, Parkinson Society Canada, Toronto, ON. Available at: http://www.parkinson.ca/atf/cf/%7B9ebd08a9-7886-4b2d-a1c4-a131e7096bf8%7D/PARKINSONSDISEASE_EN.PDF (accessed 8 May 2009).

3 National Institute of Neurological Disorders and Stroke [Internet] (2004) Parkinson's disease backgrounder. Available at: http://www.ninds.nih.gov/disorders/ parkinsons_disease/parkinsons_disease_backgrounder.htm (accessed 8 May 2009).

4 National Parkinson Foundation [Internet] About Parkinson's disease. Available at: http://www.parkinson.org/Page.aspx?pid=225 (accessed 8 May 2009).

5 de Lau, L.M. and Breteler, M.B. (2006) Epidemiology of Parkinson's disease. *Lancet Neurology*, **5**, 525–535.

6 Nussbaum, R.L. and Ellis, C.E. (2003) Alzheimer's disease and Parkinson's disease. *New England Journal of Medicine*, **348**, 1356–1364.

7 Tanner, C.M. and Goldman, S.M. (1996) Epidemiology of Parkinson's disease. *Neurology Clinics*, **14**, 317–335.

8 de Rijk, M.C., Launer, L.J., Berger, K., Breteler, M.M.B., Dartigues, J.F., Baldereschi, M., *et al.* (2000) Prevalence of Parkinson's disease in Europe: a collaborative study of population-based cohorts. *Neurology*, **54** (11) Suppl. 5, S21–S23.

List of Contributors

Paula Corabian
Institute of Health Economics
#1200, 10405 Jasper Avenue
Edmonton Alberta, T5J 3N4
Canada

Ms. Liz Dennett
Institute of Health Economics
#1200, 10405 Jasper Avenue
Edmonton Alberta T5J 3N4
Canada

Lorelei Derwent
Movement Disorders Clinic
University of Calgary, Area 3
Clinical Neurosciences
3350 Hospital Drive, NW
Calgary Alberta T2N 4N1
Canada

Shirley Heschuk
Faculty of Pharmacy &
Pharmaceutical Sciences
3126 Dentistry/Pharmacy Centre
University of Alberta
Edmonton Alberta T6G 2N8
Canada

Bin Hu
Department of Clinical Neurosciences
University of Calgary
3350 Hospital Drive, NW
Calgary Alberta T2N 4N1
Canada

Karen Hunka
Movement Disorders Clinic
University of Calgary, Area 3
Clinical Neurosciences
3350 Hospital Drive, NW
Calgary Alberta T2N 4N1
Canada

Allyson Jones
Department of Physical Therapy
2-50 Corbett Hall
University of Alberta
Edmonton Alberta T6G 2G4
Canada

Egon Jonsson
Institute of Health Economics
#1200, 10405 Jasper Avenue
Edmonton AB T5J 3N4
Canada

Parkinson Disease – A Health Policy Perspective. Edited by Wayne Martin, Oksana Suchowersky,
Katharina Kovacs Burns, and Egon Jonsson
Copyright © 2010 WILEY-VCH Verlag GmbH & Co. KGaA, Weinheim
ISBN: 978-3-527-32779-9

Kathy Kovacs Burns
Health Sciences Council
University of Alberta
305 Campus Tower
Edmonton Alberta T5G 1K8
Canada

Wayne Martin
University of Alberta
Movement Disorders Program
Edmonton Alberta T6G 0B7
Canada

Arto Ohinmaa
Institute of Health Economics
1200, 10405 Jasper Avenue
Edmonton Alberta T5J 3N4
Canada

John Petryshen
Parkinson's Society of Southern
Alberta
102, 5636 Burbank Crescent S.E.
Westech Building
Calgary Alberta T2H 1Z6
Canada

Joyce Pinckney
4015 – 77 Street NW
Edmonton Alberta T6K 0X7
Canada

Sheri L. Pohar
Canadian Agency for Drugs and
Technologies in Health
Edmonton Alberta T5J 3G1
Canada

Ranjit Ranawaya
University of Calgary
Movement Disorders Clinic
Area 3
Clinical Neurosciences
3350 Hospital Drive, NW
Calgary Alberta T2N 4N1
Canada

Cheryl Sadowski
University of Alberta
Faculty of Pharmacy and
Pharmaceutical Sciences
5068B Dentistry/Pharmacy Centre
Edmonton Alberta T6G 2N8
Canada

Oksana Suchowersky
University of Calgary
Movement Disorders Clinic Area 3
Clinical Neurosciences
3350 Hospital Drive, NW
Calgary Alberta T2N 4N1
Canada

Larry Svenson
Epidemiologic Surveillance Team
Health and Wellness
24th Floor Telus Plaza North Tower
10025 Jasper Avenue
Edmonton Alberta T5J 1S6
Canada

Marguerite Wieler
University of Alberta
Movement Disorder Clinic
Edmonton Alberta T6G 0B7
Canada

Ray Williams
Parkinson's Society of Alberta
Room 3Y18
Edmonton General
11111 Jasper Avenue
Edmonton Alberta T5K 0L4
Canada

Nikolaos Yiannakoulias
McMaster University
School of Geography and Earth Sciences
1280 Main Street West
Hamilton, Ontario L8S 4K1
Canada

Stories by (all from Alberta, Canada):

Bill Austen
Jackie Bodie
Cindy Exton
Carol Hale
Jean Harkness
Gunnar Henriksson
Linda Kenney

Georg Kriegel
Marlene Nypuik
Bill Pinckney
Elda Pinckney
Joyce Pinckney
Al Smith
Alison Wood

Part I
Parkinson Disease – Diagnosis and Treatment

Parkinson Disease – A Health Policy Perspective. Edited by Wayne Martin, Oksana Suchowersky,
Katharina Kovacs Burns, and Egon Jonsson
Copyright © 2010 WILEY-VCH Verlag GmbH & Co. KGaA, Weinheim
ISBN: 978-3-527-32779-9

A Spouse's Story

We Will Live for Today

Bill Austen

Parkinson's Disease was something I had heard of, but knew very little about. However, I was on a huge learning curve when my wife (Rose) was diagnosed with the disease in June of 2002. My initial reaction was very emotional–along with fear of the unknown and of the future. My fears proved to be unfounded after a session with Jan Hansen, the Support Services Director, of the Parkinson's Society of Southern Alberta. Rose has always had a positive attitude and looked after her physical well-being, which is important for those with Parkinson's.

At this point in time we have been very fortunate in that the disease has not had a great impact on our everyday life. Yes, some days there have to be some changes as each day is different, so we must be prepared for those changes to our schedules. Rose has days that we call "A Parkinson's Day" where she may need to rest a lot, or just need quiet time alone. There are also those days when she will drive herself to activities, while on other days she would rather not drive, so I am prepared for that change in my plans. Falling is a problem–we don't know when it will happen, where it will happen, or how serious the after-affects will be. Because of her poor balance, using the escalators in the shopping malls and department stores is a problem, so I am with her when she needs to shop. Her muscular strength has diminished somewhat, so there are physical things that she needs some help with. There are friends that we don't see as often, and that is fine as that is their way of dealing with the disease, and it has given us the opportunity to make new friends. At this point I don't consider myself a caregiver–more like the spouse who tries to support her.

I am however, familiar with the caregiver role, having been at her side while she recovered from a serious car accident. Following that accident our lives changed dramatically for several years, and I became the household engineer–cooking, cleaning, shopping, etc. It was an eye-opener into the work involved with running a household. I feel at this point that Rose and I are ready for whatever road Parkinson's takes us on. With Rose's attitude and through our support group, together with the Support Services team of the Parkinson's Society, we will live for today–but we will also be prepared for tomorrow and the future.

1
Parkinson Disease

Ray Williams

In 1817, James Parkinson, an English doctor, published *An Essay on the Shaking Palsy*, in which he characterized the symptoms he had observed in six people, some of whom were his patients, but the others he had just observed in his neighborhood. His writings described "… involuntary tremulous motion, with lessened muscular power, in parts not in action and even when supported; with a propensity to bend the trunk forwards, and to pass from a walking to a running pace; the senses and intellect being uninjured." Four decades later, the "father of clinical neurology", the French doctor Jean-Martin Charcot added symptoms to Parkinson's clinical description and attached the name Parkinson Disease to the syndrome [1].

1.1
Patient Burden

Parkinson disease (PD) is a common ailment; one in every 1000 of the population will develop the condition, and for those aged between 60 and 80 years the risk is approximately one in 100 [2]. While symptoms generally appear around age of 60, they can present in much younger people, which makes it a condition that does not recognize the boundaries of age, gender, or race.

PD is a progressive, neurologic disorder caused by a degeneration of dopaminergic neurons. Once a significant number of these neurons has been lost, that part of the brain that promotes movement no longer works effectively. As a result, people with PD experience substantial impairments in motor control and movement.

1.2
Characteristics of Parkinson Disease

PD is clinically characterized by four main features: (i) shaking back and forth when the limb is relaxed (resting tremor); (ii) slow physical movement (bradykinesia); (iii) stiffness, or resistance of the limb to passive movement when the limb

Parkinson Disease – A Health Policy Perspective. Edited by Wayne Martin, Oksana Suchowersky, Katharina Kovacs Burns, and Egon Jonsson
Copyright © 2010 WILEY-VCH Verlag GmbH & Co. KGaA, Weinheim
ISBN: 978-3-527-32779-9

is relaxed (rigidity); and (iv) poor balance (postural instability). The onset of these features is asymmetric, with one limb being affected first. The signs and symptoms then spread to the other limb on the same side, and later affect the limbs on the opposite side of the body.

Other common signs may include shuffling and freezing while walking, a stooped posture, difficulty with fine coordinated movements, difficulty in swallowing (dysphagia), small handwriting (micrographia), a soft voice (hypophonia), and a mask-like face with little expression (hypomimia).

In addition to experiencing any of these movement-related symptoms, suffering from PD impacts upon all aspects of the affected individual's life, including their emotional well-being and social functioning. For example, depression has been reported to occur in the majority of people with PD, which seems to be more frequent than in many other chronic diseases. Apathy also is experienced frequently by those living with the condition. PD-associated fatigue can be debilitating, and is an issue of growing research focus. In one study, almost half of the patients with PD claimed that fatigue was one of the three most disabling symptoms of the condition [3].

Weight loss also negatively impacts quality of life for people with PD, and can become especially marked during the advanced stages of the condition. A number of factors lead to such weight loss, including a reduced energy intake and an increased energy expenditure, a loss of appetite due to a disturbed smell and taste, a slowing of the gastrointestinal tract, as well as depression, nausea, and constipation.

Cognitive dysfunction and decline, dementia, hallucinations, and psychosis, can also occur during the advanced stages of PD. Other troubling symptoms include urinary incontinence, sleep–wake cycle dysregulation, and pain. All of these so-called "non-motor" symptoms can be particularly problematic, as there are few effective treatments.

1.3
Diagnosis of Parkinson Disease

A number of other conditions have a similar clinical presentation as PD, but at present there is no reliable technology or test that can distinguish between these ailments and PD. Rather, the diagnosis of PD is based primarily on the patient's history and a clinical examination.

1.4
Treatment for Parkinson Disease

Five classes of medications are available to treat the movement-related (motor) symptoms of PD, including: levodopa; dopaminergic agonists; anticholinergics; amantadine; and monoamine-oxidase B inhibitors.

Levodopa remains the most effective medicine, in particular for treating rigidity and slowness of movement. It is usually combined with another medication that works to prevent the rapid breakdown of levodopa in the digestive system. Most patients initially do well on levodopa. However, the treatment is associated with several side effects that people with PD may experience, such as nausea and appetite loss, involuntary movements, twisting motions and abnormal postures (dystonia), hallucinations and paranoia, and even impulse-control problems such as excessive gambling. Therefore, treatment must be adjusted individually for each patient so as to maximize the benefits and minimize the side effects.

Surgical interventions for PD were attempted as early as the 1930s, but were abandoned because of the high morbidity and mortality related to the procedures. However, in 1987, it was first shown that deep brain electric stimulation could improve tremor with PD patients. Since then, this technology has been developed for several motor symptoms in PD, although the procedure is still associated with serious side effects.

The first attempt to treat patients with PD with *cell transplantation* was made by a Swedish research group during the 1980s [4]. This involved transplanting cells from one area to another within the patient's brain, but it caused serious side effects. In recent years, attention has been focused on stem-cell research, which has shown promise but is currently still in the experimental phases.

Patients often turn to *complementary and alternative medicine* in search of therapies to help them cope. The most common reasons stated for accessing complimentary therapies are to achieve better symptom relief, to augment the effects of prescription medications, and to boost strength. However, there is limited scientific data available on the effects of most alternative therapies. This topic is explored in greater detail in Chapter 6.

There is some evidence suggesting that, with regular exercise, PD patients may experience an improvement in their motor function, gait, and balance [5].

Ongoing research in PD strives to improve available treatments and to slow the progression of the disease. In the meantime, access to multidisciplinary services and support (e.g., specialized medical care, physiotherapy, occupational therapy, speech language therapy, and community support programs) is essential for good outcomes.

New theories have emerged about the onset of PD actually occurring many years before it is currently diagnosed. This may have substantial implications for the early detection and treatment of this chronic disease.

References

1 Goetz, C.G. (2005) Jean-Martin Charcot (1825–1893). *Journal of Neurology*, **252**, 374–375.

2 de Lau, L.M. and Breteler, M.B. (2006) Epidemiology of Parkinson's disease. *Lancet Neurology*, **5**, 525–535.

3 Friedman, J. and Friedman, H. (2001) Fatigue in Parkinson's disease: a nine-year follow-up. *Movement Disorders*, **6**, 1120–1122.

4 Backlund, E.O., Granberg, P.O., Hamberger, B., Knutsson, E., Mårtensson,

A., Sedvall, G., *et al.* (1985) Transplantation of adrenal medullary tissue to striatum in parkinsonism. First clinical trials. *Journal of Neurosurgery*, **62** (2), 169–173.

5 Goodwin, V.A., Richards, S.H., Taylor, R.S., Taylor, A.H., and Campbell, J.L. (2008) The effectiveness of exercise interventions for people with Parkinson's disease: a systematic review and meta analysis. *Movement Disorders*, **23** (5), 631–640.

A Patient's Story

I Will Win My Own Race

Marlene Nypuik

In June 2002 I ran my first marathon in celebration of my 60th birthday, and as I crossed the finish line my life would change forever. Then, in May 2005, when I was diagnosed with Parkinson's Disease, my life changed forever ... again.

My first reaction to the diagnosis was "... where did I go wrong?" Over the years I've led a healthy, active lifestyle; I ran everyday and have always been very conscious of my health. One of the first things I noticed was my left hand having trouble keeping up with my right. Now I'm a person living with Parkinson's and I still live my life according to this balance.

Although I have retired after 28 years as a court reporter, I continue to train and run races. Each day I head out of the door for my morning run and I am thankful; another day, another run. Someday it may be only for a walk, but for now I run. So far, my symptoms are not pronounced and I am not on any medication. I have good days and I have better days.

Since my diagnosis I've spent a lot of time reflecting on the things that are most important in my life, like family and friends. I try to concentrate on the things that I can do instead of what I can't, and to be thankful for each day.

The Parkinson's Society of Alberta has helped me a great deal, and I appreciate their support and compassion.

And on the days when I struggle with the "what ifs", I am reminded of the words of John Bingham: "The miracle isn't that I finish. The miracle is that I have the courage to start."

2
Clinical Features of Parkinson Disease

Wayne Martin

2.1
Introduction

Parkinson disease (PD) was originally described by James Parkinson in 1817 in *An Essay on the Shaking Palsy*, based on observations of his own patients and on others that he had seen on the streets of London [1]. He accurately described the motor symptoms that form the core features of the disease, but also identified non-motor features that are now receiving increasing attention. It was Charcot, a French pioneer of neurology, who first used the term "Parkinson disease" in 1861 [2].

2.2
Cardinal Features

The principal features of PD consist of tremor, akinesia, rigidity, and postural instability; this combination of neurological features is referred to as *parkinsonism*. PD is but one cause of parkinsonism, albeit perhaps the most common cause. These features are not always present in all individuals with early PD, although they do tend to be more prevalent as the disease progresses.

Tremor is the most common initial feature, although it may be absent in up to 25% of patients with PD [3]. The tremor may be present intermittently at disease onset, and noted primarily during stress. Most commonly, the tremor is present when the limbs are at rest, and is reduced substantially by sustained posture or voluntary movement. It tends to have a supination–pronation (twisting) movement in the forearm, with alternating contraction of opposing muscle groups at a frequency of about 4–6 Hz [4]. The term "pill-rolling" is often used to describe the characteristics of the tremor. The onset of parkinsonian tremor is almost always on one side of the body, and usually in the upper limb, although in some individuals the tremor starts instead in a lower limb. The jaw or tongue may be affected, but not the head (unlike essential tremor, in which head tremor may be prominent). Although a resting tremor is most typical of PD, about 50% of affected

Parkinson Disease – A Health Policy Perspective. Edited by Wayne Martin, Oksana Suchowersky, Katharina Kovacs Burns, and Egon Jonsson
Copyright © 2010 WILEY-VCH Verlag GmbH & Co. KGaA, Weinheim
ISBN: 978-3-527-32779-9

individuals will have, in addition, an action tremor present during voluntary movement [5].

Problems related to the control of movement in PD include an impaired initiation of movement (akinesia), a reduced movement amplitude (hypokinesia), and
slowed movement (bradykinesia). These problems can affect virtually all voluntary
and many involuntary movements. In the clinic, the assessment of these features
includes observing the patient performing repeated tasks, such as tapping of the
thumb and index finger, hand opening and closing, hand pronation–supination,
and foot tapping. The parkinsonian individual will perform these movements
slowly, often with evidence of fatigability so that the repetitive movement progressively slows, with decreasing amplitude, and often with periodic arrests in movement. Other manifestations of bradykinesia/akinesia include decreased facial
expression, small handwriting (micrographia), decreased arm swing when walking,
and a tendency to take short, shuffling steps.

Rigidity refers to the increased muscle resistance to passive movement about a
joint (increased muscle tone) that is evident to the examiner during slow movements, throughout the full range of joint movement, and affecting flexors as well
as extensors. In patients with mild PD, the rigidity may be evident only with
"distraction"; that is, while repetitive movements are being performed with the
opposite limb. *Cogwheeling* (a ratchet sensation) is typically observed when testing
for rigidity in the parkinsonian individual, presumably because of an element of
tremor superimposed on the rigidity.

Postural instability (impaired balance) is usually not a problem in early PD, but
becomes very common in more advanced disease. In fact, if postural instability is
present at the onset of symptoms, then a diagnosis other than PD should be suspected [6]. With progression, posture becomes increasingly flexed, and reflexes
involved in maintaining balance become impaired. Retropulsion describes a tendency to take repeated steps backwards in response to a sudden threat to maintained balance, such as that exerted with the pull test [7].

The *diagnosis* of PD is made on the basis of the characteristic clinical features.
In a recently published door-to-door survey, up to 24% of cases were newly detected
at the time of the survey [8], indicating that underdiagnosis is common. A number
of other disorders can also masquerade as PD, leading to potential misdiagnosis.
Autopsy studies have suggested that the clinical diagnosis of PD may be incorrect
in up to 24% of cases. Clinical expertise is important in diagnosing PD, as indicated by significantly greater accuracy of diagnosis in a specialty movement disorders environment. Hughes *et al.* reported a sensitivity of 91% for the clinical
diagnosis of PD in this setting [9]. A commonly used set of clinical criteria for the
diagnosis of PD is listed in Table 2.1.

2.3
Differential Diagnosis

The features that point most strongly to a diagnosis of PD, as opposed to other
parkinsonian syndromes, include an asymmetry of clinical symptomatology, being

Table 2.1 UK Parkinson's Disease Society Brain Bank criteria for the diagnosis of PD [10].

Step 1 Diagnosis of Parkinsonian syndrome
    Bradykinesia
    At least one of the following:
        Muscular rigidity
        Rest tremor
        Postural instability
Step 2 Exclusion criteria including:
        History of repeated strokes
        History of repeated head injury
        History of definite encephalitis
        Oculogyric crises
        Neuroleptic treatment at onset of symptoms
        More than one affected relative
        Sustained remission
        Strictly unilateral features after 3 years
        Supranuclear gaze palsy
        Cerebellar signs
        Early severe autonomic involvement
        Early severe dementia with disturbances of memory, language, and praxis
        Babinski sign
        Presence of cerebral tumor or communicating hydrocephalus on CT scan
        Negative response to large doses of levodopa (if malabsorption excluded)
        MPTP exposure
Step 3 Supportive prospective criteria (at least three required):
        Unilateral onset
        Rest tremor
        Evidence of progression
        Persistent asymmetry
        Excellent response to levodopa
        Severe levodopa -induced chorea
        Levodopa response for 5+ years
        Clinical course of 10+ years

CT = computed tomography; MPTP = 1-methyl-4-phenyl-1,2,3,6-tetrahydropyridine.

worse on one side of the body than the other, the presence of a resting tremor, and a significant, ongoing symptomatic benefit from levodopa, one of the major drugs used to treat PD. It is important, however, to consider other conditions in the process of making this clinical diagnosis, including the following.

2.3.1
Essential Tremor

The tremor of PD can be confused with that of essential tremor (ET), although the characteristics of the tremor differ. In contrast to PD, the limb tremor of ET is present primarily with sustained posture and during voluntary movement, and is markedly reduced when the limbs are in a resting position. In ET, the tremor has a typical frequency of 4–12 Hz, and is in a flexion–extension direction with cocontraction of opposing muscles. The shaky handwriting that is characteristic of ET is very different from the micrographia (small handwriting) that is characteristic of PD. Patients with ET do not have parkinsonism, in that their symptoms are limited to tremor without other features such as bradykinesia or rigidity.

2.3.2
Progressive Supranuclear Palsy

Several other neurodegenerative syndromes share features with PD. Although many of these alternate diagnoses require post-mortem pathological examination for confirmation, they can often be identified with reasonable certainty with clinical examination. Progressive supranuclear palsy (PSP) is characterized by the combination of parkinsonism and abnormal eye movements. The ocular changes primarily affect rapid eye movements, particularly inhibiting attempts at downgaze. *Blepharospasm* (forced eyelid closure) and difficulties with eye opening are also common features of PSP. The clinical features of PSP tend to be relatively symmetric, although some degree of asymmetry has been described [11]. Early falls and rigidity affecting the trunk and neck are common in PSP, whereas tremor is uncommon.

2.3.3
Multiple System Atrophy

Multiple system atrophy (MSA) is a PD-like condition characterized by the combination of parkinsonism, impaired autonomic function, and a relatively poor response to levodopa. The autonomic impairment often results in blood pressure fluctuations associated with changes in posture (so that patients may faint when standing), erectile dysfunction, and bladder disturbances. Other features associated with MSA include cerebellar dysfunction, pyramidal tract signs, extreme forward neck flexion, cold mottled hands, inspiratory stridor (due to abnormal vocal cord movement), and severely slurred speech. Although individuals with MSA generally respond poorly to levodopa, there can be a good response initially in 20% of patients, and a sustained response in up to 13% [12]. Prominent involuntary facial and mouth movements in response to levodopa occur in 25% of patients with MSA.

2.3.4
Cortico-Basal Ganglionic Degeneration

An asymmetric onset of symptoms, although characteristic of PD, may also be seen in other disorders such cortico-basal ganglionic degeneration (CBGD) [13]. This is an uncommon disorder that affects the way in which the brain plans and controls voluntary movements. Typical features include a loss of the ability to perform familiar, purposeful movements in the absence of other significant motor or sensory impairment (apraxia), abnormal limb posturing, and often by the "alien-limb phenomenon," which is a tendency for the affected limb to make complex, repetitive, involuntary movements. In addition, there is often evidence of abnormal sensation and a tendency for the limbs to jerk involuntarily in response to gentle touch (stimulus-sensitive myoclonus).

2.3.5
Dementia with Lewy Bodies

The pathological hallmark of PD is the presence of abnormal structures (Lewy bodies) in neurons in the substantia nigra, seen with microscopic examination of the midbrain. In dementia with Lewy bodies (DLB), these microscopic structures are seen in a more widespread distribution, particularly affecting neurons in the cerebral cortex. DLB shares many clinical characteristics with PD, but is differentiated by the occurrence of cognitive impairment as an early rather than late feature. This is probably the second most common form of dementia after Alzheimer's disease. Spontaneous visual hallucinations and fluctuating cognition are common features of DLB. Unlike PD, rigidity is usually more prominent than bradykinesia or tremor. Patients with DLB often display pronounced sensitivity to the motor side effects of antipsychotic medications.

2.3.6
Vascular Parkinsonism

Vascular parkinsonism is typically "lower-half" parkinsonism, with a prominent gait disturbance but minimal upper-body involvement [14]. There are often additional neurological deficits consistent with multifocal cerebrovascular disease, such as pyramidal tract abnormalities, or impaired function in cerebellar symptoms. There is usually a poor response to levodopa.

2.4
Non-Dopaminergic Features of PD

Existing treatments provide significant symptom control of the cardinal motor features of PD, particularly in early disease, although motor complications (see Chapter 4) related to chronic levodopa intake can become an important source of disability. As PD progresses, the clinical picture changes somewhat from that seen in early disease. Non-dopaminergic features–that is, those that do not respond well to therapies based on activating the dopaminergic system–are now recognized as playing an important role, particularly in advanced disease, having a major negative affect on quality of life [15]. These features are introduced here and discussed in more detail in subsequent chapters. Problems such as gait and balance impairment, swallowing and speech difficulties, and autonomic disturbances such as bladder impairment and constipation, are increasingly prevalent and can be sources of significant disability in patients with advanced PD.

Although many of the motor features of PD respond well to treatment with medications acting on the dopamine system, this is not the case for all such features. Postural instability increases with disease progression and responds poorly to medication. Similarly, freezing of gait, speech abnormalities, and swallowing impairment (dysphagia) are also poorly responsive.

2.4.1
Sleep Disturbances

Sleep disruption is very common in PD, often from early in the course of the disease [16]. Broken or interrupted sleep can be primary, related to associated degeneration in sleep regulation centers in the brainstem, or may be secondary in nature, related to other problems such as excessive nocturnal urination (nocturia) or changes in motor function causing frequent arousal.

Rapid eye movement behavior disorder (RBD) is characterized by a loss of the normal inhibition of muscle tone that occurs during rapid eye movement sleep, enabling patients to physically enact their dreams. Involuntary vocalizations and abnormal movements, sometimes violent in nature, are commonly reported during sleep by bed partners of those with RBD. As many as 40% of men with RBD may eventually develop PD, with an average delay of about 12 to 13 years between the onset of RBD and the appearance of the motor features of parkinsonism [17]. Langston has suggested that the earliest description of RBD was actually in James Parkinson's original monograph, in which he stated that "… sleep becomes much disturbed. The tremulous motion of the limbs occur during sleep, and augment until they awaken the patient, and frequently with much agitation and alarm" [1, 18].

Excessive daytime sleepiness affects up to 50% of patients with PD, and can have a substantial impact [19]. An abnormally shortened period of sleep latency (<5 min) has been reported in 30% of affected individuals [20, 21]; sleep studies have indicated a transition from wakefulness to stage 2 sleep occurring within seconds, similar to that seen in narcolepsy [22]. Although it is likely that excessive daytime sleepiness has multiple causes, it is also likely that PD medications are at least partially involved [23–25].

2.4.2
Olfaction

Impaired olfactory sensation is very common in PD, with some studies suggesting abnormalities in almost all patients [26]. Patients may complain of a decline in their sense of smell long before they develop the motor features of parkinsonism. This is particularly interesting in view of Braak's suggestion that pathological changes in the olfactory pathways in the brain are observed very early in PD, preceding the development of classical PD pathology affecting the substantia nigra [27].

2.4.3
Dysautonomia

Impaired autonomic nervous system function is another feature frequently seen in patients with advanced PD. Common autonomic features include blood pressure fluctuations associated with the assumption of an upright posture (orthostatic hypotension), urinary dysfunction, constipation, and sexual dysfunction. Indeed, constipation was included in James Parkinson's original description of the disease. These features can all have a substantial negative impact on the patient's quality of life [28].

2.4.4
Neuropsychiatric Features

2.4.4.1 Dementia
Although in his original description of PD, James Parkinson stated that the intellect is spared, it is now clear that dementia is an important feature, particularly in patients with more advanced disease. Dementia refers to a significant loss of intellectual abilities that is severe enough to interfere with social or occupational functioning. It does not refer to temporary confusion or forgetfulness that might result from some other underlying illness or a side effect of medication. Dementia typically progresses over time; the intellectual abilities that are affected usually include some combinations of impairment of attention, orientation, memory, judgment, language, and motor and spatial skills [29]. Dementia occurs sixfold more frequently in elderly patients with PD than in elderly controls [30]. In a population-based survey in Norway, 28% of PD patients had dementia [31]. In patients aged over age 85 years, as many as 65% may have dementia [30]. Psychosis is often associated with dementia, and is a key factor leading to the need for nursing home placement [32]. Features of dementia in PD and DLB have recently been reviewed by Camicioli and Fisher [33].

2.4.4.2 Depression
Depression, characterized by feelings of guilt, a lack of self-esteem, sadness, and remorse, is common in PD, with up to 50% of patients suffering from clinically relevant depression at some point during the course of the illness [34]. The development of depressive features is likely related to a combination of an endogenous defect in synthesis of neurotransmitters such as dopamine, serotonin, and/or noradrenaline (norepinephrine), and to the awareness of patients that they suffer a chronic, progressive neurodegenerative disease [35]. There is a suggestion that depression may precede the motor features of PD, with 9.2% of patients reporting a previous diagnosis of depression at the time of PD diagnosis compared to 4.2%

of controls [36]. Although suicidal ideation is relatively common, deaths by suicide are rare, with the possible exception of some patients who have been treated with deep brain stimulation targeting the subthalamic nucleus [37, 38]. Anxiety disorders are common, presenting as panic attacks, phobias, or generalized anxiety disorder [39].

2.5
Natural History

Although PD is clearly a progressive disorder, studies of disease progression are somewhat confusing, not only because of the use of different clinical endpoints, but also because of the substantial symptomatic benefits of medical treatment. In a study of 100 consecutive patients who had never received levodopa, 83% progressed to needing levodopa treatment at a mean of 48 months after the initial symptoms of PD had appeared [40]. There is some evidence that those patients who are younger at the age of onset progress more rapidly than do older patients [41, 42]. A study of 800 patients followed for 13 years showed similar mortality rates to those of the general population in North America [43]. Whilst survival was not affected by the age of onset, it was affected by an increased severity and the rate at which the parkinsonism worsened, and by a decreased response to levodopa. In contrast, the results of a Norwegian study suggested a slight increase in mortality [44]. The presence of dementia shortens survival in patients with PD [45]. There appear to be PD subtypes, and there is also evidence that, with disease progression, tremor-dominant patients have less functional disability than those with disease characterized by prominent postural instability and gait impairment [46].

2.6
Conclusions

Parkinson disease is a multisystem disorder characterized not only by motor impairment but also by nonmotor features that become an increasing source of disability with disease progression. Although a patient's quality of life can be significantly impaired by PD, the appropriate management of the condition, if directed at both motor and nonmotor manifestations, can have a major impact.

References

1 Parkinson, J. (2002) An essay on the shaking palsy. *The Journal of Neuropsychiatry and Clinical Neurosciences*, **14**, 227–236.

2 Goetz, C.G., Chmura, T.A., and Lanska, D.J. (2001) The history of Parkinson's disease: part 2 of the MDS-sponsored History of Movement

Disorders Exhibit, Barcelona, June 2000. *Movement Disorders*, **16**, 156–161.

3 Hughes, A.J., Daniel, S.E., Blankson, S., and Lees, A.J. (1993) A clinicopathologic study of 100 cases of Parkinson's disease. *Archives of Neurology*, **50**, 140–148.

4 Shahani, B.T. and Young, R.R. (1976) Physiological and pharmacologic aids in the differential of tremor. *Journal of Neurology, Neurosurgery, and Psychiatry*, **39**, 772–783.

5 Lance, J.W., Schwab, R.S., and Peterson, E.A. (1963) Action tremor and the cogwheel phenomenon in PD. *Brain*, **86**, 95–110.

6 Rajput, A.H., Rozdilsky, B., and Rajput, A. (1991) Accuracy of clinical diagnosis in parkinsonism – a prospective study. *Canadian Journal of Neurological Science*, **18**, 275–278.

7 Munhoz, R.P., Li, J.-Y., Kurtinecz, M., *et al.* (2004) Evaluation of the pull test technique in assessing postural instability in Parkinson's disease. *Neurology*, **62**, 125–127.

8 de Rijk, M.C., Tzourio, C., Breteler, M.M.B., *et al.* (1997) Prevalence of parkinsonism and Parkinson's disease in Europe: the EUROPARKINSON Collaborative Study. *Journal of Neurology, Neurosurgery, and Psychiatry*, **62**, 10–15.

9 Hughes, A.J., Daniel, S.E., Ben-Shlomo, Y., and Lees, A.J. (2002) The accuracy of diagnosis of parkinsonian syndromes in a specialist movement disorder service. *Brain*, **125**, 861–870.

10 Hughs, A.J., Daniel, S.E., Kilford, L., and Lees, A.J. (1992) Accuracy of clinical diagnosis of idiopathic Parkinson's disease: a clinico-pathological study of 100 cases. *Journal of Neurology, Neurosurgery, and Psychiatry*, **55**, 181–184.

11 Barclay, C.L. and Lang, A.E. (1997) Dystonia in progressive supranuclear palsy. *Journal of Neurology, Neurosurgery, and Psychiatry*, **62**, 352–356.

12 Wenning, G.K., Ben Shlomo, Y., Magalhaes, M., Daniel, S.E., and Quinn, N.P. (1994) Clinical features and natural history of multiple system atrophy: an analysis of 100 cases. *Brain*, **117**, 835–845.

13 Lang, A.E., Riley, D.E., and Bergeron, C. (1994) Cortical-basal ganglionic degeneration, in *Neurodegenerative Diseases* (ed. D.B. Calne), W.B. Saunders, Philadelphia, pp. 877–894.

14 Elble, R.J., Cousins, R., Leffler, K., and Hughes, L. (1996) Gait initiation by patients with lower-half parkinsonism. *Brain*, **119**, 1705–1716.

15 Hely, M.A., Morris, J.G.L., Reid, W.G.J., and Trafficante, R. (2005) Sydney multicenter study of Parkinson's disease: non-L-Dopa-responsive problems dominate at 15 years. *Movement Disorders*, **20**, 190–199.

16 Garcia-Borrequero, D., Larosa, O., and Bravo, M. (2003) Parkinson's disease and sleep. *Sleep Medicine Reviews*, **7**, 115–129.

17 Schenk, C.H., Bundlie, S.R., and Mahowald, M.W. (1996) Delayed emergence of a parkinsonian disorder in 38% of 29 older men initially diagnosed with idiopathic rapid eye movement sleep behaviour disorder. *Neurology*, **46**, 388–393.

18 Langston, J.W. (2006) The Parkinson's complex: parkinsonism is just the tip of the iceberg. *Annals of Neurology*, **59**, 591–596.

19 Schapira, A.H.V. (2004) Excessive daytime sleepiness in Parkinson's disease. *Neurology*, **63**, S24–S27.

20 Tracik, F. and Ebersbach, G. (2001) Sudden daytime sleep onset in Parkinson's disease: polysomnographic recordings. *Movement Disorders*, **16**, 500–506.

21 Ulivelli, M., Rossi, S., Lombardi, C., *et al.* (2002) Polysomnographic characterization of pergolide-induced sleep attacks in idiopathic PD. *Neurology*, **58**, 462–465.

22 Rye, D.B. and Jankovic, J. (2002) Emerging views of dopamine in modulating sleep/wake state from an unlikely source: PD. *Neurology*, **58**, 341–346.

23 Ferreira, J.J., Galitzky, M., Montastruc, J.L., and Rascol, O. (2000) Sleep attacks in Parkinson's disease. *Lancet*, **355**, 1333–1334.

24 Hobson, D.E., Lange, A.E., Martin, W.R.W., Razmy, A., Rivest, J., and

Fleming, J. (2002) Excessive daytime sleepiness and sudden-onset sleep in Parkinson Disease: a survey by the Canadian Movement Disorders Group. *Journal of the American Medical Association*, **287**, 455–463.

25 Ondo, W.G., Vuong, K.D., Khan, H., Atassi, F., Kwak, C., and Jankovic, J. (2001) Daytime sleepiness and other sleep disorders in Parkinson's disease. *Neurology*, **57**, 1392–1396.

26 Muller, A., Reichmann, H., Livermore, A., and Hummel, T. (2002) Olfactory function in idiopathic Parkinson's disease (IPD): results from cross-sectional studies in IPD patients and long-term follow-up of de-novo IPD patients. *Journal of Neural Transmission*, **109**, 805–811.

27 Braak, H., Del Tredici, K., Rub, U., de Vos, R.A.I., Jansen Steur, E.N.H., and Braak, E. (2003) Staging of brain pathology related to sporadic Parkinson's disease. *Neurobiology of Aging*, **24**, 197–210.

28 Magerkurth, C., Schnitzer, R., and Braune, S. (2005) Symptoms of autonomic failure in Parkinson's disease: prevalence and impact on daily life. *Clinical Autonomic Research*, **15**, 76–82.

29 Knopman, D.S., DeKosky, S.T., Cummings, J.L., *et al.* (2001) Practice parameter: diagnosis of dementia (an evidence-based review). Report of the Quality Standards Subcommittee of the American Academy of Neurology. *Neurology*, **56**, 1143–1153.

30 Mayeux, R., Chen, J., Mirabello, E., *et al.* (1990) An estimate of the incidence of dementia in idiopathic Parkinson's disease. *Neurology*, **40**, 1513–1517.

31 Aarsland, D., Tandberg, E., Larsen, J.P., and Cummings, J.L. (1996) Frequency of dementia in Parkinson Disease. *Archives of Neurology*, **53**, 538–542.

32 Aarsland, D., Larsen, J.P., Tandberg, E., and Laake, K. (2000) Predictors of nursing home placement in Parkinson's disease: a population-based prospective study. *Journal of the American Geriatrics Society*, **48**, 938–942.

33 Camicioli, R. and Fisher, N. (2004) Parkinson's disease with dementia and dementia with Lewy bodies.

Canadian Journal of Neurological Sciences, **31**, 7–21.

34 Brown, R.G., MacCarthy, B., Gotham, A.M., Der, G.J., and Marsden, C.D. (1988) Depression and disability in Parkinson's disease: a follow-up of 132 cases. *Psychological Medicine*, **18**, 49–55.

35 Koller, W.C. and Tse, W. (2004) Unmet medical needs in Parkinson's disease. *Neurology*, **62** (Suppl. 1), S1–S8.

36 Schurmann, A.G., van de Akker, H., Ensinck, K.T.J.L., *et al.* (2002) Increased risk of Parkinson's disease after depression: a retrospective cohort study. *Neurology*, **58**, 1501–1504.

37 Myslobodsky, M., Lalonde, F.M., and Hicks, L. (2001) Are patients with Parkinson's disease suicidal? *Journal of Geriatric Psychiatry and Neurology*, **14**, 120–124.

38 Funkiewiez, A., Ardouin, C., Caputo, E., *et al.* (2004) Long-term effects of bilateral subthalamic nucleus stimulation on cognitive function, mood, and behaviour in Parkinson's disease. *Journal of Neurology, Neurosurgery, and Psychiatry*, **75**, 834–839.

39 Chaudhuri, K.R., Healy, D.G., and Schapira, A.H.V. (2006) Non-motor symptoms of Parkinson's disease: diagnosis and management. *Lancet Neurology*, **5**, 235–245.

40 Goetz, C.G., Tanner, C.M., and Shannon, K.M. (1987) Progression of Parkinson's disease without levodopa. *Neurology*, **37**, 695–698.

41 Goetz, C.G., Tanner, C.M., Stebbins, G.T., and Buchman, A.S. (1988) Risk factors for progression in Parkinson's disease. *Neurology*, **38**, 1841–1844.

42 Diamond, S.G., Markham, C.H., Hoehn, M.M., McDowell, F.H., and Muenter, M.D. (1989) Effect of age at onset on progression and mortality in Parkinson's disease. *Neurology*, **39**, 1187–1190.

43 Marras, C., McDermott, M.P., Rochon, P.A., *et al.* (2005) Survival in Parkinson Disease: thirteen-year follow-up of the DATATOP cohort. *Neurology*, **64**, 87–93.

44 Herlofson, K., Lie, S.A., Årsland, D., and Larsen, J.P. (2004) Mortality and Parkinson Disease: a community

based study. *Neurology*, **62**, 937–942.

45 Louis, E.D., Marder, K., Cote, L., Tang, M., and Mayeux, R. (1997) Mortality from Parkinson Disease. *Archives of Neurology*, **54**, 260–264.

46 Jankovic, J., McDermott, M., Carter, J., *et al.* (1990) Variable expression of Parkinson's disease: a base-line analysis of the datatop cohort. *Neurology*, **40**, 1529–1534.

A Patient's Story

Parkinson's Journey

Joyce Pinckney

Incredulous, I looked at her. She'd been my family doctor for almost 20 years. She knew me, she knew my husband, she knew my kids, she knew who I was and what I valued, what I did, and how much I loved it. She knew that I loved my project-filled life, and she knew how much of my life was movement.

For someone who had graduated at the top of her class and had come to me highly recommended by a very picky pediatrician I had worked with and respected, she had chosen a very dumb thing to say.

She had asked, in a bit of a role reversal, "Well, what did he say?" referring to the neurologist she had sent me to.

"He told me I had Parkinson's disease, early stages."

"Isn't that wonderful!" was not the response I expected – I could have flattened her on the spot. A quick scan around the examining room revealed few weapons – I could see the headlines: "Bang! Bang! Doctor's Reflex Hammer Came Down Upon Her Head" "Doctor Strangled With Her Own Stethoscope." But instead, I gave her "the look." How could she so casually sentence me to a life with Parkinson's disease and then deny my loss by calling it wonderful? I was speechless!

Even though I knew that what she meant was, having Parkinson's disease was preferable to having multiple myeloma or a brain tumor, or degenerative malignancy of the spinal cord (all of which were part of the differential diagnosis), it was still an amazingly dumb thing to say.

"The Beginning" or "Try! Just Try to Get a Diagnosis"

My first hint of problems to come was a tremble in the ring finger of my left hand. Sometimes, the fifth finger of the same hand joined in the little dance as well. If I extended my arm, the fingers trembled even more, but I could stop the movement by concentrating or smacking them. I discovered those fingers wouldn't move smoothly when I tested them, having them beat out a rhythm or pretend to march. There was a jerky lack of control and a hesitation. It seemed amusing, but even then I felt a shiver of fear. It was so unlike my body to be clumsy, to refuse to comply.

It wasn't as though I ignored the symptoms. Twice I had visited a neurologist who tested my muscle responses to electric shocks, and the reports were normal. Both times I had complained that pain was restricting my shoulder rotation. Even when I demonstrated the jerking cog-wheel movement associated with Parkinson's and asked "Could it be Parkinson's?," his comment was, "Oh, no it doesn't begin on one side." (Where was he coming from? It almost always does begin on one side.)

And so I continued with acupuncture, massage therapy, physiotherapy and the occasional chiropractic treatment. At about this time, I noticed that as people walked, their arms swung naturally by their sides, and with each arm swing synchronized with a step of the opposite foot. But my left arm was motionless, and even when I reminded it to swing it was not natural, nor did it continue to swing if I wasn't paying attention. Yet, nobody recognized the significance of this, and it should have been a dead giveaway. It was one of the first symptoms to disappear after I began taking my medications.

The next inkling was when my left arm refused to play piano properly. I was learning Oscar Peterson's *Blues of the Prairies*, and it was as though my left hand knew what to do and how to do it, but would not cooperate. That, of course, was exactly what was happening, although the hand "couldn't" cooperate rather than "wouldn't." Without the connector, "dopamine," the neural order sent by the brain reaches the muscles and is unable to instigate the appropriate movement. Like the bearer of a missive to a secured castle, the impulse cannot leap the moat to deliver the message. It is blocked, stranded without a bridge – the drawbridge dopamine. You might also think of dopamine as an interpreter who must translate the message "Major Brain" wants to give "Private Muscle" who doesn't speak "brain". The lines of communication break down at the junction of nerve and muscle.

Another Clue

In the fall of 1994, I undertook to teach belly-dancing to a group of "keeners" who had access to a school gym in Millwoods. As always, I loved it and could still summon the old charm and movements. However, I wondered about my teaching ability, for the students weren't doing as well as usual. Their left shoulder thrusts, rotations and shimmies were weak to nonexistent. I said, "You girls aren't moving your left shoulders." In a chorus the class responded, "But you're not moving yours"; and I realized they were right. My left shoulder did not move. I laughed with them and began to concentrate on my lazy shoulder. Much of the movement came back, but it was hard work!

Actually, having Parkinson's *is* hard work. There seems to be an element of forgetting how to do simple, everyday movements – habitual actions we take for granted, having mastered as children, are no longer part of our muscle memory. I find myself trapped in my coat or jacket – I can't shrug it off my shoulders and slip out. I have to remind my body that if I reach around to my back with both arms I can grasp a sleeve, and that lets me pull one side of the jacket off. Then, I do the same for the other side.

Buttons are a problem to do up, and equally to undo. More than once I've found myself totally straight-jacketed in a dress that's already over my head with long sleeve cuffs firmly fastened.

I was helped to identify what I had lost by my grandson. As he moved through the stages from babyhood to being a little boy, I realized he was learning the same things I had to re-learn. He would stand, balancing carefully, and find the safest place to put his foot to negotiate through scattered toys. Balancing an adult body on two small feet, staying upright, then moving is also a challenge if you have Parkinson's!

Trying to put shoes on a baby reminded me why I was having trouble putting on my own shoes – my feet had "forgotten" the technique, the wiggling and squiggling necessary to insert themselves into the unyielding shoes.

I had to learn again how to remove a pullover shirt or sweater. The crossing of arms, by which women remove pullovers (possibly to protect their hairdos) seemed a forgotten art.

Shopping for clothes became a triathlon:

Find it.
> Put it on.
>> Take it off.
>>> Get a gold medal.   Hooray!

After being trapped inside a too-tight article of clothing more than once in a series of fitting rooms, I created ...

Golden Maxim #1: If it's difficult to get on, it will be *impossible* to get off!

Diagnosis

The diagnosis was a long time coming. No fewer than three branches of the medical team had, under direct questioning, denied any suggestion that I had Parkinson's.

I heard "Oh, no, Parkinson's doesn't start on one side." "Parkinson's doesn't cause stiffness, it causes tremor." "You don't have a poker face, a boring voice or take those small quick stumbling steps." "You don't fall and have balance problems, do you?" And when anyone said, "Well, whatever it is it is not Parkinson's", it was exactly what I wanted to hear. However, in my heart of hearts, I knew that it was.

In 1996, when I met my present neurologist, we hit it off from the very first. When he had finished the examination he asked, "What do you think you have?"

As I said, "Parkinson's disease," my voice rose to a little girl pitch. Then, for the first time, I began to cry. Tears filled my eyes, overflowed, rolled down my cheeks, and dripped on to my silk shirt. He nodded, and silently handed me a box of tissues.

Still hoping against hope, I had one last trump card to play. I'd read in the *Reader's Digest* about a doctor in Tucson that was an expert in diagnosing early signs of Parkinson's, by using video games to test reaction times. The participant also had to identify a scent using "Scratch 'n Sniff" stickers, since one of the senses that can be lost is the sense of smell. He had designed a questionnaire to reveal the presence of depression, one of the symptoms which may precede the onset of Parkinson's disease.

Since a nursing friend of mine had moved from Edmonton to Tucson, I resolved to visit her. I called the office of Dr Erwin Montgomery and he agreed to see me free of cost. He told me to stop any medication and to come to his laboratory at the university in August, so I phoned my friend, who opened her home and her heart to me. She gave me unlimited access to her eclectic library and music collection; she showed me the sights of Tucson, and I fell in love with the Saguaros, the desert, and the town. (We now own a holiday home there. A permanent dwelling set up with Aids for Daily Living makes holidaying much more fun, as traveling becomes more challenging.)

At the university, I underwent the lab tests, and then met the doctor. He took one look at me and said, "It's Parkinson's, I'm sure, early stages. If you were my patient, I would give you a large hit of Sinemet (a dopamine replacement). If your symptoms disappear and you are less stiff, it will confirm the diagnosis."

Then I made use of my friend's library – alternating between gathering inspiration, information and crying in angry disbelief. One of the funnier quotations I found was:

> "The good thing about chronic illness is that those friends who shy away from it at first have lots of opportunity to make up for it later."

Back at home, my doctor said, "No big hit, but let's start Sinemet." And it worked. So although I finally had to believe it, I didn't accept it. Actually, 13 years later I still don't entirely accept it – I'm fighting back, every step of the way.

I believe the two most powerful defenses I have are: 1. Denial and 2. Music.

Coming Out

In 2004, when my neurologist asked if I would be interested in speaking to some second-year medical students about having Parkinson's, I was still being unrealistic – some might say "in denial." "Yes," I said, impulsively, "I think that would be fun." The image of me talking about all my experiences, as a nurse, a batik artist, belly dancer, writer, poet, jazz musician/educator, photographer, composer, and piano teacher to an admiring group of second-year medical students with artistic leanings flashed into my mind, and stayed there. It emphasized the part about my being a hero, and ignored the whole thrust of the project, which was to shed some light on how Parkinson's disease affects the person who has it, and also the people who are part of her life.

In preparing for the talk I was to give, I scarcely considered the thoughtful questions on the form they gave me: provocative questions about how Parkinson's affected me. My excuse for omitting this was that I hadn't yet dealt with it myself. I spent the first three or four years concentrating on how to hide the diagnosis from my friends. I did it so well that they were all convinced that I must be dying of cancer or some unheard-of rare malady. They wondered why no one would tell them what was going on. I was aided in this deception by the condition of my spine, as I had scoliosis, some osteoporosis, and sciatic pain in my right leg—all those million-dollar words easily distracted my friends. The actual pain from my sciatic nerve and subsequent major spinal surgeries distracted me, thus I could avoid the embarrassment, anger, despair, and horror I felt at having to share, or even relinquish my body, my vehicle for life, to this predator and master-thief, Parkinson.

In the presentation for the students, I centered on creating an exciting narrative of my life. This screened and hid away any indication of how I felt about the present and the future.

But participating in this project, called *"Art and Medicine, Beneath the Mask,"* became another milestone, because the students asked that I allow my story to be the main feature in the show. Suddenly, I was part of a display that would travel to the health facilities in Edmonton and area. So much for secrets.

Following the Path

This is a journey for me along an ambiguous path. My life is one of contradiction. I describe it as having the bedroom tidy, but inside the drawers is chaos. On the one hand, I want to do all the research about the disease, treatment and find ways to accommodate it. I speak freely and academically with apparent acceptance, while on the other hand I reject the reality of restrictions, dependence, and harbor an inner rage at the audacity of my body to have treated me in this way. This is the chaos. On the rare occasion when I allow myself to imagine a future where I'm at an advanced stage of this bizarre disease, Parkinson's, even a glimpse of what could lie ahead is too devastating for me to bear.

Though I never gave a second thought to being young and beautiful when I was, there are times when I look into the mirror and see a ravaged visage I can scarcely reconcile as representing me. In spite of the reality, I still feel young and beautiful inside. So I offer:

> Golden Maxim #2 Avoid mirrors. Just pretend. Remember a smile lifts off ten years and totally disarms the recipient.

It's very unsettling to know that I have a disease that worsens with time instead of getting better. I once remarked to a cohort, "Isn't having Parkinson's a pain?" "Well," she replied, in a tone more cheerful than resigned, "if it's not one thing, it's another."

That had as much impact on me as months of therapy with my psychiatrist. When I told him about it, my psychiatrist was so taken with the comment, he said, later "I've used that quotation with half a dozen of my patients since you told it to me."

In the same vein, my friend's mom was heard to say, "You know, if you were invited to a large gathering where everyone was told to toss their lives, with good and bad elements, into a pile in the center of the room, and everyone could choose from the pile, any life that they wished, most us would go home with our own."

Did You Say Following, or Falling?

The causes of falling are things like clutter on the floor, or having to negotiate around furniture. Once I grabbed hold of a rocking chair for stability—not recommended. Another time I threw a package forward with great energy and had a rebound backwards. I was propelled off a six-inch high step onto a patch of grass, landing on my arm, shoulder and hip—I managed to break three ribs. One or more times, I chose to wear inappropriate shoes, for vanity or fashion, and ruefully regretted it from a position on the pavement. I began to think maybe I should be fitted for a helmet.

Crashing down on my back and side are usually not so hard, but face plants are decidedly shocking and unsightly. In trying to prevent this damage to my face, I needed to retrain my arms to move up and break my fall. I spent some time practicing falling forward onto our king-size bed, being very conscious that my arms should be up and out to break my fall. I also used the pool where I had swimming therapy to try out falling and to practice balancing.

I've found as the years pass and some of my bodily functions slow, that a good quiet place for meditation is in the bathroom. The problem is, sometimes when I'm sleep-deprived, I discover I have drifted off into slumber. I awaken with a start, and realize I was asleep; or, I awaken on the floor, bleeding and sore, with black eyes pending. The last time this happened, I was aware that I had hurt the ring finger of my left hand, so I can only presume that my arm, hand, and finger must have been trying to protect my head. It's hard to describe such an accident to a sympathetic ear and still retain some sense of dignity.

I have become an expert on the art of falling. I believe I'm taking careful precautions, but then to my surprise I get caught off guard, and fall again. Once, while getting settled into a hotel room on the day of arrival, I slowly tipped over backwards and landed in my open suitcase, which was yawning on the floor behind me. It was not quite empty and so afforded some padding, but the tricky part was to get my legs out far enough that my feet reached the floor to allow me to escape. The day I was to leave I was just standing still and suddenly I tipped over sideways and ended up half inside a large wastepaper basket, with one arm propping me up. I wondered if it was a comment on where I belonged.

I believe there has been some notable progression of the disease. There are more hours when I am not able to stand proud and short than there are hours when I am able to stretch up in the torso. My pills are less dependable. I'm okay. Then suddenly I'm tip-toeing, stuttering my walk, or grabbing furniture as I pitch forward, feet stuck to the floor. I do note that I can change the direction of my fall, to land in a more comfortable place; and often, I can catch myself and re-balance before I fall.

I keep up a façade that all is well, as it sometimes is, and sometimes isn't. Above all, I try to move forward. I'm working on attitude – an attitude of accept-ance that is not acquiescence or abdication; not defeat, not surrender, but a Zen-like approach to what is, is.

3
Current Approaches to the Management of Parkinson Disease

Wayne Martin and Marguerite Wieler

3.1
Introduction

The major neurochemical abnormality in Parkinson disease (PD) is a reduction in the dopamine content of the brain. This occurs as a result of an impaired function in the neurons involved in the control of movement, projecting from the substantia nigra to the striatum. This dopamine deficiency gives rise to the major motor features of PD. The most effective current treatment strategies attempt at improving the associated motor impairment, with the primary goal being to minimize any associated disability. In patients with early PD, it is important to employ strategies that improve symptoms, while delaying the potential development of motor complications of treatment – that is, motor fluctuations and dyskinesias – as much as possible. In patients with more advanced disease, it often becomes necessary to alter treatment in order to minimize motor and/or behavioral complications that may have already developed. While pharmacological therapy is the mainstay of symptomatic treatment throughout the course of PD, neurosurgical approaches are of increasing importance in managing patients in the more advanced stages of the disease. Rehabilitation-based approaches are an essential complement to all symptomatic treatment modalities, helping to maintain function and psychosocial health. The aim of this chapter is not to provide a systematic analysis of all the management options available, but rather to review the major considerations involved in choosing the most appropriate treatment plan.

3.2
Pharmacologic Treatment

3.2.1
Symptomatic Therapy

The major pharmacological options for the symptomatic management of PD are listed in Table 3.1.

Parkinson Disease – A Health Policy Perspective. Edited by Wayne Martin, Oksana Suchowersky, Katharina Kovacs Burns, and Egon Jonsson
Copyright © 2010 WILEY-VCH Verlag GmbH & Co. KGaA, Weinheim
ISBN: 978-3-527-32779-9

Table 3.1 Major pharmacological options for the symptomatic management of PD.

Class	Drug	Usual dose range
Dopamine precursors	Levodopa/carbidopa (Sinemet®)	100/25 t.i.d. to 200/50 q.i.d.
	Levodopa/benserazide (Prolopa®)	100/25 t.i.d. to 200/50 q.i.d.
Dopamine agonists	Bromocriptine (Parlodel®)	5–15 mg t.i.d.
	Ropinirole (Requip®)	2–8 mg t.i.d.
	Pramipexole (Mirapex®)	0.5–1.5 mg t.i.d.
COMT inhibitors	Entacapone (Comtan®)	200 mg t.i.d.-q.i.d.
MAO-B inhibitors	Selegiline (Eldepryl®)	5 mg b.i.d.
	Rasgiline (Azilect®)	1 mg q.d.

COMT = catechol O-methyl transferase; MAO-B = monoamine oxidase type B.

3.2.1.1 Levodopa

Levodopa is a neutral amino acid that is initially absorbed from the small intestine and subsequently transported across the blood–brain barrier into the brain, where it is converted to dopamine. Other neutral amino acids in the gut and plasma compete for transport. Levodopa is normally administered with a peripheral decarboxylase inhibitor in order to prevent its systemic conversion to dopamine; this will also prevent the nausea and vomiting that can occur if the dopamine receptors in the medulla are activated by circulating dopamine. In Canada, levodopa is normally used in combination with the decarboxylase inhibitors carbidopa (Sinemet®) or benserazide (Prolopa®).

Levodopa has been in general use since the studies of Cotzias and his coworkers [1] during the late 1960s, and it remains the single most effective drug for the symptomatic treatment of PD. Its use is associated with decreased morbidity and mortality [2], and virtually all patients with PD experience a clinically significant benefit [3]. Although there has been concern that levodopa treatment might hasten disease progression in PD, a consensus conference concluded that there is no convincing evidence to indicate that levodopa accelerates neuronal loss in PD patients [4]. In fact, the results of a recent clinical trial suggested that levodopa might slow disease progression in early PD [5], although this interpretation is somewhat controversial.

Levodopa is generally started at a low dose, and then gradually increased until a satisfactory clinical response is obtained. By administering the compound in this fashion, acute adverse side effects such as nausea, vomiting, and postural hypotension are minimized. In early-stage PD, a daily dose of 300–400 mg levodopa is usually sufficient, given in three to four divided doses. If there is no response to higher doses of levodopa (1000 mg daily), then an alternate diagnosis rather than idiopathic PD should be suspected. These patients are unlikely to respond to higher doses or to other dopaminergic drugs. In order to fully inhibit peripheral decarboxylase (and minimize the side effects), a total intake of about 75–100 mg daily of carbidopa is required. Thus, the most appropriate preparation is usually one that contains levodopa/carbidopa (or levodopa/benserazide) in a 4:1

ratio. If nausea persists in spite of full peripheral decarboxylase inhibition, the peripheral dopamine receptor antagonist domperidone (Motilium®) can be very effective, given at 10–20 mg some 30 min before each levodopa dose. In those countries where domperidone is unavailable an alternate approach would be to administer supplemental carbidopa.

3.2.1.2 Levodopa-Induced Motor Complications

In patients with early PD, levodopa is usually well tolerated and of significant symptomatic benefit. Its chronic administration, however, can be associated with significant motor complications, to the extent that the management of patients with advanced PD may often be dominated by attempts to limit the disability related to these complications. The major motor complications include fluctuations in the motor response to levodopa, and the development of abnormal involuntary movements (dyskinesias). The prevalence of these complications increases with the duration of exposure to levodopa, and occurs in about 50% of PD patients who have received levodopa for five years [6]. These complications are more common in patients with young-onset PD [7].

Motor fluctuations consist of alternating periods of relatively good response to medication ("on" periods), and periods of significantly impaired motor function ("off" periods), in which there is a suboptimal response to medication with a reappearance of the motor features of PD. With disease progression, the response to a single intake of levodopa becomes progressively shorter, so that parkinsonian symptoms may reappear before the next dose of medication (end-of-dose deterioration, or "wearing off"). With further disease progression, some patients may experience rapid and unpredictable fluctuations between "on" and "off" periods (the "on–off" phenomenon), which are unrelated to the timing of the antiparkinsonian medication intake.

The end-of-dose deterioration is thought to be related to a reduced capacity for the storage of dopamine in presynaptic vesicles, that worsens with disease progression. With the loss of this buffering capacity, the brain dopamine levels tend to become more closely related to plasma levodopa levels, such that the clinical response becomes linked to the plasma half-life of the drug. A variable absorption and transport of levodopa across the blood–brain barrier, as well as unpredictable delays in gastric emptying, may also contribute to fluctuations in response and to the occasional "dose failure" that may be seen in more advanced disease [8].

The frequent occurrence of wearing-off with immediate-release levodopa led to the introduction of controlled-release levodopa (Sinemet CR®, Madopar HBS®) [9, 10]. By prolonging the duration of response to a single administration [11], controlled-release levodopa can decrease the disability associated with end-of-dose deterioration. As the controlled-release formulation of levodopa/carbidopa has a reduced bioavailability compared to immediate-release levodopa, a dose increase of about 20–30% is required when switching to the controlled-release preparation. Anecdotally, many Parkinson clinics have also observed that some of the newer generic preparations of controlled-release levodopa seem to control motor symptoms less predictably than does the tradename form (Sinemet CR®).

Levodopa-induced dyskinesias are abnormal involuntary movements that occur in response to levodopa administration. Although these movements are typically twisting or writhing, dystonic features (characterized by sustained muscle contraction leading to abnormal limb postures) may also be present in some affected individuals. Dyskinesias most often appear in a peak-dose pattern, evident during periods of otherwise good motor function. These movements appear to be related to an excessive stimulation of dopamine receptors, but they can also occur during "off" periods. "Off" dyskinesias are typically dystonic, and seem to be related to an inadequate activation of dopamine receptors. Dyskinesias can be diphasic, occurring as the patient is beginning to turn "on," subsiding during the peak levodopa effect, and then recurring as the patient turns "off" [12]. With disease progression, dyskinesias may persist throughout the response to a single dose of levodopa, resulting in considerable disability. Once dyskinesias have developed, they are often difficult to manage, although amantadine (Symmetrel®) has an antidyskinetic effect in some patients [13].

The underlying pathophysiology surrounding the development of these motor complications is not entirely clear. The results of animal studies have suggested that the pulsatile stimulation of striatal dopamine receptors, which occurs as a result of intermittent levodopa administration, is central to the development of levodopa-induced motor complications. It has been proposed, therefore, that the early use of controlled-release levodopa might reduce the long-term development of these complications by providing a more constant activation of the dopamine receptors. A prospective, randomized, double-blind study comparing controlled-release and immediate-release levodopa, however, showed no difference in the incidence of dyskinesias and motor fluctuations over five years [14]. There is no scientific reason, therefore, to recommend the use of controlled-release rather than regular levodopa in early PD.

3.2.1.3 Catechol-O-Methyl Transferase (COMT) Inhibitors

Levodopa is metabolized peripherally not only by decarboxylase (as described above) but also by COMT. The latter is a ubiquitous enzyme, and is sufficiently active that when levodopa is administered with a peripheral decarboxylase inhibitor, only about 10% of a given dose will reach the brain intact [15]. Entacapone (Comtan®) inhibits the peripheral metabolism of levodopa by COMT, thereby increasing its availability to the brain, and increasing the plasma levodopa elimination half-life by about 50% [16]. Double-blind, placebo-controlled trials have demonstrated increased "on" times, decreased "off" times, and improved motor scores in PD patients with motor fluctuations [17]. Unlike its predecessor tolcapone, entacapone is well tolerated, with no evidence of hepatic toxicity. However, it does have the potential to increase dopaminergic side effects due to increased levodopa availability to the brain, and can be associated with diarrhea and urine discoloration.

3.2.1.4 Monoamine Oxidase B (MAO-B) Inhibitors

Central dopamine metabolism involves both COMT and MAO-B. Entacapone does not cross the blood–brain barrier, and therefore does not impact central dopamine breakdown via COMT. However, those compounds that inhibit MAO-B centrally do have the potential to slow the breakdown of dopamine in the brain, and so will have a beneficial effect on parkinsonian symptomatology. Selegiline (Eldepryl®), at the commonly used dose of 10 mg day^{-1}, inhibits MAO-B both selectively and irreversibly, and has a modest benefit on symptom severity, delaying the need to start levodopa therapy in previously untreated patients with PD [18]. Rasagiline (Azilect®) is a potent irreversible inhibitor of monoamine oxidase with a relative selectivity for MAO-B at therapeutic doses. Rasagiline, when given at 1–2 mg daily, has been shown to be effective and well tolerated when used as monotherapy in patients with early PD. Motor function and activity of daily living (ADL) were both improved with rasagiline [19]. In levodopa-treated patients with more advanced PD who were experiencing motor fluctuations, adjunctive treatment with rasagiline at 0.5–1 mg daily led to a significant improvement that was characterized by a reduction in "off" time [20]. In general, rasagiline is well tolerated, although in theory higher doses may be associated with a sensitivity to the hypertensive effects of tyramine-containing foods. A maximum dose of 1 mg daily has therefore been recommended, although the results of tyramine challenge studies have indicated that rasagiline at a daily dose of 0.5–2 mg is not associated with clinically significant tyramine reactions [21].

3.2.1.5 Dopamine Agonists

Dopamine agonists directly stimulate the dopamine receptors, with bromocriptine (Parlodel®) and pergolide (Permax®) having been available in Canada for the treatment of PD for many years. More recently, two newer dopamine agonists – ropinirole (Requip®) and pramipexole (Mirapex®) – have become available. These differ from the older compounds in that they are not ergot derivatives, and are therefore devoid of ergot-related side effects such as retroperitoneal or pleural fibrosis. One adverse side effect of ergot-related agonists that has recently come to light is that of a carcinoid-like cardiac valvulopathy which particularly affects the tricuspid valve, although the mitral and aortic valves may also be affected [22–24]. This has resulted in pergolide being withdrawn from the market in North America. Compared to the older agonists, ropinirole and pramipexole are relatively selective in stimulating dopamine D_2 and D_3 receptors. It should be noted that the role played by the different receptors in normal motor function is unclear; however, it has been well established that D_2 receptor activation is necessary to produce an antiparkinsonian effect.

Historically, dopamine agonists have been used primarily as adjuncts to levodopa in patients who have begun to experience motor complications. Bromocriptine was the first dopamine agonist to be approved, and has a well-established utility as an adjunct to levodopa, improving parkinsonian disability while allowing a reduction in levodopa dosage [25, 26]. Placebo-controlled studies have also demonstrated antiparkinsonian and levodopa-sparing effects with ropinirole and pramipexole in levodopa-treated patients [27–30]. Other agonists available outside North America for the treatment of PD include lisuride and cabergoline. (Cabergoline is available in North America for the treatment of hyperprolactinemia, but has not been approved for PD.) Very few clinical data are available to support the use of any one agonist over another; indeed, in a comparison of pramipexole and bromocriptine Guttman *et al.* reported no statistically significant differences between the two agonists [28]. Consequently, the choice between agonists is probably best based on issues such as side effects and cost, rather than on relative efficacy.

Some evidence has been provided that dopamine agonists may be effective in early PD as an alternative to levodopa, and that the initiation of therapy with an agonist may decrease the development of motor complications. A double-blind comparison of ropinirole with levodopa indicated an absolute risk reduction for dyskinesias after five years of treatment in 26% the ropinirole-treated group [31]. Although greater proportions of patients had hallucinations (17% versus 6%), leg edema (14% versus 6%), and somnolence (27% versus 19%) in the ropinirole group, the dropout rates due to adverse events were similar in both treatment groups. Similar findings were reported in a double-blind comparison of pramipexole versus levodopa [32], with motor complications being significantly less common after pramipexole (28% versus 51%) following a two-year treatment period. The incidences of somnolence, hallucinations, and both generalized and peripheral edema were greater in the pramipexole group. In both of these studies, levodopa provided a significantly greater improvement in motor function than did the dopamine agonist, even though the study design allowed for the addition of open-label levodopa if there was insufficient symptomatic benefit from the agonist alone. A practice parameter published by the American Academy of Neurology concluded that: (i) levodopa, ropinirole, and pramipexole were all effective in ameliorating motor and ADL disability in patients with PD who required dopaminergic therapy; (ii) levodopa was more effective than ropinirole and pramipexole in treating the motor and ADL features of PD; (iii) ropinirole and pramipexole treatment resulted in fewer motor complications than levodopa after a 2.5-year follow-up; and (iv) ropinirole and pramipexole treatment was associated with more frequent adverse events that included hallucinations, somnolence, and edema [33]. Hence, the practitioner must choose between a more effective drug with a higher risk of motor complications (i.e., levodopa) and a less effective drug with a lower risk of motor complications but a higher rate of other adverse effects. This choice is best tailored to the individual patient following a full discussion of the advantages and disadvantages of the alternate approaches.

A new agonist, rotigotine (Neupro®), has recently been approved in the United States and Europe for the treatment of early-stage PD, although it is not yet available in Canada. Unlike other PD medications, rotigotine is administered as a transdermal patch that is applied to the skin once daily, providing a relatively constant plasma concentration of the medication. This new medication has been shown to be effective in placebo-controlled studies for the treatment of patients with early PD [34]. The potential adverse effects are similar to those associated with other dopamine agonists, in addition to skin reactions at the patch site. Notably, as of 2008, Schwarz Pharma has recalled Neupro in the United States because of problems with the delivery mechanism.

3.2.1.6 **Managing Drug-Induced Adverse Events**

In addition to motor complications (as discussed above), a variety of side effects is shared by all antiparkinsonian medications, due to their direct action on dopamine receptors. Consequently, levodopa and all dopamine agonists have the same general range of potential side effects. The most common side effects are nausea and vomiting, but these may be readily counteracted with domperidone (Motilium®) at 10–20 mg, given three to four times daily. In countries where domperidone is unavailable, the addition of supplementary carbidopa can be helpful. Although postural hypotension may be problematic, it can be managed with pressure stockings, increased salt intake, fludrocortisone (Florinef®) 0.1–0.2 mg daily, or the α_1-adrenergic agonist midodrine (Amatine®) 2.5–10 mg, three times daily. Ergot-derived agonists such as bromocriptine have additional potential adverse effects, including erythromelalgia, pulmonary or retroperitoneal fibrosis, and cardiac valvulopathy. The regular monitoring of these uncommon side effects is important in patients receiving these medications.

Activation of the D_2 receptor family can be associated with the development of hallucinations, these being more common with dopamine agonists than with levodopa alone. Although hallucinations are not normally an issue in early PD, they were reported in the early monotherapy studies with ropinirole and pramipexole, but were usually not severe enough for patients to withdraw from the trials [31, 32]. If hallucinations do become problematic, the first step is to rule out any other coincident medical problem, such as dehydration, electrolyte imbalance, or a febrile illness. A possible contributory role of other medications should be considered, with anticholinergic drugs such as tricyclic antidepressants, bladder antispasmodics and muscle relaxants being discontinued. Antiparkinsonian drugs such as anticholinergics, amantadine, or selegiline should also be discontinued. However, if these steps are ineffective, then the dopaminergic drug dose level may need to be reduced, starting with the dopamine agonists. Then, if the hallucinations persist or if the patient is unable to tolerate a reduced agonist dosage because of increased parkinsonism, an atypical antipsychotic can be administered. In this situation, clozapine (Clozaril®) is the neuroleptic least likely to produce extrapyramidal side effects, although its use is complicated by the need for weekly hematological monitoring due to its potential to induce agranulocytosis. Clozapine has been shown to be effective in reducing drug-induced psychosis in PD when administered at a low dose (6.25–50 mg daily) [35]. Quetiapine (Seroquel®; 12.5–50 mg daily) [36] also lacks significant extrapyramidal side effects, and may be preferable because it does not require the frequent hematological monitoring associated with clozapine. However, quetiapine has not been evaluated as extensively as clozapine in PD, and does not have the same degree of evidence-based support for its efficacy. Olanzapine (Zyprexa®) is less effective than clozapine, and has been shown to induce a worsening of parkinsonism [37]. Other neuroleptics, including risperidone, should be avoided because they are associated with significant extrapyramidal side effects.

Excessive daytime somnolence and "sleep attacks" have been reported as a potential side effect of dopamine agonists [38]. In a recent survey, the Canadian

Movement Disorders Group concluded that, although sudden-onset sleep without warning is infrequent, excessive daytime sleepiness may be present in up to 51% of independent PD patients without dementia [39]. This survey did not detect any correlation between sleepiness and a specific type of treatment, and it is uncertain whether similar symptoms may be present in PD patients who are not receiving medication. It is essential that patients be warned about this excessive sleepiness and the potential risks associated with driving.

The dopaminergic system is implicated not only in motor control, but also in various forms of addiction through the brain's reward system [40]. Pathologic gambling is an impulse control disorder defined as a failure to resist gambling impulses, despite severe personal, familial, or vocational losses. An association with dopamine agonist use in PD has been described [41], with a lifetime prevalence that may be as high as 7.2% in patients receiving dopamine agonists [42]. Patients with a younger age of disease onset, higher novelty-seeking traits, and a personal or family history of excessive alcohol use, may have a greater risk for the development of pathological gambling with dopamine agonists [43]. Other forms of impulse control disorder that have been described in association with agonist use include compulsive buying and sexual behavior [44]. Not only should patients with PD being treated with a dopamine agonist be warned with regards to the potential for excessive daytime somnolence (as noted above), but they should also be made aware of the risk of developing an impulse control disorder. These issues should be revisited on a regular basis during follow-up visits.

3.2.2
Neuroprotective Therapy

In neurodegenerative diseases such as PD, the term *neuroprotection* is used to refer to a mechanism that slows the rate of progression of the underlying disease process. An effective neuroprotective treatment may not provide significant relief of parkinsonian symptoms, but would provide a disease-altering effect, slowing the rate at which symptoms progress.

Ideally, the treatment of PD should slow disease progression; however, none of the above-described drugs has been shown to have a disease-altering effect, in spite of their significant symptomatic benefits. A neuroprotective benefit of selegiline through decreased free radical production was proposed [45] and put to clinical trial in the DATATOP (Deprenyl and Tocopherol Antioxidative Therapy of Parkinsonism) study. The trial's initial results showed that selegiline caused a 50% reduction in the risk of developing disability sufficiently severe to require levodopa therapy [18]. Although similar findings were reported by Palhagen *et al.* [46], in both of these studies functional disability in selegiline-treated patients declined during the two-month washout period; this implied that the significant symptomatic benefit of selegiline was at least partially responsible for reducing the need for levodopa. A practice parameter from the American Academy of Neurology concluded that there is no convincing clinical evidence for a neuroprotective benefit with selegiline [33]. The results of a recent study suggested that rasagiline (Azilect®) may provide a neuroprotective effect at a daily dose of 1 mg [84].

Whilst dopamine agonists have a well-established symptomatic benefit in PD (as discussed above), an additional neuroprotective effect has also been suggested. Studies utilizing functional neuroimaging as a surrogate marker of neuronal loss have suggested that both pramipexole [47] and ropinirole [48] may be associated with a slower rate of disease progression when compared to levodopa-treated patients. The relevance of these observations is uncertain, however, given the apparent lack of any significant difference between agonist and placebo in clinical measures of disease progression in these studies.

Pilot studies of creatine [49], minocycline [49], coenzyme Q10 [50, 51], and the orally active neuroimmunophyllin compound GPI-1485 [50], all have potential neuroprotective effects and are worthy of more intensive clinical trials. Large-scale clinical trials are currently underway with creatine and coenzyme Q10 to evaluate their potential role in altering the progression of PD.

3.2.3
Surgical Treatment

While pharmacological therapy provides the mainstay of treatment approaches through the course of PD, neurosurgical approaches are important in more advanced stages of the disease. Deep brain stimulation (DBS) has become an accepted adjunct to pharmacological treatment in medically refractory PD. Ablative surgery such as thalamotomy and pallidotomy has been used historically, but these procedures have given way for the most part to DBS with the permanent implantation of intracerebral electrodes connected to an implanted pulse generator. The structures most commonly targeted for DBS in patients with PD are the ventralis intermedius nucleus of the thalamus (Vim), the posteroventral portion of the globus pallidus interna (GPi), and the subthalamic nucleus (STN). Vim stimulation is effective primarily for tremor, but has little (if any) impact on rigidity and bradykinesia. In contrast, GPi and STN stimulation can be helpful for treating all of the cardinal features of PD, and also appear to be beneficial at reducing dyskinesias. A recent randomized trial comparing STN stimulation plus medication to medical management alone showed a significant benefit in motor scores and quality of life with DBS [52].

It is important to note that DBS is no more effective for parkinsonian symptoms than is levodopa when patients are in an "on" state. Indeed, the best predictor of a patient's response to DBS is the preoperative response to levodopa [53], and a failure to respond to levodopa is considered to be a contraindication to surgical treatment. In contrast, DBS can have a substantial benefit in levodopa-responsive symptoms that are present in an "off" state. Based on this observation, a major indication for DBS is the presence of medically refractory motor fluctuations. A second major indication is the presence of disabling dyskinesias. Pallidotomy or GPi stimulation has a direct benefit on contralateral dyskinesias. Pallidal surgery does not usually have a major effect on the need for medication, whereas STN surgery can reduce the requirement for PD medications, resulting in a reduction in dyskinesias secondary to the decreased dopaminergic drug dose. The relative merits of GPi versus STN stimulation are controversial, however, and a double-blind trial comparing these two targets is currently under way.

The ideal candidate for DBS surgery is the younger PD patient who is otherwise in good medical condition, does not have significant cognitive impairment, and who has disabling motor fluctuations or dyskinesias in spite of optimized medical treatment [54]. Although physiological age is a more important consideration than is chronological age, it is fair to state that, in general, older patients have a less successful outcome with more complications than do younger patients. Detailed neuropsychological testing is an important part of preoperative screening because patients with significant cognitive impairment do not tolerate the surgical procedure (which is performed in the awake patient) well, and do not have the same degree of symptomatic benefit experienced by those who are cognitively intact.

The widely perceived concept that the major clinical abnormalities of PD derive from impaired neuronal function limited to the dopaminergic system has led to attempts to replenish the dopaminergic neurons with dopamine-producing cells from other sources, such as fetal midbrain, retinal pigment epithelium, embryonic stem cells, and genetically modified cells, by neurotransplantation techniques. It is important to consider that these attempts at treatment are very much in their infancy, and that a great deal of research is required before they become generally applicable in patients with PD. It is equally important to realize that PD symptoms are not limited to those that arise from dopaminergic system dysfunction, and that nondopaminergic features have a major impact on the patient's quality of life. Any treatment that is restricted to "replacing the missing dopamine" may have a limited impact on dealing with the complexities of PD symptomatology in the long term [55].

3.2.4
Non-Pharmacologic Treatment

Although pharmacological intervention is the mainstay of symptomatic management, not all issues facing the individual living with PD are addressed by medications. The participation of a multidisciplinary team, including a neurologist specializing in movement disorders, will provide a comprehensive approach to the long-term management of issues arising in PD. Rehabilitation services, specialized nursing care and psychosocial services work together to provide on-going support, at all stages of PD. The representatives of this multidisciplinary team vary according to the needs of the individual and the family, changing with disease progression and as different issues emerge. The overall goal is to allow the individual to achieve and maintain the highest possible level of independent function–a level that will inevitably change as physical and/or cognitive abilities decline and the effectiveness of medication declines. Each team member helps educate both the patient and the family, emphasizing those issues most relevant to the stage of disability and the expertise of the discipline. It is essential that "patient-important" problems are identified, as each individual will require a slightly different approach. This will allow patients a sense of control with respect to treatment. At all stages of the disease, it is critical to emphasize that the goal of all aspects of treatment is not to achieve a "normal" state, but rather to achieve and maintain the highest possible level of independent function. Sources of reliable information should be provided, with a cautionary note made regarding uncensored information obtained from the internet.

3.3
Nursing

A nurse with specialized knowledge of PD, its treatment, and complications should be an integral member of the multidisciplinary team. Regular contact with both patient and family allows the nurse to identify needs and to act as a liaison between the patient, physician, and allied healthcare professionals, helping to reduce the "authority gap" that may otherwise exist [56]. The nurse is important in ongoing education regarding the disease process and treatment, and may deal with psychosocial concerns and difficulties managing in the home setting, especially if access to other psychosocial disciplines is not available. He/she is in a position to identify those medical concerns that are directly related to PD, compared to those that are indirectly related or unrelated and better handled by a family physician. The relationship that is established between the nurse and the patient/family often encourages candid discussions about personal, work, and family issues. The nurse frequently fields questions regarding the ability to continue working, concerns of caregivers, speech and swallowing difficulties, mobility problems, and social issues. Concerns about sexuality [57, 58] may be more comfortably broached by the nurse, who may then refer to appropriate resources as necessary. The nurse, who often is a frequent contact for the patient and the family, is invaluable in coordinating the care plan.

3.4
Rehabilitation

It might be expected that rehabilitation services would be of significant benefit in treating PD and, indeed, there is evidence that patients may benefit from physical, occupational, and speech therapy in conjunction with medications [59, 60]. However, studies of these therapies in PD all suffer from the same limitations, namely small numbers of participants, no consensus as to "best practice," and difficulties in designing large, randomized placebo-controlled trials that would fully establish the efficacy of interventions from an evidence-based perspective [60–64]. Nevertheless, the individual patient often does benefit subjectively from these services, and larger-scale scientifically rigorous studies are currently under way.

3.4.1
Physical Therapy

The role of physical therapy (PT) is to teach strategies for coping with impairment and disability, compensating and adapting as necessary [65]. The goal is to address those symptoms that are amenable to change, in order to minimize secondary complications, and to teach preventive and compensatory strategies where indicated [66, 67]. Physical therapy intervention should be tailored to the individual needs of patients at different phases of their illness and, as with other therapies, must include the goals and priorities of the patient in the management plan. Periodic reassessments ensure that, as PD progresses, appropriate additions to interventions are made. Activities are stressed that enhance the performance of functional motor tasks, including walking, turning, going from sit to stand, bed mobility, fall prevention, posture, balance, reaching, grasping and manipulating objects, in addition to general conditioning, strength and flexibility [68, 69]. Physical therapy will also assess the need for mobility devices, and recommend them if and when appropriate. It is well established that individuals with PD move more easily in the presence of external sensory cues [70–72], and it is important to incorporate these into "real-life" situations and environments. This, coupled with the principles of motor learning in task and context specific learning,[73], helps to guide interventions with PT. Detailed descriptions of these interventions are beyond the scope of this chapter, and are described elsewhere [61, 62, 74]. A recent evidence-based analysis of PT in PD has recommended that treatment be directed particularly at cueing strategies to improve gait, at cognitive movement strategies to improve transfers, at exercises to improve balance, and at the training of joint mobility and muscle power to improve physical capacity [75]. Not all PT needs to be part of a formal, hospital-based program. Rather, under the guidance of a therapist a fitness program can be implemented in community fitness facilities, especially in early PD; group exercise classes often meet the physical and social needs of people living with PD. As PD progresses and the ability to function in the home becomes increasingly compromised, a home assessment and integration of PT-specific instructions is indicated to ensure optimal independence. The inclusion of caregivers/companions/spouses in the spectrum of PT intervention often ensures better compliance, and may assist the individual with PD in problem-solving mobility difficulties in novel environments.

3.4.2
Occupational Therapy

Working together as integral members of the multidisciplinary team, the physical therapist and occupational therapist share a number of common treatment goals. A coordinated approach, where possible, will maximize the efforts of all involved. Occupational therapy (OT) tends to focus on self-care, leisure, work and activities of daily living [76], and PT intervention may overlap where these activities require strength, flexibility, and balance. The goal of OT in PD is to maintain functional independence and, with disease progression and declining abilities, to assist individuals and their families to adapt and change strategies to maximize function at the new level. Patient and family education and support are cornerstones of OT intervention at all times. One of the important roles of OT is in assessing the need for adaptive equipment. This includes assistive devices for dressing and grooming, washing and bathing, toileting, eating and drinking, and bed mobility. With increasingly compromised abilities, a home OT assessment can be helpful in promoting a safe environment, ensuring that the home is functionally optimized. The occupational therapist also advises in the areas of energy conservation, relaxation techniques, advocates the use of community resources, and assists in helping deal with the functional implications of cognitive decline.

3.4.3
Speech Therapy

The goal of the speech language pathologist (SLP) is to assist a person in improving and/or maintaining communication skills, and to assess the integrity of the mechanisms involved with swallowing. Disorders of speech and swallowing are common in PD, and these features tend to respond poorly to medication. As PD progresses, the most common problems relate to imprecise articulation (dysarthria), reduced volume and breath control, reduced facial expression and reduced control over rhythm, rate and pitch [77]. A variety of speech therapy techniques administered once or twice weekly, emphasizing rate, articulation, rhythm and pitch have been used to address these problems, often with immediate but no sustained improvement. There is evidence that the Lee Silverman Voice Therapy (LSVT®) technique, which emphasizes improving vocal adduction and overall voice and speech production, may result in longlasting benefits [78]. As with other rehabilitation therapies, SLP treatment approaches require larger and more rigorous studies to fully establish, from an evidence-based perspective, its role in the management of PD. The role of the SLP in the assessment of swallowing problems is often done in conjunction with a dietician. The risk of aspiration increases as the ability to swallow is compromised in later stages of PD.

3.5
Nutrition

The importance of nutritional needs in PD is often overlooked. In early PD, no special care is usually required beyond stressing a well-balanced diet. However, in disease progression dysphagia is common, with aspiration becoming a risk during the later stages. At this point, the patient may be referred to a dietician and/or SLP for nutritional counseling and advice on food preparation. In later stages, when the response to medication becomes unpredictable, a low-protein diet may be beneficial, as there is evidence that levodopa absorption is impeded by dietary protein [79, 80]. It is important to involve a dietician if such dietary manipulations are being considered to ensure that nutritional requirements are met. Adequate hydration must be stressed, particularly in more advanced disease.

3.6
Psychosocial Issues

The diagnosis of PD, and the prospect of dealing with a chronic progressive disease, usually presents a significant challenge for both the patient and family. Although, the need for formal psychosocial support will vary between individuals, referral to a professional should be considered to assist in equipping the patient and family with coping strategies and maintaining realistic expectations with respect to abilities and limitations secondary to PD. Routine screening for depression with standard rating scales during regular office visits may identify problems in the early stages and facilitate timely intervention. Anxiety, mental and physical fatigue and sleep disturbances are often present in PD, all of which will impact on the quality of life [81]. All patients will benefit from ongoing assessment and treatment of emotional, social, and psychological needs.

With disease progression, the emotional, mental and physical strain placed on family members and caregivers is increased. It is important to ensure that the caregivers' needs are being met as part of the overall patient management. A patient's ability to cope in the face of decreasing independence is greatly affected by the ability of the caregiver to deal with the demands of daily life. The ability to cope can be affected by sleep deprivation, economic/financial concerns, and the physical stress of caring for a dependent person, as well as the need for home care and respite and the stress associated with the need for nursing home/continuing care placement [82]. Access to community support services will better enable the caregiver and, by extension, the patient to cope with a progressive, neurological condition.

An important source of social and psychological support can be found in support groups to help meet the needs of both the person with PD and his or her family. The ability to interact with others who have similar experiences has been shown to be beneficial at all stages of the disease [83].

3.7
Conclusions

Parkinson disease is a progressive disorder that demands an holistic approach to treatment. Pharmacologic, surgical, and nonpharmacologic interventions all play important roles in the comprehensive management of people living with PD, and their families. These interventions must be tailored to the individual and modified as the disease progresses, with the goal of minimizing significant functional disability and maximizing the quality of life as much as possible.

References

1 Cotzias, G.C., Van Woert, M.H., and Schiffer, L.M. (1967) Aromatic amino acids and modification of parkinsonism. *New England Journal of Medicine*, **276**, 374–379.

2 Diamond, S.G., Markham, C.H., Hoehn, M.M., McDowell, F.H., and Muenter, M.D. (1989) Effect of age at onset on progression and mortality in Parkinson's disease. *Neurology*, **39**, 1187–1190.

3 Hughes, A.J., Ben-Shlomo, Y., Daniel, S.E., and Lees, A.J. (1992) What features improve the accuracy of clinical diagnosis in Parkinson's disease: a clinicopathologic study. *Neurology*, **42**, 1142–1146.

4 Agid, Y., Chase, T., and Marsden, D. (1998) Adverse reactions to levodopa: drug toxicity or progression of disease? *Lancet*, **351**, 851–852.

5 Fahn, S., Oakes, D., Shoulson, I., *et al.* (2004) Levodopa and the progression of Parkinson's disease. *New England Journal of Medicine*, **351**, 2498–2508.

6 Lang, A.E. and Lozano, A.M. (1998) Parkinson's disease. *New England Journal of Medicine*, **339**, 1044–1053.

7 Kostic, V., Przedborski, S., Flaster, E., and Sternic, N. (1991) Early develop- ment of levodopa-induced dyskinesias and response fluctuations in young- onset Parkinson's disease. *Neurology*, **41**, 202–205.

8 Djaldetti, R., Baron, J., Ziv, I., and Melamed, E. (1996) Gastric emptying in Parkinson's disease: patients with and without response fluctuations. *Neurology*, **46**, 1051–1054.

9 Nutt, J.G. (1987) On-off phenomenon: relation to levodopa pharmacokinetics and pharmacodynamics. *Annals of Neurology*, **22**, 535–540.

10 Chase, T.N., Engler, T.M., and Mouradian, M.M. (1994) Palliative and prophylactic benefits of continuously administered dopaminomimetics in Parkinson's disease. *Neurology*, **44** (Suppl. 6), S15–S18.

11 Ahlskog, J.E., Muenter, M.D., McManis, P.G., Bell, G.N., and Bailey P.A. (1988) Controlled-release Sinemet (CR-4): a double-blind crossover study in patients with fluctuating Parkinson's disease. *Mayo Clinic Proceedings*, **63**, 876–886.

12 Muenter, M.D., Sharpless, N.S., Tyce, G.M., and Darley, F.L. (1977) Patterns of dystonia ("I-D-I" and "D-I-D") in response to l-dopa therapy for Parkinson's disease. *Mayo Clinic Proceedings*, **52**, 163–174.

13 Metman, L.V., Del Dotto, P., LePoole, K., Konitsiotis, S., Fang, J., and Chase, T.N. (1999) Amantadine for levodopa- induced dyskinesias: a 1-year follow-up study. *Archives of Neurology*, **56**, 1383–1386.

14 Koller, W.C., Hutton, J.T., Tolosa, E., *et al.* (1999) Immediate-release and controlled-release carbidopa/levodopa in PD: a 5 year randomized multicenter study. Carbidopa/Levodopa Study Group. *Neurology*, **53**, 1012–1019.

15 Kurth, M.C. and Adler, C.H. (1998) COMT inhibition: a new treatment strategy for Parkinson's disease. *Neurology*, **50** (Suppl. 5), S3–S14.

16 Ruottinen, H.M. and Rinne, U.K. (1996) Entacapone prolongs levodopa response in a one month double blind study in parkinsonian patients with levodopa related fluctuations. *Journal of Neurology, Neurosurgery, and Psychiatry*, **60**, 36–40.

17 Parkinson Study Group (1997) Entacapone improved motor fluctuations in levodopa-treated Parkinson's disease patients. *Annals of Neurology*, **42**, 747–755.

18 Parkinson Study Group (1989) Effect of deprenyl on the progression of disability in early Parkinson's disease. *New England Journal of Medicine*, **321**, 1364–1371.

19 Parkinson Study Group (2002) A controlled trial of rasagiline in early Parkinson Disease: the TEMPO Study. *Archives of Neurology*, **59**, 1937–1943.

20 Parkinson Study Group (2005) A randomized placebo-controlled trial of rasagiline in levodopa-treated patients with Parkinson Disease and motor fluctuations: the PRESTO study. *Archives of Neurology*, **62**, 241–248.

21 de Marcaida, J.A., Schwid, S.R., White, W.B., *et al.* (2006) Effects of tyramine administration in Parkinson's disease patients treated with selective MAO-B inhibitor rasagiline. *Movement Disorders*, **21**, 1716–1721.

22 Van Camp, G., Flamez, A., Cosyns, B., *et al.* (2004) Treatment of Parkinson's disease with pergolide and relation to restrictive valvular heart disease. *Lancet*, **363**, 1179–1183.

23 Baseman, D.G., O'Suilleabhain, P.E., Reimold, S., Laskar, S.R., Baseman, J.G., and Dewey, R.B., Jr. (2004) Pergolide use in Parkinson disease is associated with cardiac valve regurgitation. *Neurology*, **63**, 301–304.

24 Zanettini, R., Antonini, A., Gatto, G., Gentile, R., Tesei, S., and Pezzoli, G. (2007) Valvular heart disease and the use of dopamine agonists for Parkinson's disease. *New England Journal of Medicine*, **356**, 39–46.

25 Calne, D.B., Teychenne, P.F., Claveria, L.E., Eastman, R., Greenacre, J.K., and Petrie, A. (1974) Bromocriptine in parkinsonism. *British Medical Journal*, **4**, 442–444.

26 Lieberman, A., Kupersmith, M., Estey, E., and Goldstein, M. (1976) Treatment of Parkinson's disease with bromocriptine. *New England Journal of Medicine*, **295**, 1400–1404.

27 Lieberman, A., Ranhosky, A., and Korts, D. (1997) Clinical evaluation of pramipexole in advanced Parkinson's disease: results of a double-blind, placebo-controlled, parallel-group study. *Neurology*, **49**, 162–168.

28 Guttman, M., and the International Pramipexole-Bromocriptine Study Group (1997) Double-blind comparison of pramipexole and bromocriptine treatment with placebo in advanced Parkinson's disease. *Neurology*, **49**, 1060–1065.

29 Lieberman, A., Olanow, C.W., Sethi, K., *et al.* (1998) A multicenter trial of ropinirole as adjunct treatment for Parkinson's disease. *Neurology*, **51**, 1057–1062.

30 Rascol, O., Lees, A.J., Senard, J.M., Pirtosek, Z., Montastruc, J.L., and Fuell, D. (1996) Ropinirole in the treatment of levodopa-induced motor fluctuations in patients with Parkinson's disease. *Clinical Neuropharmacology*, **19**, 234–245.

31 Rascol, O., Brooks, D.J., Korczyn, A.D., *et al.* (2000) A five-year study of dyskinesias in patients with early Parkinson's disease who were treated with ropinirole or levodopa. *New England Journal of Medicine*, **342**, 1484–1491.

32 Parkinson Study Group (2000) Pramipexole versus levodopa as initial treatment for Parkinson's disease. *Journal of the American Medical Association*, **284**, 1931–1938.

33 Miyasaki, J.M., Martin, W., Suchowersky, O., Weiner, W.J., and Lang, A.E. (2002) Practice parameter: initiation of treatment for Parkinson's disease: an evidence-based review. *Neurology*, **58**, 11–17.

34 Watts, R.L., Jankovic, J., Waters, C., Rajput, A., Boroojerdi, B., and Rao, J. (2007) Randomized, blind, controlled trial of transdermal rotigotine in early Parkinson Disease. *Neurology*, **68**, 272–276.

35 Parkinson Study Group (1999) Low-dose clozapine for the treatment of drug-induced psychosis in Parkinson's disease. *New England Journal of Medicine*, **340**, 757–763.

36 Fernandez, H.H., Friedman, J.H., Jacques, C., and Rosenfeld, M. (1999) Quetiapine for the treatment of drug-induced psychosis in Parkinson's disease. *Movement Disorders*, **14**, 484–487.

37 Goetz, C.G., Blasucci, L.M., Leurgans, S., and Pappert, E.J. (2000) Olanzapine and clozapine. Comparative effects on motor function in hallucinating PD patients. *Neurology*, **55**, 789–794.

38 Frucht, S., Rogers, J.D., Greene, P.E., Gordon, M.F., and Fahn, S. (1999) Falling sleep at the wheel: motor vehicle mishaps in persons taking pramipexole and ropinirole. *Neurology*, **52**, 1908–1910.

39 Hobson, D.E., Lang, A.E., Martin, W.R.W., Razmy, A., Rivest, J., and Fleming, J. (2002) Excessive daytime sleepiness and sudden-onset sleep in Parkinson Disease. A survey by the Canadian Movement Disorders Group.

Journal of the American Medical Association, **287**, 455–463.

40 Lawrence, A.D., Evans, A.H., and Lees, A.J. (2003) Compulsive use of dopamine replacement therapy in Parkinson's disease: reward systems gone awry? *Lancet Neurology*, **66**, 845–851.

41 Dodd, M.L., Klos, K.J., Bower, J.H., Geda, Y.E., Josephs, K.A., and Ahlskog, J.E. (2005) Pathological gambling caused by drugs used to treat Parkinson Disease. *Archives of Neurology*, **62**, 1377–1381.

42 Voon, V., Hassan, K., Zurowski, M., Duff-Canning, S., de Souza, M., Fox, S., Lang, A.E., and Miyasaki, J. (2006) Prospective prevalence of pathologic gambling and medication association in Parkinson Disease. *Neurology*, **66**, 1750–1752.

43 Voon, V., Thomsen, T., Miyasaki, J.M., *et al.* (2007) Factors associated with dopaminergic drug-related pathological gambling in Parkinson Disease. *Archives of Neurology*, **64**, 212–216.

44 Weintraub, D., Siderowf, A.D., Potenza, M.N., *et al.* (2006) Association of dopamine agonist use with impulse control disorders in Parkinson Disease. *Archives of Neurology*, **63**, 969–973.

45 Mytilineou, C. and Cohen, G. (1985) Deprenyl protects dopamine neurons from the neurotoxic effect of 1-methyl-4-phenyl-pyridinium ion. *Journal of Neurochemistry*, **45**, 1951–1953.

46 Palhagen, S., Heinonen, E.H., Hagglung, J., *et al.* (1998) Selegiline delays the onset of disability in de novo parkinsonian patients. *Neurology*, **51**, 520–525.

47 Parkinson Study Group (2002) Dopamine transporter brain imaging to assess the effects of pramipexole vs. levodopa on Parkinson Disease progression. *Journal of the American Medical Association*, **287**, 1653–1661.

48 Whone, A.L., Watts, R.L., Stoessl, A.J., *et al.* (2003) Slower progression of Parkinson's disease with ropinirole versus levodopa: the real-pet study. *Annals of Neurology*, **54**, 93–101.

49 NINDS NET-PD Investigators (2006) A randomized, double-blind, futility clinical trial of creatine and minocycline in early Parkinson Disease. *Neurology*, **66**, 664–671.

50 NINDS NET-PD Investigators (2007) A randomized clinical trial of coenzyme Q10 and GPI-1485 in early Parkinson Disease. *Neurology*, **68**, 20–28.

51 Shults, C.W., Oakes, D., Kieburtz, K., *et al.* (2002) Effects of coenzyme Q10 in early Parkinson Disease: evidence of slowing of the functional decline. *Archives of Neurology*, **59**, 1541–1550.

52 Deuschl, G., Schade-Brittinger, C., Krack, P., *et al.* (2006) A randomized trial of deep-brain stimulation for Parkinson's disease. *New England Journal of Medicine*, **355**, 896–908.

53 Charles, P.D., Van Blercom, N., Krack, P., *et al.* (2002) Predictors of effective bilateral subthalamic nucleus stimulation for PD. *Neurology*, **59**, 932–934.

54 Weaver, F.M., Stern, M.B., and Follett, K. (2006) Deep-brain stimulation in Parkinson's disease. *Lancet Neurology*, **5**, 900–901.

55 Lang, A.E. and Obeso, J.A. (2004) Challenges in Parkinson Disease: restoration of the nigrostriatal dopamine system is not enough. *Lancet Neurology*, **3**, 309–316.

56 MacMahon, D.G. (1999) Parkinson's disease nurse specialists: an important role in disease management. *Neurology*, **57** (Suppl. 3), S21–S25.

57 Jacobs, H., Vieregge, A., and Vieregge, P. (2000) Sexuality in young patients with Parkinson's disease: a population based comparison with healthy controls. *Journal of Neurology, Neurosurgery, and Psychiatry*, **69**, 550–552.

58 Welsh, M., Hung, L., and Waters, C.H. (1997) Sexuality in women with Parkinson's disease. *Movement Disorders*, **12**, 923–927.

59 de Goede, C.J.T., Keus, S.H.J., Kwakkel, G., and Wagenaar, R.C. (2001) The effects of Physical Therapy in Parkinson's disease: a research synthesis. *Archives of Physical Medicine and Rehabilitation*, **82**, 508–515.

60 Goetz, C.G., Koller, W.C., Poewe, W., Rascol, O., Sampaio, C., *et al.* (2002) Management of Parkinson's disease: an evidence-based review. *Movement Disorders*, **17** (Suppl. 4), S156–S159.

61 Deane, K.H., Jones, D., Playford, E.D., Ben-Shlomo, Y., and Clarke, C.E. (2002) Physiotherapy versus placebo or no intervention in Parkinson's disease. *Cochrane Database of Systematic Reviews*, Issue **3**.

62 Deane, K.H., Jones, D., Ellis-Hill, C., Clarke, C., Playford, E.D., and Ben-Shlomo, Y. (2002) Physiotherapy for Parkinson's disease: a comparison of techniques. *Cochrane Database of Systematic Reviews*, Issue **1**.

63 Deane, K.H., Whurr, R., Playford, E.D., Ben-Shlomo, Y., and Clarke, C. (2002) Speech and language therapy versus placebo or no intervention for dysarthria in Parkinson's disease. *Cochrane Database of Systematic Reviews*, Issue **2**.

64 Deane, K.H., Whurr, R., Playford, E.D., Ben-Shlomo, Y., and Clarke, C. (2002) Speech and language therapy for dysarthria in Parkinson's disease: a comparison of techniques. *Cochrane Database of Systematic Reviews*, Issue **2**.

65 American Physical Therapy Association (1997) Guide to physical therapy practice. *Physical Therapy*, **77**, 1163–1650.

66 Schenkman, M. and Butler, R.B. (1989) A model for multisystem evaluation treatment of individuals with Parkinson's disease. *Physical Therapy*, **69**, 944–955.

67 Schenkman, M., Donovan, J., Tsubota, J., *et al.* (1989) Management of individuals with Parkinson's disease: rationale and case studies. *Physical Therapy*, **69**, 944–955.

68 Morris, M.E. (2000) Movement disorders in people with Parkinson's disease: a model for physical therapy. *Physical Therapy*, **80**, 578–597.

69 Scandalis, T.A., Bosak, A., Berliner, J.C., Helman, L.L., and Wells, M.R. (2001) Resistance training and gait function in patients with Parkinson's disease. *American Journal of Physical Medicine and Rehabilitation*, **80**, 38–43.

70 Morris, M.E., Iansek, R., Matyas, T.A., and Summers, J.J. (1994) Ability to modulate walking cadence remains intact in Parkinson's disease. *Journal of Neurology, Neurosurgery, and Psychiatry*, **57**, 1532–1534.

71 Marchese, R., Diverio, M., Zucchi, F., Lentino, C., and Abbruzzese, G. (2000) The role of sensory cues in the rehabilitation of Parkinson's patients: a comparison of two physical therapy protocols. *Movement Disorders*, **15**, 879–883.

72 Behrman, A.L., Teitelbaum, P., and Cauraugh, J.H. (1998) Verbal instructional set normalise the temporal and spatial gait variables in Parkinson's disease. *Journal of Neurology, Neurosurgery, and Psychiatry*, **65**, 580–582.

73 Schmidt, R.A. (1999) *Motor Control and Learning: A Behavioral Emphasis*, 3rd edn, Human Kinetics Inc, Champaign, Illinois.

74 Morris, M.E. and Iansek, R. (1997) An interprofessional team approach to rehabilitation in Parkinson's disease. *European Journal of Physical and Rehabilitation Medicine*, **6**, 166–170.

75 Keus, S.H.J., Bloem, B.R., Hendriks, E.J.M., Bredero-Cohen, A.B., and Munneke, M. (2007) Evidence-based analysis of physical therapy in Parkinson's disease with recommendations for practice and research. *Movement Disorders*, **22**, 451–460.

76 Turner, A., Foster, M., Johnson, S.E., Stewart, A.M. (eds) (1996) *Occupational Therapy and Physical Dysfunction*, 4th edn, Churchill Livingstone Inc., New York, pp. 549–569.

77 Ramig, L.O., Sapir, S., Fox, C., and Countryman, S. (2001) Changes in vocal loudness following intensive treatment (LSVT() in individuals with Parkinson's disease: a comparison with untreated patients and normal age-matched controls. *Movement Disorders*, **16**, 79–83.

78 Ramig, L.O., Sapir, S., Fox, C., Countryman, S., Pawlas, A.A., O'Brien, C., Hoehn, M., and Thompson, L.L. (2001) Intensive voice treatment (LSVT) for patients with Parkinson's disease: a 2 year follow up. *Journal of Neurology, Neurosurgery, and Psychiatry*, **71**, 493–498.

79 Karstaedt, P.J. and Pincus, J.H. (1992) Protein redistribution diet remains effective in patients with fluctuating parkinsonism. *Archives of Neurology*, **49**, 149–151.

80 Koller, W.C. (2002) Treatment of early Parkinson's disease. *Neurology*, **58** (Suppl. 1), S79–S86.

81 Shulman, L.M., Taback, R.L., Rabinstein, A.A., and Weiner, W.J. (2002) Non-recognition of depression an other non-motor symptoms in Parkinson's disease. *Parkinsonism and Related Disorders*, **8**, 193–197.

82 Carter, J.H., *et al.* (1998) Living with a person who has Parkinson's disease: the spouse's perspective by stage of disease. *Movement Disorders*, **13**, 20–28.

83 Olanow, C.W. and Koller, W.C. (eds) (1998) An algorithm (decision tree) for the management of Parkinson's disease: treatment guidelines. *Neurology*, **50** (Suppl. 3), S1–S57.

84 Olanow, C.W., Rascol, O., Hauser, R., *et al.* (2009) A double-blind, delayed-start trial of rasagiline in Parkinson's disease. *New England Journal of Medicine*, **361**, 1268–1278.

A Patient's Story

Happiness is a Choice

Jean Harkness

Reflecting on the past few years it has very much been an emotional and physical roller-coaster; but I know I am fortunate in comparison to so many who have Parkinson's. I am very blessed to have a strong support system in the way of family and friends. These folk show great concern for my well-being and for where I'm at in life—not just how can they help, but what the professionals are saying, such as prescription changes, and so on.

My first real indication that something was dreadfully wrong came in 2001 when, at our youngest son's wedding he asked me to dance, and there was no way my feet would move. Before this I had had some tingling and what I thought to be minor concerns. I was referred to the Movement Disorder Clinic in 2002, where they determined I had a mild case of Parkinson's. Since that day there have been changes in my condition. Stiffness, rigidity, tremor, dyskinesia and, uncertainty in everything. You can say in one minute that you are fine—it's a good day, and so on—and the next you're shaking like a leaf (tremors) or plainly moving in an uncontrolled fashion. This is when we (husband, family, and I) have had to learn to laugh a lot! For instance, when getting out of the car I may need a little push, or some help putting on my jewelry. So I can't definitely say good days and bad—it's more often good times and not so good. But you have to do your best to develop a positive mental attitude and find a side of life that perhaps has been evading you.

There are many things that can be a challenge for me, even the simple ordinary everyday tasks may be very difficult and often impossible for me to do. Things that require coordination and/or a little bit of strength will often evade me. These times can create feelings of helplessness, and this is when I reach out for help. I try not to get myself into pressured or time-sensitive situations, as this only results in frustration, uncertainty, increased tremor, and slowness. By allowing sufficient time to do things—like getting ready to go out or preparing dinner—I can have a rest or ask for help.

The decision to stop driving was most hurtful for me, as I always enjoyed driving and the independence that I always had. I was able to share this capability with others. But when I couldn't keep a steady pressure on the gas and brake pedals I decided that it was the right time to give up driving. My family and friends have stepped up to the plate, and for this I am very grateful, even though it is so difficult to be dependent.

Who did I reach out to?

- Family first, then close friends
- The medical profession—that is, the family doctor and referral to the Movement Disorder Clinic at University of Calgary Foothills Hospital.

- The Parkinson's Society of Southern Alberta: I can't say enough good about this society and their extremely professional staff. They are there to serve you ... I urge you to use the services of PSSA, to consider becoming a member, and to support it both through volunteering and financially whenever possible.
- The Church
- Clubs and associations

The feelings of dependency, helplessness, and discomfort can create a sense of loneliness. I have found that you can't stick your head in the sand—you have to push on, and you have to reach out.

I realize that my life will never be the same as it used to be, but if I continue to believe that happiness is a choice, then life is great.

4
Treatment of Non-Motor Symptoms of Parkinson Disease

Ranjit Ranawaya and Oksana Suchowersky

Parkinson disease (PD) is more than just a disorder of dopamine. A variety of other neurotransmitter systems are involved with a loss of serotonin, norepine-phrine, acetylcholine, cholecystokinin octapeptide (CCK-8) and somatostatin due to gradual widespread neuronal degeneration in the cortex, brainstem, and spinal cord [1]. This leads to a wide variety of non-motor manifestations, including autonomic, cognitive, psychiatric, and vegetative that become more apparent with disease progression and frequently lead to significant morbidity and loss of quality of life in advanced disease. Recognition and treatment of the condition are as important as medical control of the motor symptoms. Unfortunately, it has been shown in a previous study that the recognition and correct diagnosis of these symptoms by neurologists during office visits is generally poor [2].

In Chapter 3, some of the non-dopaminergic (non-motor) features associated with PD were briefly described. In this chapter, the details of these features will be expanded and their management described. The non-motor symptoms of PD are listed in Table 4.1.

4.1
Sleep Disturbances

Many PD patients complain of poor sleep, and the cause is usually multifactorial [3]. As these patients fall within the age range in which sleep disturbances are common among the general population, it is important to consider alternative causes for the sleep disturbance, such as sleep apnea or restless leg syndrome, before ascribing these to the patient's PD. In men, nocturia should be investigated to exclude urinary tract infection, detrusor hyperactivity, or prostatism.

Once the above possibilities have been excluded, the first step is to determine the possible PD-related causes such as medication effects, nocturnal wearing off and dystonia, and nocturia. For example, selegiline has metamphetamine breakdown products and should be scheduled in the morning as a single daily dose. Sedative drugs should be avoided in the daytime. If the patient is experiencing early morning wakening due to "off" dystonia, then a sustained-release levodopa

Parkinson Disease – A Health Policy Perspective. Edited by Wayne Martin, Oksana Suchowersky,
Katharina Kovacs Burns, and Egon Jonsson
Copyright © 2010 WILEY-VCH Verlag GmbH & Co. KGaA, Weinheim
ISBN: 978-3-527-32779-9

Table 4.1 Non-motor symptoms of Parkinson disease.

Sleep disorders
   Sleep fragmentation and insomnia
   REM sleep behavior disorder
   Periodic movements in sleep/restless legs syndrome
   Excessive daytime somnolence
Autonomic dysfunction
Orthostatic hypotension
   Urinary dysfunction
   Constipation
   Other gastrointestinal abnormalities (nausea, bloating, cramping)
   Sweating and flushing
   Sexual dysfunction
   Drooling
   Seborrhea
   Dyspnea
Neuropsychiatric problems
   Mood disorders (depression)
   Anxiety
   Apathy and anhedonia
   Medication-related (impulse control disorders, punding, hypersexuality)
   Frontal executive dysfunction
   Hallucinations
   Psychosis
   Dementia
Sensory symptoms
   Olfactory dysfunction
   Visual abnormalities
   Dysesthesia
   Pain
Other problems
   Eye movement abnormalities
   Fatigue

preparation can be added at bedtime. Alternatively, the patient may wish to keep a tablet of the rapid-acting levodopa at the bedside to take should he or she awake with stiffness or painful cramps. The following of good sleep hygiene practices is also important.

If none of these is effective then hypnotic medications may need to be prescribed. For example, tricyclic antidepressants taken at low dose at bedtime may be useful, as they are sedating, and may reduce the nocturia that many of the patients experience, that is related to autonomic dysfunction. In more severe cases – and particularly in the setting of evening hallucinations and/or cognitive dysfunction – the use of atypical neuroleptics such as quetiapine or clozapine may be required. Rapid eye movement (REM) sleep disorders may be treated with additional dopaminergic therapy, or by the use of clonazepam.

In patients with poor sleep, *daytime somnolence* is a frequent complaint. It is important to recognize that this can also be a side effect of the dopaminergic agonists. The daytime somnolence can be so severe as to result in sudden sleep attacks [4], and in this situation either a reduction in the dose or a substitution with another dopamine agonist may be considered. If, despite this, daytime somnolence persists, the addition of modafinil has been shown to be helpful [5].

4.2
Autonomic Dysfunction

Autonomic dysfunction is a common feature in PD, and is estimated to occur in up to 80% of patients within 10–15 years of disease onset [6]. The variety of symptoms seen is listed in Table 4.1, while details of treatment are summarized in Table 4.2.

4.2.1
Orthostatic (Postural) Hypotension

This is defined as a fall in systolic blood pressure of at least 20 mmHg. Patients will complain of dizziness or feeling faint on standing, particularly after a large meal or with prolonged standing. Rarely, the drop in blood pressure may be so severe that the patient loses consciousness. In addition to the primary autonomic insufficiency, contributing factors include: treatment with levodopa and dopamine agonists, the use of antihypertensives or diuretics, and poor nutrition and decreased fluid intake. Management includes regular blood pressure monitoring lying and

Table 4.2 Treatment of autonomic dysfunction in Parkinson disease.

Postural hypotension	↑ fluid/salt intake
	Discontinue antihypertensives
	Fludrocortisone
	Midodrine
Urinary urgency/frequency	Amitriptyline
	Oxybutinin
	Desmopressin
Constipation	↑ fluid, ↑ exercise
	Stool softeners
Gastrointestinal abnormalities	Domperidone, ondansetron
Nausea	
Bloating	
Cramping	
Sialorrhea	Anticholinergics
	Amitriptyline
	1% atropine solution
	Botulinum toxin injections
Seborrhea	Steroid cream
	Ketoconazole cream
Sexual dysfunction	Sildenafil
	Yohimbine

standing, discontinuation of antihypertensives and diuretics, stressing the importance of adequate fluid and salt intake, and the use of waist-high support stockings (if tolerated). Patients should be counseled to sit or lie down immediately should they feel dizzy or faint in order to prevent falls. If conservative measures fail, the addition of fludrocortisone or midodrine may be required [7, 8].

4.2.2
Urinary Dysfunction

Urinary dysfunction, including frequency, urgency and nocturia are frequently reported in PD [9, 10]. Detrusor hyperreflexia is the predominant abnormality of bladder dysfunction which results in bladder contractions. It is important to rule out other causes of bladder dysfunction, such as prostatic hypertrophy in males, before empiric trials of anticholinergic drugs are undertaken [11]. As tolterodine is less lipophilic, it may be more suitable than other anticholinergics for patients with cognitive impairment [12].

4.2.3
Gastrointestinal Dysfunction

Gastrointestinal dysfunction affects the whole gastrointestinal system. Symptoms can result in significant discomfort; recognition leads to earlier and more effective intervention [13, 14].

4.2.3.1 Dysphagia
Dysphagia is present in the majority of patients; documented abnormalities include a prolongation of triggering of the swallowing reflex, a reduced rate of swallowing, and slowness of sequential muscle movements. Aspiration can result in more severe cases. The formal evaluation of swallowing abilities is indicated in patients with complaints of coughing with eating, or food sticking in the throat.

4.2.3.2 Gastroparesis
Gastroparesis is characterized by symptoms of discomfort or bloating after meals, early satiety, and nausea. Gastric emptying time has been shown to be slowed in PD, and of note, is even slower in levodopa-treated individuals [14]. Treatment involves eating small and frequent meals, the discontinuation of medications such as anticholinergics that impede gastric emptying, and the use of domperidone, a peripheral dopamine antagonist which does not cross the blood–brain barrier.

4.2.3.3 Constipation
Constipation occurs in 20% of patients, if the current definition of less than three bowel movements per week is used. A reduced colonic transit time has been described to occur, and may worsen with disease progression. Megacolon and pseudo-obstruction can be uncommon complications. A graduated approach to treatment is recommended, beginning with addition of fiber and fiber supple-

ments, followed by stool softeners, and osmotic laxatives. Little is known about small bowel dysfunction, but it is postulated that dysmotility may also be present.

4.2.3.4 Anorectal Dysfunction
Anorectal dysfunction has also been noted, with disordered contraction and relaxation of muscles of defecation resulting in excessive straining and sense of incomplete evacuation.

4.2.4
Weight Loss

Weight loss may occur, due to decreased caloric intake secondary to gastrointestinal dysfunction, or increased energy expenditure due to the PD. However, the fact that some patients have weight loss even when caloric intake is adequate suggests that this may be an intrinsic component of the disease process.

4.2.5
Sweating Disturbances

Sweating disturbances, and in particular *hyperhidrosis*, were reported in 64% of PD patients, compared to 12.5% of controls in one study [15]. The patterns of sweating abnormalities were often localized and asymmetric, and they occur predominantly during "off" periods and "on" periods with dyskinesia. In some patients sweating may respond to the addition of dopamine agonists [16].

4.2.6
Sexual Dysfunction

Sexual dysfunction is relatively common in patients with PD, with 81% of men and 43% of women reporting reduced sexual activity [17]. Some PD patients develop hypersexuality due to PD medications (see impulse control disorders). Counseling to help the couple understand and deal with problems with sexuality is recommended, but unfortunately sexuality specialists are few and far between. Only one randomized controlled study with sildenafil has been conducted in a relatively small number of PD patients [18]. The results indicated that sildenafil was efficacious and relatively safe in both PD and multiple system atrophy (MSA) patients with erectile dysfunction. A worsening of postural hypotension was a possible side effect.

4.2.7
Sialorrhea

Sialorrhea (drooling) is a distressing and embarrassing problem for many PD patients. It is the result of decreased swallowing, rather than an excess production of saliva. The use of atropine drops applied sublingually has been reported to be effective in one open-label study [19]. For severe drooling, the injection of botuli-num toxin into the salivary glands can be helpful [20].

4.2.8
Dyspnea

Dyspnea is not an infrequent complaint. Ventilation problems have been described, but the clinical significance is unclear. Occasionally, stridor can occur as an "off" phenomenon.

It should be recognized that many symptoms of autonomic dysfunction will occur concurrently, and significantly impact on quality of life. In particular, bladder, bowel, and sexual dysfunction will frequently coexist in the same patient.

4.3
Neuropsychiatric Problems

4.3.1
Depression

Depression represents the most common psychiatric complication of PD. Psycho-social support, counseling, and psychotherapy play an important part in its man-agement, particularly when it is related to depressive reactions at the time of diagnosis. Since depression in PD is associated with neurotransmitter changes and is not only to a reaction to the disease process, specific pharmacological treat-ment may be required [21]. Tricyclic antidepressants (TCAs) – in particular amitriptyline – have been shown to be effective in treating depression in PD in randomized controlled trials [22]. However, as treatment with TCAs is often limited by adverse effects, selective serotonin reuptake inhibitors (SSRIs) are cur-rently the most widely used class of drugs to treat depression in PD. Although there are a number of open-label and case reports supportive of the effectiveness of SSRIs, no controlled trials assessing their efficacy and safety are as yet available [22]. Rarely, SSRIs can result in a deterioration of PD.

MAO-A inhibitors should not be coprescribed with levodopa because of the potential risk of developing severe hypertension and/or serotonin syndrome. The risk of serotonin syndrome with the combined use of SSRIs and MAO-B inhibitors (e.g., selegiline, rasagiline) appears to be low [23].

4.3.2
Anxiety

Anxiety is characterized by apprehension, and may be associated with autonomic features such as hyperventilation and palpitations. It has been estimated to occur in up to 25% of PD patients [24]. As anxiety and depression can increase during "off" periods, and may even precede akinetic states, these patients should first be treated with a dopamine replacement (see below). If it is a chronic problem, psychiatric assessment with the use of antidepressants or benzodiazepines with a short half-life (e.g., alprazolam, lorazepam or oxazepam) is recommended.

4.3.3
Apathy

Apathy may coexist with depression, but may also occur as an independent symptom in PD. In the latter situation, it usually remains resistant to treatment and impacts significantly on the patient's quality of life.

4.3.4
Medication-Related Psychiatric Problems

These can occur in a variety of forms as a result of the dopamine replacement therapies used for treatment of PD motor symptoms. These include impulse control disorders (ICDs) [25], hypomania, dopa dysregulation syndrome [26], or hypersexuality and aberrant sexual behaviors [27].

4.3.5
Impulse Control Disorders

Impulse control disorders have received a great deal of attention recently. These are characterized by excessive or poorly controlled preoccupations, urges, or behaviors, and include pathologic gambling, compulsive shopping, and sexual preoccupation. Although the exact prevalence is unknown, it is postulated that ICDs may occur in up to 10% of PD patients. They appear to be more commonly associated with use of dopamine agonists rather than levodopa. The most carefully studied of the ICDs has been *pathological gambling*, which has been shown to be associated with an earlier PD onset, higher novelty-seeking traits, and a personal or family history of alcoholism [25, 28]. In a UK study of 388 patients taking anti-Parkinson medication, 17 (4.4%) developed pathological gambling, all of whom were prescribed dopamine agonists. Thus, 8% of patients taking dopamine agonists had pathological gambling [29]. The reduction or stopping of dopamine agonists may improve the pathological gambling behavior [30].

4.3.6
Dopamine Dysregulation Syndrome

This may occur in a small percentage of patients, manifesting as behavioral abnormalities such as hypomania and an overuse of dopamine replacement therapy [26].

4.3.7
Punding Behavior

Punding behavior is a stereotypical motor behavior characterized by an intense fascination with the repetitive manipulation, examination, cataloging, and endless sorting of objects of common use [31]. It is observed in a minority of PD patients. There are similarities between punding and obsessive-compulsive disorder (OCD) such as purposelessness, and a feeling of calm after performing of the act; however, punding is not associated with obsessive compulsiveness. Even though the patients acknowledge that the behavior is inappropriate and unproductive, attempts by the family to forcefully interrupt the behavior leads to irritability and dysphoria. Those patients who pund are usually receiving higher doses of dopamine replacement therapy, and have more severe dyskinesias than patients who do not pund [32]. Punding may be improved with a reduction of anti-PD medications.

4.3.8
Hypersexuality

Hypersexuality has been reported as a complication of treatment with dopamine agonists [27] , and has also described following high-frequency subthalamic deep brain stimulation [33]. Multidisciplinary care with psychiatric intervention is required. The hypersexuality may resolve after stopping the dopamine agonist or adjusting the stimulation parameters; in more severe cases, the addition of an antipsychotic (e.g., quetiapine) may help. Antihormone therapies with drugs such as cyproterone are currently being investigated.

4.3.9
Dementia

Dementia will develop with time in over 70% of the PD population, and is a major precipitant of nursing home placement. Although, at least in part, this is due to the spread of Lewy bodies to the cerebral cortex, its development likely is multifactorial, with contributing factors being advanced age and comorbidities (notably lacunar infarcts) [22].

4.3.10
Psychosis

Psychosis affects nearly one-third of patients with PD, and is a predictor of cognitive deterioration. Manifestations include hallucinations, delusions, and confusional psychosis. Hallucinations may occur in two settings. Superimposed medical illness such as urinary or respiratory infection and dehydration [35] can trigger hallucinations and confusion; these patients are usually also confused and agitated. When PD patients present with hallucinations or confusion, medical causes should be sought and treated aggressively. If no secondary causes are found, the cause is likely PD-related, as PD patients receiving chronic dopaminergic therapy may develop visual hallucinations. In this case, a careful assessment of all medications that the patient is taking is indicated, and a strategy focused on the reduction of polypharmacy should be developed. Although, all anti-Parkinson medications can cause psychiatric side effects, some are more prone to these side effects than others [36]. Anticholinergics are more likely to cause confusion and psychosis, followed by selegiline, amantadine, and long-acting dopamine agonists. Standard levodopa may be better tolerated than controlled-release preparations. Therefore, when simplifying anti-parkinsonian therapy these drugs should be discontinued in the order mentioned above, and patients maintained on the lowest doses of regular-acting levodopa required. If the reduction of anti-Parkinson drugs is likely to markedly worsen mobility and activities of daily living, then the cautious use of atypical neuroleptics such as clozapine and quetiapine may be warranted. These agents should be initiated at low doses, as PD patients typically respond to very low doses and are very sensitive to side effects [37].

For cognitive deterioration, treatment with cholinesterase inhibitors might be helpful. Only donepezil and rivastigmine, have shown some benefit in the treatment of dementia in PD [22, 38].

4.4
Sensory Symptoms and Pain

4.4.1
Pain

Pain is very common in PD, and may be due to secondary causes such as radicular problems, stiffness of the shoulders and neck, early morning foot dystonia, or muscle cramps. However, painful sensations unrelated to any apparent disorders, usually localized in the most affected side, have been reported. A positron emission tomography (PET) study, in which pain threshold before and after the administration of levodopa was compared in PD patients and in controls, showed the nociceptive threshold to be lower in PD patients and to return to normal ranges after levodopa administration. It was hypothesized that the basal ganglia and the dopaminergic system participate in processing nociceptive information [39]. However, clinical experience has indicated that central pain seems to be poorly responsive to dopaminergic treatments, and often requires specific treatments.

Very recently, it has been suggested that contributing to pain in PD patients may be an increased incidence of peripheral neuropathy, as a complication of chronic levodopa administration. This may be the result of a B vitamin deficiency [45].

4.4.2
Olfactory Dysfunction

Olfactory dysfunction is a common abnormality in PD, and typically precedes the onset of motor PD symptoms. As up to one-third of these patients are unaware of their loss of smell, any evaluation needs to involve objective measures [40]. Currently, the most popular method is the Pennsylvania Smell Identification Test

(UPSIT), in which approximately 80% of PD patients will score abnormally, with the deficit being unrelated to either disease duration or the use of dopaminergic agents. As olfactory dysfunction can predate motor symptoms by a number of years, this has stimulated interest in olfactory evaluation being used for presymptomatic PD detection. Olfaction is either normal or mildly impaired in essential tremor, progressive supranuclear palsy, corticobasal degeneration and multisystem atrophy; hence, the testing of smell may help to distinguish these disorders from PD in diagnostically challenging cases [34].

4.5
Other Problems

4.5.1
Eye Movement Abnormalities

Eye movement abnormalities have been shown to occur in over 75% of PD patients. These include saccadic latency, hypometric saccades, slowing of smooth pursuit, and upgaze abnormalities [41]. The most distressing to patients is convergence insufficiency, which results in diplopia with reading and other activities requiring near vision. Eye movement abnormalities may worsen as an "off" phenomenon; in these cases improvement will be seen with dopaminergic therapy. Reduced levels of dopamine in the dopamine-containing amacrine cells leads to decreased color vision, which also improves with dopaminergic therapy [42]. It has been postulated that visual problems may contribute to cognitive dysfunction [46].

4.5.2
Fatigue

Fatigue has, until recently, been an unrecognized symptom in PD. However, the results of recent studies have shown that up to 50% of patients report significant fatigue – twice the number of matched controls. No association was found with pain or sleep problems, but fatigue increased in severity as the disease advanced [43], and this had a significant impact on the patient's quality of life. As yet, no specific treatment has been developed for this problem.

4.6
Non-Motor Fluctuations

Until recently, end of dose fluctuations have been thought of as primarily involving motor symptoms, but attention has now been drawn to the frequency of non-motor symptoms occurring as wearing-off phenomena. It has been shown that between 20% and 70% of fluctuating patients exhibit end-of-dose non-motor symptoms [44]; these are as disabling as motor "offs" in many patients, and in some cases are much more distressing. These symptoms can be grouped into three primary categories: cognitive/psychiatric; sensory; and autonomic. In the cognitive/psychiatric category, anxiety, slowness of thinking and fatigue are the most common symptoms, occurring in approximately 60% of patients. The most frequent sensory phenomena include akathesia and dysesthesia, in about 50% of cases. Common autonomic symptoms are drenching sweats, flushing, and dyspnea. Treatment involves recognition, explanation and reassurance, as well as the optimal adjustment of medication to reduce any fluctuating levels of dopaminergic medications.

4.7
Conclusions

Non-motor symptoms in Parkinson disease are a major source of disability. It is important that these be recognized early so that appropriate treatment will lead to an improvement in the quality of life for these patients.

References

1 Braak, H., Braak, E., Yilmazer, D., Schultz, C., de Vos, R.A., and Jansen, E.N. (1995) Nigral and extranigral pathology in Parkinson's disease. *Journal of Neural Transmission Supplement*, **46**, 15–31.

2 Shulman, L.M.., Taback, R.L., Rabinstein, A.A., and Weiner, W.J. (2002) Non-recognition of depression and other non-motor symptoms in Parkinson's disease. *Parkinson-Related Disorders*, **8**, 193–197.

3 Lees, A.J., Blackburn, N.A., and Campbell, V.L. (1998) The nighttime problems of Parkinson's disease. *Clinical Neuropharmacology*, **11**, 512–519.

4 Hobson, D.E., Lang, A.E., Martin, W.R., Razmy, A., Rivest, J., and Fleming, J. (2002) Excessive daytime sleepiness and sudden-onset sleep in Parkinson's disease. *Journal of the American Medical Association*, **287**, 455–463.

5 Adler, C.H., Caviness, J.N., Hentz, J.G., Lind, M., and Tiede, J. (2003) Randomized trial of modafinil for treating subjective daytime sleepiness in patients with Parkinson's disease. *Movement Disorders*, **18**, 287–293.

6 Wenning, G.K., Scherfler, C., Granata, R., *et al.* (1999) Time course of symptomatic orthostatic hypotension and urinary incontinence in patients with postmortem confirmed parkinsonian syndromes: a clinicopathological study. *Journal of Neurology, Neurosurgery, and Psychiatry*, **67**, 620–623.

7 Jankovic, J., Gilden, J.L., Hiner, B.C., Kaufmann, H., Brown, D.C., Coghlan, C.H., *et al.* (1993) Neurogenic orthostatic hypotension: a double-blind, placebo-controlled study with midodrine. *Israel Medical Journal*, **95**, 38–48.

8 Low, P.A., Gilden, J.L., Freeman, R., Sheng, K.N., and McElligott, M.A. (1997) Efficacy of midodrine vs. placebo in neurogenic orthostatic hypotension. A randomized, double-blind multicenter study. Midodrine Study Group. *Journal of the American Medical Association*, **277**, 1046–1051.

9 Campos-Sousa, R.N., Quagliato, E., da Silva, B.B., de Carvalho, R.M., Jr, Ribeiro, S.C., and de Carvalho, D.F. (2003) Urinary symptoms in Parkinson's disease: prevalence and associated

factors. *Arquivos de Neuro-psiquiatria*, **61**, 359–363.

10 Winge, K. and Fowler, C.J. (2006) Bladder dysfunction in Parkinsonism: mechanisms, prevalence, symptoms, and management. *Movement Disorders*, **21**, 737–745.

11 Andersson, K.E. (2000) Treatment of overactive bladder: other drug mechanisms. *Urology*, **55** (Suppl. 5A), 51–57.

12 Todorova, A., Vonderheid-Guth, B., and Dimpfel, W. (2001) Effects of tolterodine, trospium chloride, and oxybutynin on the central nervous system. *Journal of Clinical Pharmacology*, **41**, 636–644.

13 Pfeiffer, R.F. (2003) Gastrointestinal dysfunction in Parkinson's disease. *Lancet Neurology*, **2**, 107–116.

14 Jost, W.H., *et al.* (1997) Gastrointestinal mobility problems in patients with Parkinson's disease. Effects of antiparkinsonian treatment and guidelines for management. *Drugs and Aging*, **10**, 249–258.

15 Swinn, L., Schrag, A., Viswanathan, R., Bloem, B.R., Lees, A., and Quinn, N. (2003) Sweating dysfunction in Parkinson's disease. *Movement Disorders*, **18**, 1459–1463.

16 Sage, J.I. and Mark, M.H. (1995) Drenching sweats as an off phenomenon in Parkinson's disease: treatment and relation to plasma levodopa profile. *Annals of Neurology*, **37**, 120–122.

17 Yu, M., Roane, D.M., Miner, C.R., Fleming, M., and Rogers, J.D. (2004) Dimensions of sexual dysfunction in Parkinson Disease. *American Journal of Geriatric Psychiatry*, **12**, 221–226.

18 Hussain, I.F., Brady, C.M., Swinn, M.J., Mathias, C.J., and Fowler, C.J. (2001) Treatment of erectile dysfunction with sildenafil citrate (Viagra) in parkinsonism due to Parkinson's disease or multiple system atrophy with observations on orthostatic hypotension. *Journal of Neurology, Neurosurgery, and Psychiatry*, **71**, 371–374.

19 Hyson, H.C., Johnson, A.M., and Jog, M.S. (2002) Sublingual atropine for sialorrhea secondary to parkinsonism: a pilot study. *Movement Disorders*, **17**, 1318–1320.

20 Lagalla, G., Millevolte, M., Capecci, M., Provinciali, L., and Ceravolo, M.G. (2006) Botulinum toxin type A for drooling in Parkinson's disease: a double blind, randomized, placebo-controlled study. *Movement Disorders*, **21**, 704–707.

21 Mayberg, H.S. and Solomon, D.H. (1995) Depression in Parkinson's disease: a biochemical and organic viewpoint. *Advances in Neurology*, **65**, 49–60.

22 Miyasaki, J.M., Shannon, K., Voon, V., Ravina, B., Kleiner-Fisman, G., Anderson, K., *et al.* (2006) Practice parameter: evaluation and treatment of depression, psychosis, and dementia in Parkinson Disease (an evidence-based review): report of the Quality Standards Subcommittee of the American Academy of Neurology. *Neurology*, **66**, 996–1002.

23 Richard, I.H., *et al.* (1997) Serotonin syndrome and the combined use of deprenyl and an antidepressant in Parkinson's disease. *Neurology*, **48**, 1070–1077.

24 Trew, M. and Suchowersky, O. (2005) Anxiety and Parkinson's disease, in *Parkinson's Disease* (eds M. Ebadi and R.F. Pfeiffer), CRC Press, pp. 339–346.

25 Voon, V., Hassan, K., Zurowski, M., Duff-Canning, S., de Souza, M., Fox, S., *et al.* (2006) Prospective prevalence of pathologic gambling and medication association in Parkinson Disease. *Neurology*, **66**, 1750–1752.

26 Evans, A.H. and Lees, A.J. (2004) Dopamine dysregulation syndrome in Parkinson's disease. *Current Opinion in Neurology*, **17**, 393–398.

27 Klos, K.J., Bower, J.H., Josephs, K.A., Matsumoto, J.Y., and Ahlskog, J.E. (2005) Pathological hypersexuality predominantly linked to adjuvant dopamine agonist therapy in Parkinson's disease and multiple system atrophy. *Parkinsonism and Related Disorders*, **11**, 381–386.

28 Crockford, D., Quickfall, J., Currie, S., *et al.* (2008) Prevalence of problem and pathological gambling in Parkinson's disease. *Journal of Gambling Studies*, **24**, 411–422.

29 Grosset, K.A., Macphee, G., Pal, G., Stewart, D., Watt, A., Davie, J., *et al.* (2006) Problematic gambling on dopamine agonists: not such a rarity. *Movement Disorders*, **21**, 2206–2208.

30 Dodd, M.L., Klos, K.J., Bower, J.H., Geda, Y.E., Josephs, K.A., and Ahlskog, J.E. (2005) Pathological gambling caused by drugs used to treat Parkinson Disease. *Archives of Neurology*, **62**, 1377–1381.

31 Evans, A.H., Katzenschlager, R., Paviour, D., O'Sullivan, J.D., Appel, S., Lawrence, A.D., *et al.* (2004) Punding in Parkinson's disease: its relation to the dopamine dysregulation syndrome. *Movement Disorders*, **19**, 397–405.

32 Silveira-Moriyama, L., Evans, A.H., Katzenschlager, R., and Lees, A.J. (2006) Punding and dyskinesias. *Movement Disorders*, **21**, 2214–2217.

33 Romito, L.M., Raja, M., Daniele, A., Contarino, M.F., Bentivoglio, A.R., Barbier, A., *et al.* (2002) Transient mania with hypersexuality after surgery for high frequency stimulation of the subthalamic nucleus in Parkinson's disease. *Movement Disorders*, **17**, 1371–1374.

34 Suchowersky, O., Reich, S., Perlmutter, J., *et al.* (2006) Practice parameter: diagnosis and prognosis of new onset Parkinson's disease (an evidence based review). *Neurology*, **66**, 968–975.

35 Thomsen, T., Pannisset, M., Suchowersky, O., *et al.* (2008) Impact of standard of care for psychosis in Parkinson Disease. *Journal of Neurology, Neurosurgery, and Psychiatry*, **79**, 1413–1415.

36 Schrag, A. (2004) Psychiatric aspects of Parkinson's disease: an update. *Neurology*, **251**, 795–804.

37 Juncos, J.L., *et al.* (2004) Quetiapine improves psychotic symptoms and cognition in Parkinson's disease. *Movement Disorders*, **19**, 29–35.

38 Bullock, R. and Cameron, A. (2002) Rivastigmine for the treatment of dementia and visual hallucinations associated with Parkinson's disease: a case series. *Current Medical Research and Opinion*, **18**, 258–264.

39 Brefel-Courbon, C., Payoux, P., Thalamas, C., Ory, F., Quelven, I., Chollet, F., *et al.* (2005) Effect of levodopa on pain threshold in Parkinson's disease: a clinical and positron emission tomography study. *Movement Disorders*, **20** (12), 1557–1563.

40 Hawkes, C.H., *et al.* (1997) Olfactory dysfunction in Parkinson's disease. *Journal of Neurology, Neurosurgery, and Psychiatry*, **62**, 436–446.

41 Briand, K.A., *et al.* (1999) Control of voluntary and reflexive saccades in Parkinson's disease. *Experimental Brain Research*, **129**, 38–48.

42 Müller, T., Woitalla, D., Peters, S., Kohla, S., and Przuntek, H. (2002) Progress of visual dysfunction in Parkinson's disease. *Acta Neurologica Scandinavica*, **105** (4), 256–260.

43 Herlofson, K. and Larsen, J.P. (2002) Measuring fatigue in patients with Parkinson's disease – the Fatigue Severity Scale. *European Journal of Neurology*, **9**, 595–600.

44 Witjas, T., *et al.* (2002) Nonmotor fluctuations in Parkinson's disease: frequent and disabling. *Neurology*, **59**, 408–413.

45 Toth, C., *et al.* (2008) Neuropathy as a potential complication of levodopa use in Parkinson's disease. *Movement Disorders*, **187**, 852–832.

46 Bodis-Wollner, I. (1999) Visual and visual cognitive dysfunction in Parkinson's disease: spatial and chromatic vision. *Advances in Neurology*, **80**, 383–388.

A Patient's Story

Unlucky Woman

Linda Kenney

Well, there it was – the call for my story. What am I going to say – that I am a lucky woman that I have this disease? No, I can't say that, even though I respect Michael J. Fox's terminology. That was his story – this is mine.

I cannot – and will not – accept this thing in my body that is trying to take over. Not on your life! I am not going to sugar-coat it – I hate it – I don't want any part of it. But I have no choice, it is here to stay, like it or not.

That pretty much sums up my feelings on Parkinson's. Me, with a chronic illness? The one who took good care of herself, ate the right foods, and exercised. I feel cheated! My friends used to say, "how could she have a disease – she always took such good care of herself." Well, life comes with no guarantees.

My first recollection that there was something wrong was when I was driving to work on day and I noticed that the fingers on my left hand had a tremor. I was stressed more than usual at that time with work, my mother's illness and the fact that my husband had just lost his job. I didn't know much about Parkinson's, but that was the first thing that came to mind. A local neurologist confirmed that it was Parkinson's, wrote out a prescription for Sinemet, and told me to come back in six weeks. I asked my family doctor for a second opinion, and approximately six months later the original diagnosis was confirmed by a doctor at the Movement Disorder Clinic in Calgary. Other than my husband I told no one, and I wanted to keep it that way. I enjoyed my very demanding but rewarding position as Executive Assistant to the Superintendent of Schools, and I was able to hide the symptoms and carry on with my work for at least five years, even though the lack of sleep and adjustment to medications made it very difficult. But then the day of reckoning came. The stresses of work, lack of sleep, and so on eventually took a toll on my body and I crashed. My doctor said I could not go back – just like that, no adjustment! My 35 years of working was over. That was my identity! What was I going to do to fill my time and to meet my need for accomplishment? I cried for three months.

But, I never was one to sit around. Well, here we are six years later, and I don't have enough time to do all I want to do. I am always being told to slow down, but that's almost impossible for me – it's just the way I am. In addition to my daily exercise routine, which is most important for all – but especially those of us with Parkinson's – I walk, do pilates, stretches, whatever it takes to keep my muscles strong and supple. I also have several other commitments, such as home computer services, marshaling on a local golf course, house and yard sitting, and several other activities that may just arise.

It is now about 12 years since my diagnosis, and my medication keeps it pretty much under control, but unfortunately my body is showing signs of having taken the medicines for so long. I seem to be battling infections of one kind or another, which in turn means I need to take more medicine to kill the infection. My joints and muscles ache more often, and I am always tired, no matter how much sleep I get. There is a constant battle between me and "Parky" (this thing inside of me) – I am fighting it, but my defenses seem to be wearing me down.

But there are always positives to every story. Yes, I have Parkinson's, but I'm grateful that mine has been slow in progressing, because that has allowed me to do much more than most people affected with this debilitating disease. There are many people out there just like me who have not yet "come out of the closet." I understand their fear – fear of losing their jobs, of looking different, of being ridiculed, and fear of the unknown. The disease never ceases to surprise me – just when I think I've got it under control the tremors and anxiety start. Then, the more I try to stop it, the more tremor there is. And then when I expect the symptoms to appear, they do not. No wonder they call it the "unpredictable disease."

What is very important is that the emotional well-being of the patient is addressed, with depression being one of the biggest and most common challenges that we face. But what is visible is not always the whole picture. I'm still waiting for a cure, but the reality of that happening in my lifetime seems rather slim. So I continue with my life, taking on its challenges and sometimes, just sometimes, I can pretend that I don't have this thing in my body – that I didn't invite.

Yet, I've met some wonderful people through this journey. My volunteer work with the Balance Research Laboratory at the University of Lethbridge is very rewarding, and I'm presently involved in a research project exploring new ways to manage the movement difficulties associated with Parkinson's disease. The goal of this research is to try and develop improved physical therapies for patients with the disease. They are investigating whether listening to music will help to overcome the walking difficulties often experienced by people with Parkinson's.

I'll continue to help out where I can, and try to make a difference, but it's getting harder each day to hide the physical symptoms of my Parkinson's, and I am forever working on my mental wellness. We all face challenges in life, some more than others, and we can give into them and do nothing, or we can choose to deal with them and make the best of them. One thing for sure, I do know at this time, I am not going to give up on it.

5
Palliative Care and End-of-Life Issues with Parkinson Disease

Lorelei Derwent, Karen Hunka, and Oksana Suchowersky

Parkinson disease (PD) can be divided into three stages: early, moderate, and advanced. With each stage there is a progression of disability, with increasing complexity of care required to manage motor and non-motor symptoms [1], and these have been addressed in the previous chapters of this book. In the advanced stages of PD, the emphasis of care needs to be shifted from a more aggressive medical approach such as increasing PD medications or stereotactic surgery, to providing comfort and support when mobility, physical, and cognitive functions decline, and when the non-motor features of PD become more problematic [2].

Unfortunately, little information is available with respect to palliative care in PD. Although, traditionally, palliative care services have mostly focused on cancer, there is a clear need to develop palliative care strategies for chronic progressive neurode-generative conditions such as PD. In the past, quality end-of-life care for patients with PD has been impeded by a lack of studies investigating the prevalence and severity of its disabling psychological and physical symptoms, as well as evidence-based treatment guidelines [3]. Whilst, previously, this may have been partly due to PD not having been thought of as a "terminal" disease, it is now accepted that PD results in not only substantial morbidity but also a shortened lifespan [4].

5.1
Challenges in Advanced-Stage PD

In advanced-stage PD, both the patients and families must be allowed time to come to terms with the fact the disease has reached a stage where no more can be done to alleviate the motor symptoms, despite the best medical/surgical care having been provided [1, 2]. At this stage, the primary goal for both the patient and physician becomes the palliative management of non-motor complications, so as to provide comfort and to enhance the patient's quality of life as much as possible [5]. Management by healthcare professionals within a multidisciplinary setting that involves neurology, nursing, psychiatry, psychology, physiotherapy, speech therapy, occupational therapy, and social work, is recommended to allow the patients, caregivers, and family members time to come to terms with their loss

Parkinson Disease – A Health Policy Perspective. Edited by Wayne Martin, Oksana Suchowersky,
Katharina Kovacs Burns, and Egon Jonsson
Copyright © 2010 WILEY-VCH Verlag GmbH & Co. KGaA, Weinheim
ISBN: 978-3-527-32779-9

of independence, both physically and mentally, and the eventual need for the patient to be placed in assisted-living facilities. In this respect, using the counseling resources provided by the Parkinson support societies can also be very helpful.

Since it is very important to respect the wishes of both the patient and their family as to how much intervention he or she desires during the later stages of the disease, the development of a living will (personal directive) and frank discussions regarding the situation are recommended, before any severe symptoms and cognitive dysfunction actually develop.

5.2
The Most Common Causes of Death in PD

Strangely enough, death in PD occurs most often from complications rather than from the disease itself. Fluctuations in motor function, such as unpredictable "off" periods alternating with dyskinesia, freezing of gait, and postural instability, can cause falls that result in fractures (particularly of the hip) and head injuries (such as subdural hematomas) [2]. *Orthostatic hypotension* – a significant drop in blood pressure related to positional change – as well as a decreased muscle strength due to immobility, can also contribute to falls.

Swallowing problems and an ineffective cough reflex contribute to aspiration pneumonia, and other chest infections. Swallowing problems may also contribute to poor nutrition and weight loss due to a decreased dietary intake [2].

Complications of *immobility* include chest infections, urinary tract infections and impaired skin integrity (pressure sores) [2, 6]. Immobility may also exacerbate other conditions such as chronic obstructive pulmonary disease (COPD) and heart disease, and may also contribute to the development of deep-vein thrombosis (DVT; i.e., blood clots) and pulmonary emboli [2].

5.3
Specific Problems in the Advanced-PD Patient

Non-motor problems lead to increasing disability in advanced disease, and have been shown to result in more morbidity than do motor symptoms. The recognition and treatment of such problems is important, and have been addressed in detail in the previous chapters. Consequently, they will be discussed only briefly at this point.

5.3.1
Pain

Pain remains an underappreciated symptom in the advanced stages of PD [2, 5], and can occur in 40–50% of patients [6]. The pain is generally related to PD symptoms of stiffness, rigidity, and "off" dystonia, but it can also result from severe dyskinesias due to excessive dopaminergic therapy. The stooped posture in advanced PD patients can cause back pain and spasm [5]. Pain may also result from complications of immobility such as pressure sores, musculoskeletal aches and pains, cramps or spasms, and contractures. Comorbidities such as arthritis and neuropathic pain may aggravate or contribute to pain. As a result of pain, sleep disruption occurs in up to 90% of patients [6]. In a survey of caregivers of PD patients, pain was reported as a common complaint and was also under-treated, especially in those patients not receiving palliative/hospice or skilled nursing care [3].

5.3.2
Cognitive Decline

Dementia affects 30–40% of patients, with the most important risk factors being a long duration of illness and older age. The development of dementia is a clear marker of a poor prognosis, and suggests that the disease is entering its last stages [2, 5]. Behavioral problems such as wandering, sundowning (i.e., evening agitation with worsening confusion), agitation, and combativeness are common. These behavioral symptoms can be difficult for families to manage in the community, and frequently lead to patients being placed in long-term care facilities [1].

Hallucinations and *delusions* are the most common psychotic symptoms experienced. Although they are related to the use of dopaminergic medications, their development is usually a precursor of the development of cognitive decline. Hallucinations often involve complex scenes, and may include small animals or insects and sometimes deformed, aggressive, or hostile people. Deceased people from the patient's past can also be present [6]. Hallucinations can be very disturbing for the patient, particularly as insight into them is lost with cognitive decline. Hallucinations also result in the caregiver encountering difficulties when managing the patient.

5.3.3
Other Psychiatric Complications

Depression and anxiety occur in up to 40% of all patients with PD. The prevalence may be higher at the end stage as the motor and non-motor symptoms worsen. A worsening depression predicts a worsening disability [5], and is often part of the terminal decline. It may be manifest by increased anxiety, mood change, changes in sleep patterns, or physical decline [2].

5.3.4
Speech and Swallowing Difficulties

The impairment of swallowing and a fear of choking can be distressing for both the patient and caregiver. These lead to inadequate nutritional and fluid intake, compromising the patient's health and challenging the maintenance of body weight. The inability to ingest adequate nutrients may also be due to the patient's loss of independence and depression [6]. When patients can no longer take their PD medications by mouth or maintain an adequate food intake, it may be appropriate to consider providing nutrition and hydration through a feeding tube [2].

Communication between patients and caregivers may become impaired due to *hypophonia* (quiet, soft voice), an inability to articulate clearly, speech initiation failure, and problems associated with cognitive decline (impaired executive functioning, decision making, and memory problems). In this situation, PD sufferers and families have identified feelings of psychological and social isolation, and feel that they have to struggle to "stay connected" to each other and their social networks [4].

5.3.5
Bowel and Bladder Dysfunction

Bowel and bladder dysfunction is universal in the advanced stages of PD [4]. *Constipation* is typically a major problem due to immobility, decreased oral food and fluid intake, poor gut motility, and the side effects of medications. The complications that arise from constipation include hemorrhoids, fecal impaction, fatigue and headache, confusion, and increased hallucinations [6]. Severe impaction can even result in hospitalization for bowel obstruction. Occasionally, patients have required surgical management with permanent colostomy [2].

Bladder problems experienced in advanced PD include urinary frequency, urgency, nocturia, dribbling, and incontinence [1]. These problems are not easily solved and contribute to significant care requirements. Incontinence of the bowel and bladder often prompt a referral to long-term care facilities, and can be the "last straw" for caregivers.

5.3.6
Sleep Disturbances

Sleep disturbances are common in PD, and increase in frequency and severity with progression of the disease. Common sleep disorders include rapid eye movement (REM) behavior disorder (RBD), restless leg syndrome [5], and sleep fragmentation (difficulty maintaining sleep). Patients frequently complain of nightmares and may act out their dreams, sometimes resulting in injuries to their sleeping partners.

5.4
Caregiver Burden

The care needs of the advanced PD patient takes its toll on those who form the support network. Caregiver burden in PD is significantly associated with the patient's increasing physical and cognitive disability. Caregivers themselves report suffering from depression, anxiety, fear of the future, fatigue, sleep disruption and financial difficulties as they cope with caring for their loved one [5].

In a study of caregivers and PD patients in Australia, examining unmet needs, the caregivers stated that the declining health of the person receiving care, which included: (i) the development of dementia, depression, and behavioral problems, (ii) care needs becoming too specialized, and (iii) care being required from more than one caregiver, were the main reasons that prevented them from continuing in their caregiving role. It should also be remembered that caregivers tend to be older and have their own health issues, as well as limited incomes and resources, which lead in turn to an inability to care for the PD patient at home. Financial issues such as giving up employment to be a caregiver, the cost of services, financial commitments, having to continue to work to provide for the family, or having to return to work for financial reasons, all impacted on the caregivers' ability to care for the patient at home versus placement in long-term care or hospice facilities [7].

The reasons given by patients as to what would prevent them from remaining at home, primarily concerned issues relating to their own health and care capabilities, disease progression, and lack of mobility. Patients also identified concerns regarding their caregiver, including the latter not coping or managing due to illness, loss of functional abilities, loss of spouse or income, or increasing expenses. Patients indicated that they preferred to remain at home with their family for as long as is possible, but if placement was being considered, then they should be able to move into a facility of their own choice [7].

Suggestions for improved support for caregivers in this study included:

- Improved financial support through government and insurance agencies.
- Increased access to respite.
- Increased access to home support services, such as housekeeping assistance and social or recreational activities for caregivers.
- Assistance with transportation.
- Better access to allied health professionals such as social workers, physiotherapists, dieticians, and occupational therapists.
- Increased services in rural areas.
- Improved training and education for healthcare staff in providing supportive and palliative care.

5.4.1
Placement in Long-Term Care Facilities

The provision of appropriate services for people with PD involves many agencies and departments across acute, community and long-term care sectors [7]. According to an epidemiological study of nursing home residents in the United States, almost 20% of older patients with PD eventually require long-term care. Moreover, almost half of these patients came from an acute care hospital, while another 16% were admitted from another long-term care facility. Approximately 60% of the PD patients resided in an assisted living or long-term care facility for five years, or longer [8].

Based on the assumption that long-term care accessibility for people with PD in the Canadian and United States healthcare systems are similar, and using the prevalence figures for PD in Alberta (see Chapter 2), it is conservatively estimated that some 1500 persons with PD currently require an assisted living environment in Alberta.

In a Norwegian study, it was noted that one in ten nursing home residents had a diagnosis of PD, with evidence of both undertreatment and overtreatment of PD identified. Only 50% of these patients were judged to be receiving optimal medical management [9].

Currently, there is a significant limitation of resources to care adequately for a PD patient over a long period of time, both in the community and in long-term care. In particular, physical therapy, occupational therapy, speech therapy and dietician services are limited.

The lack of trained professionals in long-term care facilities to care for PD patients, along with staff shortages and a high turnover of staff, are all barriers against PD patients receiving the support and care that they need.

Ongoing medical review and education, provided by interdisciplinary clinics specializing in PD, are recommended to assist in optimizing PD patient care. However, these clinics face limited resources such as financial, physical space and personnel (Movement Disorder Specialists, nurses, physiotherapists, occupational therapists, dieticians, speech therapists, and social workers) to optimally meet the needs of the PD population.

Advanced-PD patients living in areas far from PD clinics (usually located in major urban centers) have additional difficulties in traveling to appointments. Hence, novel ways of providing ongoing specialized medical care should be developed that may include reviewing patients by videoconference, or multidisciplinary case conferencing via the telephone.

5.4.2
The Case for Palliative Care in PD

As stated by Bunting [1]:

> "The end of the patient's life is often arduous for the patient and family. The caregiver may be exhausted from providing years of physical and emotional care. Many caregivers have invested so much of themselves in the caregiving role that they are socially isolated and have few support systems to assist them in the advanced stage through to bereavement."

Palliative care is defined by the World Health Organization as:

> "An approach that improves the quality of life of patients and families facing the problems associated with life threatening illness, through the

prevention and relief of suffering by means of early identification and impeccable assessment and treatment of pain and other problems, physical, psychosocial and spiritual" [10].

In June 2000, a federal Canadian report by the Standing Senate Committee on Social Affairs, Science and Technology [11] emphasized the need for integrated, accessible, and adequate funding of services that could support PD patients and families, both in institutional and home settings in rural and urban communities. Expanded and properly funded end-of-life home care and hospice services should include: (i) financial coverage for drugs; (ii) access to both professional and supportive care services; (iii) access to community day programs; (iv) 24 h palliative teams; and (v) support for families for respite care and bereavement follow-up. End-of-life care should be interdisciplinary and skilled, and include community participation in the planning, implementation, and evaluation of programs and services [11].

People with PD and their families have experiences and needs that are similar to other palliative care populations (most commonly, advanced cancer patients). Cancer and PD patients share challenges in managing physical changes, and concerns regarding the practical aspects of care, safety and adjustments to symptoms were shown to be numerous in both groups [5].

As mentioned above, one major difference between PD and the usual palliative care populations relates to uncertainty about whether PD should be considered a terminal disease, as it is difficult to predict the lifespan of PD patients [4]. Traditionally, the management of PD patients has focused on drug treatment and multidisciplinary care of what was considered to be a long-term, slowly progressive disorder. Palliative care specialists have not been involved routinely. Because of the difficulties in predicting the time of death and the long duration of the disease, hospices and palliative care centers have generally refused referral of PD patients for admission [2]. Thus, patients with neurodegenerative conditions and their caregivers have not automatically been associated with palliative and hospice care, even in the terminal stage of the disease [12].

The need to change the current model of care delivery for patients with PD is being influenced by the growth of the elderly population. As the post-World War II "baby boomers" in Canada continue to age, it is clear that the staggering increase in PD and other neurodegenerative disorders related to aging will place a huge strain on healthcare resources, and in turn alter the traditional models of healthcare delivery [1].

5.4.3
The Need for Advanced Care Planning

Advance directives are best seen as part of a planning and communication process that help people prepare for death, in consultation with their loved ones. The preparation of an advanced care directive should initiate discussions between PD patients and their family, and provide guidance and support for substitute decision makers who must make the difficult decisions regarding life-sustaining treatment.

If loved ones and medical professionals have participated in a process of serious communication, then the problems associated with the interpretation and application of advanced directives are likely to be much reduced [11].

End-of-life choices, including advance care planning with open and frank discussions with the patient of what constitutes a "good death" (either at home or elsewhere, and the value of palliative/hospice care), and who should be designated the agent, should be initiated early in the disease process, before the patient's increasing problems impair their ability to decide about their care. In this way, the stress on families and designated agents forced to make difficult decisions can be greatly reduced [5].

5.5
Summary

Parkinson disease is a progressive neurodegenerative disorder that presents unique challenges in the management of motor and non-motor symptoms when in its advanced stages. Both, caregiver burdens and limited resources in the community and in institutional settings fuel the need to incorporate palliative care across the healthcare continuum.

As stated in the report by the Standing Senate Committee on Social Affairs, Science and Technology [11]:

> "Quality end-of-life care must become an entrenched core value of Canada's healthcare system. Each person is entitled to die in relative comfort, as free as possible from physical, emotional, psychosocial, and spiritual distress. Each Canadian is entitled to access skilled, compassionate, and respectful care at the end of life".

References

1 Bunting-Perry, L.K. (2006) Palliative care in Parkinson's disease: implications for neuroscience nursing. *Journal of Neuroscience Nursing*, **38** (2), 106–113.

2 Voltz, R., Bernat, J.L., Borasio, G.D., Maddocks, I., Oliver, D., and Portenoy, R.K. (2004) *Palliative Care in Neurology*, Oxford University Press, New York, Oxford, pp. 48–57, and 338.

3 Goy, E., Carter, J., and Ganzini, L. (2007) Parkinson disease at the end of life: Caregiver perspectives. *Neurology*, **69**, 611–612.

4 Hudson, P.L., Toye, C., and Kristjanson, L.J. (2006) Would people with Parkin-son's disease benefit from palliative care? *Palliative Medicine*, **20**, 87–94.

5 Elman, L.B., Houghton, D.J., Wu, G.F., Hurtig, H.I., Markowitz, C.E., and McCluskey, L. (2007) Palliative care in amyotrophic lateral sclerosis, Parkinson's disease, and multiple sclerosis. *Journal of Palliative Medicine*, **10** (2), 440–444.

6 Thomas, S. and MacMahon, D. (2004) Parkinson's disease, palliative care and older people. *Nursing Older People*, **16** (2), 22–26.

7 Aoun, S., Kristjanson, L., and Oldham, L. (2006) The challenges and unmet needs of people with neurodegenerative

conditions and their carers. *Journal of Community Nurses*, **11** (1), 17–20.

8 Buchanan, R., Wang, S., Huang, C., Simpson, P., and Manyam, B. (2002) Analyses of nursing home residents with Parkinson's disease using the minimum data set. *Parkinsonism and Related Disorders*, **8** (5), 369–380.

9 Thomas, S. and MacMahon, D. (2002) Managing Parkinson's disease in long-term care. *Nursing Older People*, **14** (9), 23–29.

10 World Health Organization Europe (2004) *Better Palliative Care for Older People*, WHO Regional Office for Europe, pp. 6–37.

11 Standing Senate Committee on Social Affairs, Science and Technology (2000) Quality end of life care: the right of every Canadian. Available at: http://www.parl.gc.ca/36/2/parlbus/commbus/senate/Com-e/upda-e/rep-e/repfinjun00-e.htm (accessed 31 October 2008).

12 Kristjanson, L.J., Aoun, S.M., and Oldham, L. (2005) Palliative care and support for people with neurodegenerative conditions and their carers. *International Journal of Palliative Nursing*, **12** (8), 368–377.

A Caregiver's Story

A Husband's Point of View

Bill Pinckney

"So", you ask, "how has Parkinson's affected me?" Well, let me say, it has simply upended my life. It is a cruel and nasty disease, and our lives have been altered beyond belief. I can accept that our future is uncertain, but the biggest trouble for me is my inability to do anything to fix the problem. I'm a fixer, and it just drives me crazy to see Joyce suffering, and to be helpless to change that.

We dreamed of a carefree retirement filled with travel. I saw us strolling along some far-off beach, traveling to wonderful old cities of Europe, drinking tea in Japan, exploring the byways of fascinating places. All this is gone. Did I imagine myself caring for someone in a wheelchair, walker, a cane wielder? No way.

Add to this some of the more bizarre features of Parkinson's, such as poker face (my wife's wonderful smile disappearing), sleep disturbances, the slowness; all that can, with work, be accepted. But, in addition, there is a change in personality. From someone who climbed every mountain and needed no reassurance of her worth, she has become one who doesn't try the molehills, and wants constant reassurance. That's a big thing to adjust to.

I depended on her, and now she's not as dependable. I am holding this family of two afloat in ocean waves that nearly pull me under.

There is a paranoia that is cruel and painful to live with. She doesn't trust me. My privacy is totally invaded. It doesn't seem fair.

I've had to concentrate on trying to finance a long and expensive old age. Her needs will not diminish, but likely escalate, and I'm not sure I can handle it. I never thought I'd be acting as a nursemaid to someone. But I still love the person she was, and still mostly is. And I'm loyal.

I am consumed with worry that there will not be enough money for our retirement, and that neither of us will be able to make more. She blithely says, "No problem," and then spends money wastefully–not usually in large amounts, but a constant drain.

I have to worry about keeping strong and well; about not having a heart attack, or a stroke, or being too fat. Everything is work. Not much joyful play when I come home.

She wants more than I can give–she wants something I don't understand. As long as she was completely self-sufficient, I wasn't asked to provide it. That was better.

But then there are happy times. Times when she asks for help in plain English, and I can do something. I'd happily (well, maybe not happily) take her place in Parkinson's grip. If I could, I would accept the disease, to spare her the pain and the physical changes that so erode her sense of worth. It is tiresome to have to endlessly build someone up, especially when she is doing pretty damn well.

Sometimes it seems she still does enough to tire out any normal person. It does seem hard to believe. She won't rest, drives herself until she almost drops, falls asleep standing up. I don't get it.

But, I feel quite proud of how well I have learned to cope: in the kitchen, in the grocery store, doing the laundry and housekeeping. Not many guys are legitimate princes.

We still tell great stories together, create pleasing (to us) music together, and put on a hell of a party or gourmet meal. Together, we are more than twice each of us. We complement and entertain each other, our guests and friends. People like to be near us. And we are still in love.

Maybe someday, I'll feel less furious with fate for dealing this blow, and find that the positive growth has been worth it. But for now, it's one day at a time.

6
Natural Health Products in Parkinson Disease

Cheryl Sadowski and Shirley Heschuk

6.1
Introduction

There is an increasing trend in the use of complementary and alternative medicine (CAM) to treat illness and promote health [1]. "Complementary" means the therapy that is used in tandem with conventional treatments, whereas "alternative" includes therapies that generally replace or substitute for a conventional treatment. CAM includes traditional therapies (Traditional Chinese Medicine, Ayurveda, Native American), mind–body–spirit practices such as prayer, massage, chiropractic, therapeutic touch, energy healing, music therapy (see Chapter 7), acupuncture, homeopathy, and the use of botanicals and nutritional supplements [Natural Health Products (NHPs) in Canada]. These practices are not usually reimbursed by medical insurance companies, and in general patients pay for them out-of-pocket.

To date, whilst there is substantial literature on the use of CAM among the general population, there is very little available in specific disease state populations, such as Parkinson disease (PD), where there is only symptomatic, noncurable treatment. As many of the treatments available for PD have debilitating adverse effects, patients may be motivated to seek treatment for their condition, or to try to ameliorate the adverse effects caused by their prescribed therapy. When Ryan and Johnson [2] surveyed patients coming to a neurology clinic in the US, they found that about 18.5% took alternative therapies, compared to 42.1% of the general population [1]. When broken down into disease states, 46% of the patients with PD had used alternative medications [2]. The most frequently taken alternative medications were vitamins E and C, followed by St John's wort (for depression), ginkgo biloba (for memory loss), and ginseng (for immune stimulation). A survey of 201 PD patients showed that 40% of them used at least one alternative therapy, and 23.4% used at least one vitamin or herb [3]. The most common alternative therapies were massage and acupuncture, while the most common alternative medications were vitamin E (68% of those using vitamins and herbs), coenzyme Q10 (15%), multivitamins (11%), vitamin C (8.5%), and ginkgo biloba (8.5%). In a UK study, 54% of patients with PD reported

Parkinson Disease – A Health Policy Perspective. Edited by Wayne Martin, Oksana Suchowersky,
Katharina Kovacs Burns, and Egon Jonsson
Copyright © 2010 WILEY-VCH Verlag GmbH & Co. KGaA, Weinheim
ISBN: 978-3-527-32779-9

using at least one form of complementary therapy for their condition, or some other indication [4].

To date, very few investigations have been conducted on massage therapy or acupuncture treatment for PD. A pilot study of therapeutic massage for PD patients found that, in addition to enjoying the massage, individuals showed improvements in self-confidence, well-being, walking and activities of daily living [5]. A recent systematic review detailing the effectiveness of acupuncture for PD found that the evidence from 11 randomized controlled trials was not convincing, as the number (and quality) of the trials, as well as their total sample size, were too small to draw any firm conclusions [6].

Further research has been conducted on the use of complementary/alternative medications (NHPs) in PD patients, and these will be discussed in detail for selected products later in this chapter.

Health Canada has developed new regulations for NHPs which came into effect on 1st January 2004. These NHPs include:

- Plant or plant materials (botanicals, herbals)
- Algae
- Bacteria and probiotics
- Fungi
- Nonhuman animal materials
- Isolates and extracts
- Vitamins, amino acids, fatty acids, and minerals
- Synthetic duplicates of the above materials.

These products form a subset of the drug category, and the regulations are meant to ensure that Canadians have access to safe and efficacious products. By 2010, manufacturers selling products in Canada under this category will be required to provide proof of good manufacturing practices, and will be issued a natural product number (NPN). Label claims will depend on the level of evidence of efficacy. These regulations do not apply to loose herbs. Additional information can be found on the Health Canada website: http://www.hc-sc.gc.ca/hpfb-dgpsa/nhpd-dspn/index_e.html.

Because these products are thought of as "natural," they are viewed as safe or innocuous. However, as many of the people using these therapies are also using "mainstream" medicines, there may be a concern about adverse reactions by causing or aggravating a health problem, or by interacting pharmacokinetically or pharmacodynamically with the patient's prescribed therapy. Mallet and colleagues [7] recently reviewed the challenges of managing drug interactions in older adults. Unfortunately, many physicians do not have accurate records with regards to a medication history, even when only conventional pharmaceutical products are considered. Because of the changes in pharmacodynamics and pharmacokinetics, older people are particularly at risk of drug interactions. Herbal products and dietary supplements contribute to significant interactions, which may increase the risk of adverse events [8]. Some of the more common and well-documented interactions are listed in Table 6.1.

Table 6.1 Pharmaceuticals used for PD: possible harmful interactions with NHPs.

Pharmaceutical	NHP (use)	Interaction
Levodopa/carbidopa combination	5-HTP (for depression)	Possible increased risk of scleroderma-like syndrome [9]
	Kava (for anxiety)	Impairs effectiveness of levodopa/carbidopa [10]
Levodopa or Levodopa/carbidopa combination	L-methionine, D-phenylalanine (for PD)	Possible impaired action of drug based on amino acid/levodopa interaction [11]
	Iron (for anemia)	Absorption interference [12]–iron decreases the absorption of levodopa or levodopa/carbidopa combination
	Policosanol (for hyperlipidemia)	Possible potentiation of dyskinesia side effect [13]
	SAMe (for depression, osteoarthritis)	Possible increased "wearing off" effects of levodopa [14]
	Vitamin B6 (for PD)	Impairs effectiveness of levodopa taken alone, but does not interact with levodopa/carbidopa combination [15]
Prolactin-inhibitors, bromocriptine, pergolide	Chasteberry (for menopausal symptoms)	Possible potentiation of drug action [16]
Selegiline	5-HTP, SAMe, St. John's wort (for depression)	Possible risk of serotonin syndrome (tachycardia, hypertension, confusion, agitation, tremor, coma, seizures)
	Ephedra, green tea, guarana (for weight loss)	Monoamine oxidase inhibitor (MAOI) interaction – risk of hypertensive crisis [17]

These risks are compounded by the fact that patients do not necessarily report the use of CAMs to their healthcare professional. In a recent survey in the US [1], only 38.5% of subjects with a physician reported the use of alternative therapy to that physician. The physician or other clinician may also fail to inquire about CAM use from the patient. In the US, when the American Association for Retired Persons (AARP) conducted a telephone survey of 1559 seniors aged 50 years or more [18], 42% were found to be using supplements, while 63% reported using one or more NHP in the past. Of those who used NHPs, 69% did not discuss this with their physician; when asked "why?", 42% said the physician never asked, 30% were unaware that they should have, and 19% said that there was not enough time during the office visit. Not surprisingly, 74% of the respondents indicated they were already taking prescription medications. It was interesting to note that, in all age groups, the majority of patients using NHPs did so to treat a specific condition, although specific conditions were not addressed in the AARP report. Unfortunately, many physicians say they feel unprepared to discuss NHPs with patients [19]; whilst many are aware that NHPs exist, and that the patients use them, they do not include such questions in routine discussions with patients [20].

Chung [21] recently reviewed a series of nine studies examining the safety and efficacy of herbal medicines for the treatment of PD. Although, unfortunately, there was insufficient evidence for a thorough review, it was interesting to note the high rates of NHP use among this vulnerable population.

There is a significant interest in identifying a neuroprotective treatment for PD, as no cure is available at the present time. Hence, the National Institute of Neurology Disorders and Stroke have formed the Committee to Identify Neuroprotective Agents in Parkinson's (CINAPS) [22], and are currently considering 12 compounds. These products included caffeine and coenzyme Q10, in addition to prescription drugs (e.g., pramipexole, selegiline) and products not yet available commercially, such as trophic or nutritional factors. In 2006, the American Academy of Neurology released the Practice Parameters for Parkinson Disease, among which was one Practice Parameter that dealt specifically with neuroprotective and alternative therapies [23]. At the time of this review, there were no alternative treatments that had demonstrated any evidence of impacting upon disease progression.

In this chapter, attention will be focused on NHPs which have evidence of use in PD, namely: ashwagandha, caffeine, choline, coenzyme Q10, creatine, fava beans, green tea, melatonin, and vitamin E.

6.2
Methods

In order to select the NHPs for review, products were identified from the Natural Standard Database and the Natural Medicines Comprehensive Database. These databases were reviewed in February 2007 for the products with the highest level of evidence for treatment of PD.

For the Natural Standard Database, no product had sufficient evidence to be rated as grade A or B; however, ashwagandha, choline, coenzyme Q10, melatonin, and vitamin E were designated as grade C, which was the highest level of evidence for products used to treat PD. Grade C is defined as "unclear of conflicting scientific evidence."

For the Natural Medicines Comprehensive Database, products that were "possibly effective" were identified. In addition to products included in the Natural Standard Database, caffeine and green tea were identified as products of interest for this search.

Thus, the final seven products to be investigated included ashwagandha, choline, coenzyme Q10 (CoQ10), melatonin, vitamin E, caffeine, and green tea.

Further searches were conducted in Medline (1950–September 2008) and Embase (1988–September 2008). A combination of subject headings and keywords pertaining to herbal medicine in general, and to specific types of NHP, were used. Relevant

MeSH headings included: Medicine, Herbal; Plants, Medicinal; Homeopathy; Parkinson Disease; and Parkinsonian Disorders. Two additional popular products, creatine and fava beans, were identified and included in the investigations.

6.2.1
Ashwagandha *(Withania somnifera)*

Ashwagandha, a traditional Indian (Ayurvedic) medical herb, is thought of as "Indian ginseng." It is often marketed simply as "Withania," and is also called winter cherry or Dunal. The berries, fruits, and roots have been used traditionally, whilst in Western herbal medicine most preparations are made from the root of the shrub. Ashwagandha is considered to be a general promoter of health, and is purported to have adaptogenic, anti-stress and anti-inflammatory effects.

6.2.1.1 Pharmacology
Over 35 compounds have been identified in ashwagandha, including steroidal lactones and alkaloids that are together called *withanolides* (particularly withaferin A). Preparations are often standardized to their percentage contents of withanolides. A number of animal/*in vitro* studies have demonstrated anti-inflammatory, antifungal, antioxidant, and thyroid-stimulation effects, as well as cancer inhibition. Ashwangandha has been known to upregulate cholinergic receptor functions in the brain, which could adversely affect some of the Parkinsonian syndromes, such as a worsening of excessive salivation [24].

6.2.1.2 Dosing
Normally, 1–6 g of the whole herb is administered orally each day, either in capsules or in the form of a tea. The tea is prepared by boiling ashwagandha roots in water for 15 min and cooling the infusion; the normal dose is three cups per day. Tincture or fluid extracts can be dosed at 2–4 ml, three times daily.

6.2.1.3 Adverse Effects
When given orally, ashwagandha is well tolerated at normal doses. However, large doses may cause gastrointestinal upset, diarrhea, and vomiting secondary to irritation of the mucous and serous membranes.

6.2.1.4 Precautions
Care should be taken when administering ashwagandha in the presence of the following conditions:

- Diabetes: due to its possible hypoglycemic properties.
- Peptic ulcer disease: due to a possible irritation of the mucous and serous membranes.
- Thyroid disorders: due to possible thyroid stimulatory properties.

6.2.1.5 Drug Interactions
Possible interactions of ashwagandha with other drugs are listed in Table 6.2.

6.2.1.6 **Clinical Evidence**

Nagashayana *et al.* [25] completed a prospective study to evaluate the efficacy of *Ayurveda* treatment (a concoction in cow's milk of powdered *Mucuna pruriens* and *Hyoscyamus reticulates* seeds and *Withania somnifera* and *Sida cordifolia* roots) in PD patients. *Mucuna pruriens* is reported to contain levodopa as one of its constituents. PD patients who underwent this treatment showed improvements in symptoms such as stiffness, tremor, bradykinesia and cramp-like pain in the lower limbs. The improvement observed in this study may be due to the levodopa contained in the herbal medication.

6.2.1.7 **Conclusion**

There is insufficient scientific evidence to recommend the use of ashwagandha in the management of PD. *Withania somnifera* (ashwagandha) has been studied only in a herbal combination treatment, where one of the herbs used (*Mucuna pruriens*) contained levodopa, which is believed to have provided the benefit seen. The contribution of ashwagandha to the management of PD is unclear.

6.2.2
Caffeine

Caffeine (1,3,7-trimethylxanthine) is mainly derived from coffee beans, which are used make a stimulating drink.

6.2.2.1 **Pharmacology**

Caffeine is a central nervous system (CNS) stimulant, and also has anorectic, thermogenic, and diuretic properties. Caffeine may counter the suppressive effect of adenosine on brain dopaminergic transmission by the direct downregulation

Table 6.2 The interaction of ashwagandha with other drugs.

Drug class	Clinical effect
Central nervous system depressants: (benzodiaepines, sedatives, anxiolytics)	Increased depressant effects and toxicity
Anticoagulants	Increased coagulation time–additive effect
Antihyperglycemic drugs/insulin	Increased hypoglycemic effect
Antihypertensive drugs	Increased hypotensive effect
Thyroid drugs	Ashwagandha may cause hyperthyroidism and may interact with drugs for hyperthyroidism or hypothyroidism
Immunosuppressants (azathioprine, cyclosporine, prednisone, etc.)	Ashwagandha has potential immune-stimulating effects, and would therefore decrease the effectiveness of immunosuppressants

of adenosine A2A receptors, and may inhibit neurotoxicity induced by 1-methyl-4-phenyl-1,2,3,6-tetrahydropyridine (MPTP), a toxin known to cause parkinsonism [26]. Several studies have shown an inverse relationship between the consumption of caffeine and PD [27]. Caffeine from non-coffee sources (e.g., tea, cola beverages, chocolate) is also inversely associated with PD [28]. Therefore, the more caffeine one consumes either from coffee or other sources of caffeine (e.g., tea, cola beverages, chocolate) the lower the risk of developing Parkinson Disease. Of course this would be within a limit as 1–3 cups of coffee/day is considered moderate use. Higher amounts could cause adverse effects. Caffeine may also modify the genetic effect in families with PD [29]. For instance, nitric oxide synthases genes are associated with PD and potentially interact with caffeine and this would necessitate analysis of effect modification [29]. Within a family portraying these genes, the effect (risk of developing PD) of those who drink caffeinated beverages could be compared with those members of the family who do not.

6.2.2.2 Dosing
A moderate daily intake of caffeine (200–600 mg) equates to one to three cups of coffee.

6.2.2.3 Adverse Effects
Caffeine may cause insomnia, nervousness, restlessness, gastric irritation, nausea, vomiting, tachycardia, quickened respiration, tremors, delirium, convulsions, and diuresis. Large doses can produce headache, anxiety, agitation, ringing in the ears, premature heartbeat, and arrhythmia.

6.2.2.4 Precautions
Alternative sources of caffeine include the following [30]:

- Coffee (bean): 1–2% caffeine (1 cup brewed = 200 mg caffeine)
- Mate (leaf and stem): 0.2–2% caffeine
- Guarana (seed): 2.5–7% caffeine
- Cocoa (bean): 0.07–0.36% caffeine
- Green tea: 2–4% caffeine (1 cup = 10–80 mg)
- Kola nut (cola nut): 1–2.5% caffeine
- Cola soft drinks: up to 75 mg caffeine per 350 ml.

6.2.2.5 Drug Interactions
Possible interactions of caffeine with other drugs are listed in Table 6.3.

6.2.2.6 Clinical Evidence

Neuroprotection

Meta-Analysis: Hernan *et al.* [27] conducted a systematic review to summarize the epidemiological evidence on the association between cigarette smoking, coffee drinking, and the risk of PD. Some case-control and cohort studies were included.

Table 6.3 The interaction of caffeine with drugs and other NHPs.

Drug class	Clinical effect
Caffeine-containing herbs: see Section 6.2.2.4	Additive effect, increased risk of adverse effects
Calcium	High caffeine intake increases urinary calcium excretion and also decreases absorption of calcium
Ephedra (Ma Huang)	Use of caffeine and ephedra together (common for weight loss) increases the risk of serious life-threatening adverse effects: hypertension, myocardial infarction, stroke, seizures, and death.
Stimulant drugs diethylpropion, epinephrine, phentermine, pseudoephedrine, MAOIs	Increase the risk of adverse effects.
Oral contraceptives	May decrease the rate of caffeine clearance by 40–65%
Quinolone antibiotics	Quinolones decrease caffeine clearance

The results indicated that the risk of PD is 30% lower among coffee drinkers than among non-coffee drinkers. Each additional cup of coffee per day is associated with a risk reduction of 10%, although the magnitude of this reduction may differ by gender. The Nurses' Health Study that included only women found a virtually null linear relationship.

Case-Control Study: Hancock *et al.* [29] used a family-based case-control data set for genetics association between PD and three factors inversely associated with PD in prior studies, namely smoking, caffeine, and NSAIDs (nonsteroidal anti-inflammatory drugs). The conclusion was that smoking and caffeine would possibly modify genetic effects in families with PD, and should be considered as effect modifiers in conducting gene studies for PD.

Prospective Study: Ascherio *et al.* [28] examined the relationship of coffee and caffeine consumption on the risk of PD among participants in two ongoing cohorts: the Health Professionals' Follow-Up Study (HPFS) and the Nurses' Health Study. The study population comprised 47 351 men and 88 565 women who were free of PD, stroke, or cancer at baseline. The results showed a strong inverse association between caffeine consumption and risk of PD in men. An inverse association was also observed with the consumption of coffee, caffeine from non-coffee sources, and tea, but not in decaffeinated coffee. Among women, the relationship between caffeine or coffee intake and risk of PD was U-shaped, with the lowest risk observed at moderate intakes (one to three cups of coffee per day). These associations are consistent with a protective effect of moderate caffeine consumption against PD, but the possibility of a nonlinear relationship in women requires further evaluation as hormonal (e.g., estrogen) interactions may play a role.

Treatment

Case-Control Study: Kitagawa *et al.* [31] observed the beneficial effects of 100 mg of caffeine in patients of "total akinesia"-type of freezing of gait. The results showed that low doses of caffeine could improve the inability of heel-off of the first swing leg at gait initiation. Not all patients responded to the effects of caffeine. However, the inability to regulate the stride-to-stride variations and impairment of toe-off at the stance–swing transition were not influenced by caffeine. The chronic administration of caffeine resulted in the development of tolerance to the effects on freezing of gait (FOG) within a few months.

Caffeine in Combination with Levodopa

Double-Blind, Randomized, Cross-Over Study: Deleu *et al.* [32] studied the acute effects of caffeine on the nature and magnitude of the levodopa pharmacokinetics and pharmacodynamics in patients with idiopathic Parkinson disease (IPD). The findings indicated that caffeine shortened the maximal plasma concentration of levodopa, decreased the latency to levodopa walking and tapping motor response, and increased the magnitude of walking response. This supports the idea that low-dose caffeine (200 mg) administered 15 min before levodopa may be a useful synergistic adjunct to conventional anti-Parkinson agents in some patients with IPD.

6.2.2.7 Conclusion

Animal studies have confirmed that caffeine prevents akinesia in dopamine-depleted mice, most likely by inhibiting the suppressive effect of adenosine on dopaminergic transmission. The results of recent animal studies have suggested that, in addition to their acute locomotor effects, caffeine and other A2A antagonists may protect from environmental or endogenous MPTP-like toxin-induced neurotoxicity, which have been implicated in the etiology of PD. Clinical trials in men have identified a strong inverse association between caffeine consumption and risk of PD, but the possibility of a nonlinear relationship in women requires further evaluation. The results of recent studies [31, 32] have shown that caffeine might serve as a useful synergistic adjunct to conventional anti-Parkinson agents in some PD patients.

6.2.3
Choline

Because it is synthesized in the human body, choline is not considered to be a vitamin (in the past, it was classified as a B vitamin). Choline is produced in the liver, and may also be ingested from foods such as liver, muscle meats, fish, nuts, beans, peas, and eggs. It is also readily available in a typical diet.

6.2.3.1 Pharmacology

Choline and its metabolites are used for the synthesis of cell membrane phospholipids; it may also act as a methyl-group donor for other compounds, for example in the methylation of homocysteine to form methionine. Choline also acts as a precursor for the neurotransmitter, acetylcholine. Because choline is purported to have certain anti-inflammatory effects, it has been used to treat asthma and hepatitis.

Choline, when administered as cytidine 5′-diphosphocholine (CDP-choline), has been shown to increase dopamine levels in the CNS [33]. Several studies have identified reduced levels of choline in the CNS of patients with neurologic disorders, including PD [34, 35].

6.2.3.2 Dosing

An average diet is estimated to provide between 200 and 600 mg of choline on a daily basis. In order to treat inflammatory conditions, choline doses of between 500 and 1000 mg, given three times daily, are required. Doses of up to 3.5 g per day in adults appear to be tolerated, although adverse effects are more pronounced at this high dose level. Among other products that release choline upon dissolution are included CDP-choline [33].

6.2.3.3 Adverse Effects

The most significant adverse effects of choline include gastrointestinal upset, vomiting, and diarrhea at higher doses; this may be a result of the steatorrhea caused by high dosing. Some patients have reported sweating, with a fishy body odor [36], while others have suffered dizziness, insomnia, and headaches. Patients have also reported agitation, depression, paranoia, and epilepsy; however, choline has been used to treat these conditions.

6.2.3.4 Precautions

No precautions have been reported for choline administration.

6.2.3.5 Drug Interactions

Possible interactions of choline with other drugs are listed in Table 6.4. Choline has also been associated with decreased plasma homocysteine levels, which may be evidenced through laboratory monitoring.

6.2.3.6 Clinical Evidence

Pilot Study 1: Twenty patients with PD each received CDP-choline intramuscularly at 1000 mg per day for 15 days, and then 500 mg daily for a further 15 days [37].

Table 6.4 The interaction of choline with drugs and other NHPs.

Drug class	Clinical effect
Carnitine	Choline reduces carnitine elimination through the urine
Levodopa	Choline causes an increased concentration of dopa
Methotrexate	Reduced levels of choline
Succinylcholine	Theoretically enhances the effect of succinylcholine

After 30 days, there were improvements in a number of measures, including walking times, rigidity, and handwriting.

Pilot Study 2: Eighty-five patients with PD were randomized to receive CDP-choline (1200 mg daily) plus their usual dose of levodopa, or CDP-choline plus half their usual dose of levodopa [38]. After 4 weeks of treatment there were no significant differences between the groups on a variety of measures. The authors suggested that choline could be further studied as a means of reducing the dose of levodopa.

Pilot Study 3: Thirty patients with PD were treated with CDP-choline (500 mg daily) for 30 days [39]. Electrophysiologic parameters and contractions were observed, and the authors reported a stabilization of neurologic signs. Although an increase in dyskinesias was noted, this was decreased when the dose of levodopa was reduced by one-third.

Pilot Study 4: This double-blind cross-over study with CDP-choline in PD patients demonstrated benefits in both bradykinesia and rigidity [40].

Pilot Study 5: A recent trial using magnetic resonance spectroscopy found that, over 4 weeks, there was no difference in concentrations of choline containing compounds, including metabolites such as phosphorylcholine, myoinositol, or glycerophosphorylcholine [41].

6.2.3.7 Conclusion
Given the limited and dated nature of the data acquired, and the fact that only pilot studies were conducted, choline appears to be unsuitable for the treatment of PD.

6.2.4
Coenzyme Q10 (CoQ10)

CoQ10, also known as *ubiquinone* or *ubiquinol*, is naturally occurring and found in high concentrations in mitochondria, particularly in the myocardium. It is found in small amounts in the diet in meats and seafood. As the body produces adequate amounts of CoQ10, it is not considered a vitamin. Levels in the body are highest during the first 20 years of life, and decline with age.

6.2.4.1 Pharmacology
CoQ10 has antioxidant effects and plays a role in adenosine triphosphate (ATP) production. It has been found to be present in low levels in patients with heart conditions (congestive heart failure and hypertension), muscular dystrophies, PD, cancer, diabetes, and HIV/AIDS.

In experimental models of PD, cerebral concentrations of CoQ10 led to a reduced loss of dopaminergic neurons [42]. CoQ10 is thought to affect the mitochondrial electron transport chain, which leads to a preservation of dopaminergic neurons.

6.2.4.2 Dosing

In PD, the most common dosage is 100 mg per day, given in divided amounts, although daily oral doses of between 300 and 1200 mg have been studied for the treatment of PD. CoQ10 should be taken with meals that contain some fat, so as to increase its absorption.

6.2.4.3 Adverse Effects

Adverse effects associated with CoQ10 administration are typically mild and transient; they include nausea, stomach upset, increased light sensitivity of the eyes, and dizziness. Some debate persists regarding the effects that CoQ10 may have on patients with diabetes. In some clinical trials CoQ10 has been shown to have no adverse effect on blood glucose levels, although others have demonstrated a reduction in hemoglobin A_{1C} levels.

6.2.4.4 Precautions

CoQ10 treatment may need to be restricted in patients with diabetes (see Section 6.2.5.3).

6.2.4.5 Drug Interactions

Possible interactions of CoQ10 with other drugs are listed in Table 6.5. Some concern has also been expressed that CoQ10 may interact with chemotherapeutics, such as doxorubicin, cyclophosphamide, and also radiation therapy. However, this may be due to its effect as an antioxidant.

CoQ10 may interact with other NHPs, such as L-carnitine and red yeast. As L-carnitine plays a role with mitochondrial energy production, it is possible that a synergistic effect may occur. As red yeast includes a statin-like constituent, the interactions may be similar to those with statins (see Table 6.5).

Table 6.5 The interactions of CoQ10 with drugs.

Drug class	Clinical effect
Antidiabetic drugs	CoQ10 causes hypoglycemia (low blood sugar); therefore blood glucose levels should be monitored and doses adjusted
Statins	Lower CoQ10 levels (CoQ10 is dependent on HMG-CoA reductase for its synthesis; statins inhibit this enzyme and cause a decrease in CoQ10 production)
Antihypertensive drugs	CoQ10 will have additive effects with antihypertensive drugs. This is of particular concern in patients with PD, as orthostasis and falls are problematic
Warfarin	CoQ10 is chemically similar to vitamin K, and may have vitamin K-like procoagulant effects, thereby reducing the anticoagulation effects of warfarin

6.2.4.6 Clinical Evidence

Randomized Placebo-Controlled Double Blind Trials

Study 1: This double-blind, placebo-controlled, randomized trial included 131 patients with PD [43]. The participants had no motor fluctuations and were receiving stable anti-parkinsonian treatment. The patients were assigned randomly to nanoparticular CoQ10 (100 mg, three times daily) or placebo, for 3 months. The primary outcome was the change in the Unified Parkinson Disease Rating Scale (UPDRS) parts II and III between baseline and three months. There were no differences in the primary outcome, nor in any secondary clinical outcomes. The authors noted that the product was well tolerated, but displayed no symptomatic effects.

Study 2: This double-blind, placebo-controlled, randomized trial included 80 patients with early PD [44]. The participants were assigned randomly to CoQ10 treatment, with daily doses of 300, 600, or 1200 mg, or placebo. The study ran for 16 months, with the primary endpoint being the change in UPDRS score between baseline and final visit. Those patients receiving the highest CoQ10 dose (1200 mg per day) had less deterioration on UPDRS scores than did those receiving the placebo. The activity of daily living (ADL) scores improved significantly for the drug-treated patients. However, this symptomatic improvement, which was not anticipated, has led to criticism about the interpretation of the study. It should also be noted that those in the 1200 mg per day arm did not show any delay in their need for dopaminergic therapy.

Study 3: This double-blind, placebo-controlled trial involved 28 patients administered CoQ10 at 360 mg per day for 4 weeks [45]. There was a slight, but statistically significant, improvement in PD symptoms, as measured by the Farnsworth–Munsell 100 Hue test (FMT).

Open-Label Studies

Study 1: This open-label pilot study involved 17 patients with PD [46]. The focal point of the study was safety and tolerability, with subjects given escalating doses of CoQ10 (1200, 1800, 2400, and 3000 mg per day) with vitamin E 1200 IU per day. Only 13 of the 17 patients achieved the highest dose level, and the CoQ10 blood levels did not differ between the 2400 and 300 mg dose groups. Overall, CoQ10 was well tolerated.

Study 2: This open-label study involved only 12 patients, with CoQ10 dosed at 500 mg twice daily for 3 months, followed by 500 mg three times daily for 3 months (total 6 months).[47] Although there was some improvement in the patients' movement, this was not statistically significant.

Study 3: This pilot study involved only 15 subjects assigned to 200 mg CoQ10 twice daily, three times daily, or four times daily [42]. The patients also received vitamin E (400 IU daily), as concern had been expressed about formation of the ubisemiquinone-10 radical. Whilst there were no statistically significant improvements in motor scores, at the highest dose (800 mg per day) two patients had a small number of casts in their urine, which was of unknown significance.

Study 4: This open-label pilot study involved 10 patients with PD who were treated with CoQ10 100 mg twice daily for 3 months [48]. Following treatment, there were no significant differences in the UPDRS or motor tests.

6.2.4.7 Conclusion

Some promise was noted that a degree of symptomatic benefit was noted in the larger, higher-dose clinical trials with CoQ10, although these benefits were not especially large. Overall, CoQ10 was well tolerated, although further studies are required to determine if its purported neuroprotective effect exists.

6.2.5
Creatine (N-Aminoiminomethyl-N Methyl Glycine)

Creatine is a naturally occurring compound produced by the liver, kidneys, and pancreas from the amino acids glycine, arginine, and methionine. Most individuals also consume 1–2 g of exogenous creatine daily, mainly from meat and fish. It is found primarily in skeletal muscle (95%), and has gained popularity as a natural ergogenic supplement to enhance athletic performance and build lean body mass.

6.2.5.1 Pharmacology

Creatine plays an important role in energy production in the mitochondria, where it is converted to phosphocreatine that is able to transfer a phosphoryl group to ADP (adenosine diphosphate) so as to produce ATP, an "energy molecule." The ingestion of higher levels of creatine is thought to provide a larger total pool of creatine in the skeletal muscle, and to enhance the ability to renew ATP. Creatine administration has been shown to be beneficial for certain types of high-intensity exercises (e.g., weight lifting, sprinting), but has not demonstrated any benefit in endurance performance (e.g., cycling, cross-country running) [49, 50]. Creatine supplementation in the PD patient may help to increase muscle fitness and lead to an improved functional status, thus maintaining independence and preventing disability [51].

Both, *in vitro* and *in vivo* studies have indicated neuoprotective effects of creatine in several animal models of neurodegenerative diseases such as PD [52]. The oral supplementation of creatine in mice has been shown to protect against striatal dopamine depletion and a loss of substantia nigra tyrosine hydroxlase immunoreactive neurons [53].

6.2.5.2 Dosing

Currently, many different forms of creatine, in varying concentrations, are available commercially; these include creatine monohydrate and creatine monophosphate. The doses range from 10–30 g for 4–6 days, followed by a maintenance dose of 2–5 g for up to 140 days.

It is recommended that creatine be taken with carbohydrates (so as to enhance its absorption), and also to maintain good hydration during its use.

6.2.5.3 Adverse Effects
Adverse effects related to creatine treatment include muscle cramps, dehydration, possible weight gain, and impaired renal function (there is inconclusive evidence for the latter point).

6.2.5.4 Precautions
Creatine should be *avoided* in patients with:

- impaired renal function or dehydration
- bipolar disorder (this may result in hypermania).

Creatine should be *used with caution* in patients with:

- diabetes (unknown effect on kidneys and blood glucose levels);
- seizures (potential to cause seizures);
- arrhythmias (potential for increased symptoms);
- deep vein thrombosis (potential for increased symptoms); and
- kidney stones (potential for increased symptoms).

6.2.5.5 Drug Interactions
Possible interactions of creatine with other drugs are listed in Table 6.6.

6.2.5.6 Clinical Evidence

Randomized Controlled Trials

Study 1: This study included 60 patients with PD who were enrolled in blinded fashion and given either creatine ($n = 40$) or placebo ($n = 20$) over 2 years [54].

Table 6.6 The interactions of creatine with drugs and other NHPs.

Drug class	Clinical effect
Antidiabetics	Decreased glucose levels
Anti-inflammatory	Impaired renal function
Antilipidemic	Increased lipid lowering
Caffeine	Decreased exercise benefit
Diuretics	Increased diuretic effect
Ephedra	Risk of ischemic stroke
Nephrotoxic drugs (cyclosporine, aminoglycosides)	Increased nephrotoxic effect

Patients were loaded with creatine at 20 g per day for 6 days, followed by 2 g per day for 6 months, and then 4 g per day for the remainder of the study. Creatine improved patient mood and led to a smaller dose increase of dopaminergic therapy but had no effect on overall unified Parkinson's Disease Rating Scale scores or dopamine transporter SPECT.

Study 2: The primary objective of this study was to evaluate the therapeutic effects of resistance training with or without creatine supplementation in patients with mild to moderate PD [55] . Twenty patients were enrolled and randomized to receive resistance training + creatine or resistance training + placebo, using a double-blind methodology. Creatine was supplemented at 20 g per day for the first 5 days, and 3 g per day thereafter. Both groups participated in resistance training twice weekly. The muscular endurance was found to have improved in both groups, although the creatine group showed a greater improvement in chest press strength and biceps curl strength.

Study 3: The patients in study 1 [54] were evaluated, using laboratory blood and urine tests, for potential side effects of creatine with a special focus on renal function [56]. At one year, the serum creatin levels were higher in the treatment group, but this difference was not noted between 12 and 24 months. Although there was no evidence of any renal damage (as indicated by renal markers), the creatine-treated group reported more gastrointestinal complaints.

Study 4: In this study, the aim of the National Institute of Neurological Disorders and Stroke Neuroprotection Exploratory Trials in Parkinson's Disease (NINDS NET-PD) investigators aimed to determine if creatine and minocycline had the potential to alter the short-term course of early PD and impact the progression of the disease [57]. A total of 200 patients was enrolled and randomized to either creatine (10 g per day), minocycline (200 mg per day), or placebo for 12 months. The futility threshold was set at a 30% reduction in the UPDRS progression. Neither creatine nor minocycline could be rejected as futile. The aim was to use the results of this study to inform further trials testing minocycline or creatine about PD progression.

6.2.5.7 Conclusion
Although the early clinical trials with creatine showed much promise, very little evidence was acquired to support its routine use. The patients appeared to tolerate creatine fairly well and, in some cases, this improved their muscle strength and endurance. However, further investigations with creatine are essential.

6.2.6
Fava Bean *(Vicia faba)*

The fava bean is a legume, also known as broad bean, faba, and horse bean. It is native to North Africa and southwest Asia and extensively cultivated elsewhere.

Fava beans have been eaten for thousands of years throughout the world, especially in the Mediterranean region, and are also used medically in the treatment of PD, as they are rich in levodopa.

6.2.6.1 Pharmacology

The entire fava plant, including the leaves, stems, pods, and immature beans, contain levodopa. The young pod and the immature (green) beans inside the pod contain the greatest amount of levodopa, and the mature or dried bean the least. One-half cup of fresh green fava beans, or 100 g of canned green fava beans, when drained, may contain about 50–100 mg of levodopa.

6.2.6.2 Dosing

The amount of levodopa in the fava bean can vary greatly, depending on the species of fava, the area where it is grown, the soil conditions, rainfall, and other factors. Thus, it is possible to ingest either too much or too little levodopa.

The use of faba should be discussed with physician. Typically, treatment should be started with a small amount, perhaps 28 g or two tablespoons of whole beans per day for about one week, after which any effect should be determined. Some people have reported that a half-cup (ca. 110 g) of fava per day, or even every other day, gives good results. If the fava beans reduce PD symptoms, the physician may need to adjust any other concurrent PD medications.

6.2.6.3 Adverse Effects

Typical adverse effects include: (i) *allergy*, which may manifest as a rash or gastrointestinal upset and, occasionally, as coma; and (ii) *favism*, a rare inherited disease in the enzyme glucose-6-phosphate dehydrogenase G6PD) is lacking. If a patient with this condition eats fava beans, then hemolytic anemia can occur whereby the red blood cells break down such that the debris blocks the blood vessels, resulting in possible kidney failure and even death.

6.2.6.4 Precautions

See Section 6.2.7.3.

6.2.6.5 Drug Interactions

Possible interactions of faba with other drugs are listed in Table 6.7.

Table 6.7 The interactions of fava bean with drugs.

Drug class	Clinical effect
Monoamine oxidase inhibitor (MAOI) – isocarboxazide, phenelzine, tranylcypromine, selegiline	Hypertensive crisis due to increased amount of dopamine produced

6.2.6.6 Clinical Evidence

Case-Control Studies

Study 1: Five healthy volunteers (serving as controls) and six PD patients (no treatment for 12 h) each ate 250 g of cooked broad beans (*Vicia faba*) at 1 h after a breakfast which consisted of tea or coffee with biscuits or a slice of bread [58, 59]. Blood samples were obtained before eating the fava beans (time 0) and every 30 min thereafter for 4 h. Clinical evaluation was scored according to the Webster scale. In the PD patients, a substantial clinical improvement was noted over the next 4 h, three patients showed severe dyskinesias (similar to that occurring after a dose of levodopa), and the plasma levodopa concentrations rose. T he five volunteers also showed an increase in plasma levodopa levels after eating broad beans, but the levels were lower than in the PD patients. Five days later, the PD patients were given oral levodopa (125 mg) plus carbidopa (12.5 mg) at time 0, and at 30 min intervals thereafter for 4 h. Both, the plasma levels of levodopa and clinical improvement in the patients was similar to that experienced after ingesting fava beans. It was concluded that these findings may have implications for fava beans in the treatment of PD, especially in patients with mild symptoms.

Open-Label Trial Eight patients who previously had reported favorable motor effects from broad bean ingestion were asked to eat 250 g of cooked broad beans at least twice daily, without otherwise altering their dietary habits [60], and during which time their medical treatment was maintained. Only three patients completed the required daily diary recording the times and durations of "on" and "off" periods as well as sleep. A baseline assessment (before broad bean supplementation) was made for 5–7 days, and again corresponding to the 1–3 months during broad bean administration. All three patients observed a strikingly prolonged "on" time and a shortened "off" time, while one patient reported an increase in sleep time. These preliminary results suggested that broad bean meals may be efficacious as a means of reducing levodopa off-period disability.

6.2.6.7 Conclusion
There is preliminary evidence, albeit in small-scale studies, suggesting that the ingestion of fava beans may serve as an effective complementary treatment to levodopa. However, controlled clinical trials are required to confirm these findings, and also to explore the underlying mechanisms.

6.2.7
Green Tea *(Camellia sinensis)*

There are three categories of tea: black, oolong, and green, all of which are obtained from *Camellia sinensis*, which is native to Southeast Asia. *Black tea* leaves are fermented and contain mostly theaflavins and thearubigins as the active ingredients. *Green tea* is a nonoxidized, nonfermented tea, which contains polyphenolic compounds such as epicatechin, epicatechin gallate, epigallocatechin and epigallocatechin gallate (EGCG), whereas *oolong tea* is partially oxidized and contains a considerable amount of polyphenols. Tea polyphenols have been found to be powerful antioxidants, to possess iron-chelating properties, and be capable of crossing the blood–brain barrier.

Green tea is also a source of caffeine; one cup of tea contains 10–80 mg (average ca. 50 mg) of caffeine, depending on the strength and size of the cup (by comparison, coffee contains ca. 200 mg caffeine per cup).

6.2.7.1 Pharmacology

Green tea contains polyphenols (flavonoids), which may prevent dopaminergic neurodegeneration, such as found in PD. Both, *in vivo* and *in vitro* studies have shown that polyphenols block the dopamine transporter, which may increase the concentration of synaptic dopamine, and/or decrease the uptake of neurotoxins [61]. It has been shown in both mouse and human cell lines that (−)-EGCG is a potent inhibitor of microglial activation, which is believed to play a pivotal role in the selective neuronal injury associated with PD [62]. Because EGCG can penetrate the brain [63, 64], and in light of its potent action against microglial activation, EGCG may represent a prospective candidate to alleviate microglial-mediated dopaminergic neuronal injury in PD. Green tea also contains 2–4% caffeine (10–80 mg caffeine per cup), which may block adenosine receptors and thus prevent the inhibition by adenosine of dopaminergic transmission [65]. Decaffeinated green tea would possess the polyphenol effect, but not the caffeine effect.

6.2.7.2 Dosing

When dosed as a tea, one cup would contain approximately 50 mg of caffeine and 80–100 mg of polyphenols (depending on the strength and cup size). The daily consumption of five cups or less is considered to be safe.

When dosed as an extract in capsules the amount per capsule may vary considerably, from 100 to 750 mg.

6.2.7.3 Adverse Effects

Adverse effects are mainly due to the caffeine content (see Section 6.2.2), which may cause insomnia, nervousness, restlessness, gastric irritation, nausea, vomiting, tachycardia, quickened respiration, tremors, delirium, convulsions, and diuresis. Large doses can produce headache, anxiety, agitation, ringing in the ears, premature heartbeat, and arrhythmia.

Nausea, vomiting, abdominal bloating and pain, dyspepsia, flatulence, and diarrhea have been noted with green tea intake.

Tannins can cause constipation.

6.2.7.4 Precautions

Patients who are *allergic* to either caffeine or tannin should avoid drinking green tea. In *diabetics*, hyperglycemia may occur after drinking green tea containing 200 mg caffeine. The safety of green tea ingestion in *pregnant* and *breastfeeding* women has not been investigated; hence, the ingestion of green tea would best be avoided in this group.

6.2.7.5 Drug Interactions

Possible drug interactions of green tea are due to its caffeine content (see Section 6.2.2). Green tea may also contain vitamin K, which can reduce the anticoagulant effects of warfarin.

6.2.7.6 Clinical Evidence

Prospective Study   A prospective cohort of 63 257 Chinese men and women identified 157 incident PD cases [66]. The total caffeine intake was inversely related to PD risk (P for trend = 0.002). Black tea, a caffeine-containing beverage, showed an inverse association with PD that was not confounded by total caffeine intake or tobacco smoking (P for trend = 0.0006). Green tea drinking was unrelated to PD risk. The ingredients of black tea, other than caffeine, appear to be responsible for the beverage's inverse association with PD.

Prevention/Neuroprotection

Case-Control Study 1: This matched case-control study in the Limousin Region, France, found that first-degree relative and tea drinking were the main risk factors for developing PD [67]. The authors maintained that further research is needed to validate that tea consumption increases the risk of PD.

Case-Control Study 2: This epidemiological case-control study did not confirm any inverse association for either coffee or total caffeine consumption, but demonstrated reduced risks related to the consumption of tea and cola [68]. These findings were suggestive of protective effects from beverage components other than caffeine.

Case-Control Study 3: This aim of this case-control study was to identify possible environmental risk factors for PD [69]. However, no association was found between the risk for PD and coffee- and tea-drinking habits.

6.2.7.7 Conclusion

The results of preclinical (animal) studies have suggested that green tea polyphenols may play a role in the prevention or treatment of PD, although human data to support this proposal are lacking. There is also conflicting evidence on the effect of consuming two or more cups of green tea daily; some studies showed an inverse correlation between tea consumption of and the development of PD [68], others showed either an increased risk of PD [67] or no effect on the development of the disease [69]. A recent study [66] examined the differential effects of black versus green tea on the risk of PD in the Singapore Chinese Health Study; the results indicated that black tea, but not green tea, lowered the risk of PD. Ingredients in the black tea other than caffeine appeared to be responsible for the beverage's inverse association with PD.

6.2.8
Melatonin (N-Acetyl-5-Methoxytryptamine)

Melatonin is a neurohormone produced in the brain by the pineal gland, from the amino acid tryptophan. The synthesis and release of melatonin are stimulated by darkness and suppressed by light, suggesting the involvement of melatonin in circadian rhythm and the regulation of diverse body functions. Levels of melatonin in the blood are highest prior to bedtime. Melatonin secretion also changes with advancing age, with the highest night-time concentrations ($\sim$250 pg ml^{-1}) in children aged between 1 and 3 years. The average night-time concentration in older children (8–15 years) is approximately 120 pg ml^{-1}, and this begins to decline to approximately 20 pg ml^{-1} in older adults (50–70 years). Melatonin is most often administered to treat insomnia and "jet lag."

6.2.8.1 Pharmacology

Melatonin has been found to prevent cell death and methylphenyltretahyropyridine (MPTP)-induced damage to the substantia nigra and dopaminergic neurons in experimental parkinsonism, thus preventing disease progression in these animals [70]. The etiology of dopaminergic neuron death is not known, although the involvement of oxidative stress [71, 72] and increased iron (a pro-oxidant) levels [73] has been reported. Melatonin is an antioxidant which easily passes the blood–brain barrier and also lacks any relevant adverse side effects.

6.2.8.2 Dosing

Various studies have indicated that the administration of 0.1–0.3 mg melatonin may produce blood levels within the normal physiologic range at night-time, which may be sufficient especially for the elderly. Pharmacological doses of melatonin (>0.3 mg) typically do not increase effects above those achieved by physiological doses, and might even be less effective. "Quick-release" melatonin may be more effective than sustained-release formulations.

In children, there is limited evidence of the benefits of melatonin, and its safety has not been established. Some studies have suggested that 2.5–10 mg, taken nightly at the desired bedtime, may be effective under certain circumstances (e.g., blind, seizure disorder, mental retardation).

No dosing of melatonin has yet been established in regard to PD.

6.2.8.3 Adverse Effects

Although melatonin is generally regarded as safe in recommended doses for short-term use (e.g., as for insomnia), some typical adverse effects may include:

- An increased risk of blood clots and disorientation with overdose.
- Fatigue, dizziness, headache, irritability, and sleepiness.
- A reduction in blood pressure.
- Mild gastrointestinal effects, such as nausea, vomiting, or cramping.
- Hormonal effects, such as increases or decreases based on underlying patient characteristics.

- Visual system; there may be an increased sensitivity of photoreceptors to light.

6.2.8.4 Precautions

Precautions should be taken when administering melatonin to patients with glaucoma, as the ocular pressure may be increased. Likewise, there may be a risk of inducing seizures. Diabetic patients may also suffer hyperglycemic episodes (elevated blood sugar levels).

6.2.8.5 Drug Interactions

Possible interactions of melatonin with other drugs are listed in Table 6.8.

Table 6.8 The interactions of melatonin with drugs.

Drug class	Clinical effect
Cytochrome P450 1A2 inhibitors: – Cimetidine – Clarithromycin – Fluvoxamine – Isoniazid – Ketoconazole – Levofloxacin – Paroxetine	P450 1A2 metabolizes melatonin; therefore, drugs that inhibit or reduce this enzyme can increase levels of melatonin in the body
Cytochrome P450 1A2 inducers: – Phenobarbital – Phenytoin – Rifampin – Ritonavir – Smoking	P450 1A2 metabolizes melatonin; therefore, drugs that induce this enzyme can decrease levels of melatonin in the body
Zolpidem and other sedative drugs	Increased daytime drowsiness is reported when melatonin is used at the same time
Warfarin	Decreases the effect of warfarin – increased risk of blood clots
Non-steroidal anti-inflammatory drugs	Reduce production or secretion of melatonin
Beta-blockers	
Oral contraceptives	
Antiseizure drugs	Melatonin may lower seizure threshold and increase the risk of seizure
Antihypertensives	Melatonin causes a drop in blood pressure
Diabetes medications	Melatonin causes elevated blood glucose levels

6.2.8.6 Clinical Evidence

Observational Study   An observational study was conducted to compare the melatonin secretion pattern in untreated patients with PD and in those with PD receiving a dopaminergic treatment but without levodopa-related motor complications (LDRMCs), as well as in patients with PD receiving a dopaminergic treatment and with LDRMCs [74]. There was a significant ($P < 0.05$) phase advance in plasma melatonin secretion in patients receiving a dopaminergic treatment compared to untreated patients. The circadian secretion pattern of melatonin is modified in patients with LDRMCs. It is postulated that there may be melatonin-induced changes in dopamine receptor sensitivity by interaction with striatal melatonin receptors. Further studies are required to determine the mechanisms involved in changes in melatonin secretion patterns observed in this study.

6.2.8.7 Conclusion
Due to very limited studies conducted to date, no recommendation can be made for or against the use of melatonin in PD. Better-designed investigations must be carried out before any firm conclusions can be reached in this respect.

6.2.9
Vitamin E

Vitamin E, a fat-soluble vitamin with antioxidant properties, comprises four tocopherols (α, β, γ, and δ-tocopherol) and four tocotrienols. $R,R,R,$-α-tocopherol (formerly D-α-tocopherol) is the naturally occurring, most biologically active form. Synthetic vitamin E, which is all-rac-α-tocopherol (formerly D,L-α-tocopherol), has been proposed for the prevention or treatment of numerous health conditions, often based on its antioxidant properties. However, aside from the treatment of vitamin E deficiency (which is rare), there are no clearly proven medicinal uses of vitamin E supplementation beyond the recommended daily allowance. There is ongoing research in numerous diseases, particularly in cancer and heart disease.

Dietary sources of vitamin E include eggs, fortified cereals, fruit, green leafy vegetables (e.g., spinach), meat, nuts/nut oils, poultry, vegetable oils (corn, cottonseed, safflower, soybean, sunflower), wheat germ oil, and whole grains. Cooking and storage may destroy some of the vitamin E in foods.

6.2.9.1 Pharmacology
Vitamin E is a dietary compound that functions as an antioxidant scavenging toxic free radicals.

6.2.9.2 Dosing
Vitamin E supplements are available in either natural or synthetic forms. The natural forms are usually labeled with the letter "d" (e.g., d-gamma-tocopherol), whereas synthetic forms are labeled "dl" (e.g., dl-alpha-tocopherol).

The recommended daily allowance (RDA) for vitamin E in adults is usually expressed as alpha-tocopherol equivalents (ATE) in order to account for the different biological activities of the various forms of vitamin E, as well as in International Units (IU), which are often used for foods and supplements. (To convert between these, 1 mg ATE = 1.5 IU.) The RDA for males and females aged over 14 years is 15 mg (22.5 IU), for pregnant women of any age it is 15 mg (22.5 IU), and for breastfeeding women of any age it is 19 mg (28.5 IU).

For supplementary α-tocopherol, the tolerable upper intake level (UL) for adults aged >18 years, as recommended by the US Institute of Medicine, is 1000 mg per day (equivalent to 1500 IU). This recommended limit is not altered during pregnancy or breastfeeding.

6.2.9.3 Adverse Effects

Typically, there is an increased risk of bleeding with Vitamin E, especially with high doses (>400 IU per day) (see Section 6.2.10.4).

6.2.9.4 Precautions

Recently acquired evidence has suggested that the regular use of high-dose vitamin E supplements (≥400 IU per day) may increase the risk of death (from "all causes") by a small degree [75].

High doses of vitamin E (>400 units) might increase the risk of bleeding, due to an inhibition of platelet aggregation and antagonism of vitamin K-dependent clotting factors (particularly in patients with vitamin K deficiency).

6.2.9.5 Drug Interactions

Possible interactions of vitamin E with other drugs are listed in Table 6.9.

6.2.9.6 Clinical Evidence

Prevention/Neuroprotection

Meta-analysis 1: This meta-analysis included eight studies evaluating the effects of vitamin C, vitamin E, and beta-carotene on the risk of PD [76]. Vitamin E was

Table 6.9 The interactions of vitamin E with drugs.

Drug class	Clinical effect
Anticoagulant/antiplatelet drugs	Increased risk of bleeding
Chemotherapy	Antioxidants may interfere with some chemotherapeutic agents (e.g., alkylating agents, anthracyclines, or platinums), which themselves can depend on oxidative damage to tumor cells for their anticancer effects
Orlistat	May prevent the absorption of vitamin E

found to be protective against PD when consumed at a moderate intake (second and third quartile of the distribution).

Meta-analysis 2: This analysis combined two large cohort studies, the Nurses' Health Study, and the Health Professionals Follow-up Study [77]. The study aim was to evaluate the dietary intake and use of supplements, with over 120 000 participants completing questionnaires. The intake of vitamin E was not associated with the risk of developing PD; however, if patients were in the highest quartile for dietary intake of vitamin E there was a significant reduction in developing PD.

Randomized Placebo-Controlled Trial The Deprenyl and Tocopherol Antioxidative Therapy of Parkinsonism (DATATOP) trial was initiated in 1987 to determine if selegiline or vitamin E could delay the progression of PD [78]. A total of 800 patients with PD was randomized to receive either vitamin E plus selegiline, placebo plus selegiline, vitamin E plus placebo, or placebo plus placebo. Selegiline was dosed at 5 mg twice daily, and vitamin E at 1000 IU twice daily. Vitamin E failed to prevent the progression of disease, whether combined with selegiline or placebo, over the 10-year trial.

6.2.9.7 Conclusions

While the DATATOP trial demonstrated no benefit, some debate has emerged regarding the benefit of consuming higher amounts of dietary tocopherol versus high doses of supplements [79, 80]. Some observational evidence has been acquired that vitamin E might be protective, although the largest randomized trial, DATATOP, has refuted the benefits of using vitamin E to prevent the progression of PD. Due to recent reports of increased mortality, vitamin E is not recommended for the prevention or treatment of PD.

6.3
Conclusions

Parkinson disease patients use NHPs to either prevent or treat their disease, and also to ameliorate any adverse effects that may be caused by their prescribed therapy. However, the body of evidence supporting the use of NHPs for the management of PD is weak, and it seems that data are available for very few of these materials with regards to the prevention or treatment of PD. Moreover, most of these data have originated from small, short-term pilot studies.

Often, PD patients will use NHPs not realizing that interactions may occur between them and conventional pharmaceutical products. In this case, the patients should be made aware that such interaction may either lessen or increase the effects of their prescribed therapy, or increase the risk of adverse reactions. It is of the utmost importance that patients inform their healthcare practitioners of any NHP use, and that the healthcare practitioner in turn enquires about such usage when conducting medication reviews. It is the responsibility of healthcare professionals to maintain an awareness of NHPs and of relevant research studies.

Patients should not forego any proven therapies to take NHPs, as this might not only delay treatment but also result in an effective therapy being replaced.

Unfortunately, at present there is little evidence available to indicate that NHPs should be used routinely in clinical practice, despite their widespread use. The extensive use of CAM therapies and medications in PD requires attention to be directed towards testing the safety and efficacy of NHPs, as well as informing both the healthcare providers and patients about the potential benefits, costs, limitations, and risks. Clearly, further research is required to determine the benefit of NHPs on the prevention and treatment of PD.

References

1 Eisenberg, D.M., Davis, R.E., Ettner, S.L., *et al.* (1998) Trends in alternative medicine use in the US, 1990–1997: results of a follow up national survey. *Journal of the American Medical Association*, **280**, 1569–1575.

2 Ryan, M. and Johnson, M.S. (2002) Use of alternative medications in patients with neurologic disorders. *Annals of Pharmacotherapy*, **36**, 1540–1545.

3 Rajendran, P.R., Thompson, R.E., and Reich, S.G. (2001) The use of alternative therapies by patients with Parkinson's disease. *Neurology*, **57**, 790–794.

4 Ferry, P., Johnson, M., and Walliw, P. (2002) Use of complementary therapies and non-prescribed medication in patients with Parkinson's disease. *Postgraduate Medical Journal*, **78**, 612–614.

5 Paterson, C., Allen, J.A., Browning, M., *et al.* (2005) A pilot study of therapeutic massage for people with Parkinson's disease: the added value of user involvement. *Complementary Therapies in Clinical Practice*, **11** (3), 161–171.

6 Lee, M.S., Shin, B.C., Kong, J.C., *et al.* (2008) Effectiveness of acupuncture for Parkinson Disease: a systematic review. *Movement Disorders*, **23** (11), 1505–1515.

7 Mallet, L., Spinewine, A., and Huang, A. (2007) The challenge of managing drug interactions in elderly people. *Lancet*, **370**, 185–191.

8 McCabe, B.J. (2004) Prevention of food-drug interactions with special emphasis on older adults. *Current Opinion in Clinical Nutrition and Metabolic Care*, **7**, 21–26.

9 Joly, P., Lampert, A., Thomine, E., *et al.* (1991) Development of pseudobullous morphea and scleroderma-like illness during therapy with L-5-hydroxotryptophan and carbidopa. *Journal of the American Academy of Dermatology*, **25**, 332–333.

10 Schelosky, L., Raffauf, C., Jendroska, K., *et al.* (1995) Kava and dopamine antagonism. *Journal of Neurosurgery and Psychiatry*, **58**, 639–640.

11 Nutt, J.G., Woodward, W.R., Hammerstad, J.P., *et al.* (1984) The «on-off» phenomenon in Parkinson Disease. Relation to levodopa absorption and transport. *New England Journal of Medicine*, **310**, 483–488.

12 Campbell, N.R. and Hasinoff, B.B. (1991) Iron supplements: a common cause of drug interactions. *British Journal of Clinical Pharmacology*, **31**, 251–255.

13 Powers, K.M., Smith-Weller, T., Franklin, G.M., *et al.* (2003) Parkinson's disease risks associated with dietary iron, manganese, and other nutrient intakes. *Neurology*, **60**, 1761–1766.

14 Liu, X., Lamango, N., and Charlton, C. (1998) L-dopa depletes S-adenosylmethionine and increases S-adenosyl homocysteine: relationship to the wearing-off effects. *Abstracts – Society of Neuroscience*, **24**, 1469.

15 Hardman, J.G. and Limbird, L.E. (eds) (2001) *Goodman & Gilman's the Pharmacologic Basis of Therapeutics*, 10th edn, McGraw-Hill Medical Publishing Division.

16 Jarry, H., Leonhardt, S., Wuttke, W., *et al.* (1994) *In vitro* prolactin but not LH and FSH release is inhibited by compounds in extracts of *Agnus-castus*: direct evidence for a dopaminergic principle by the dopamine receptor assay. *Experimental and Clinical Endocrinology*, **102**, 448–454.

17 Hansten, P.D. (2008) *Drug Interactions Analysis and Management*, Wolters Kluwer Health.

18 AARP (2007) *Complementary and Alternative Medicine. What People 50 and Older are Using and Discussing with Their Physicians*, AARP, http://assets.aarp.org/rgcenter/health/cam_2007.pdf (accessed April 1, 2009).

19 Milden, S.P. and Stokols, D. (2004) Physicians' attitudes and practices regarding complementary and alternative medicine. *Behavioural Medicine*, **30** (2), 73–82.

20 Corbin Winslow, L. and Shapiro, H. (2002) Physicians want education about complementary and alternative medicine to enhance communication with their patients. *Archives of Internal Medicine*, **162** (10), 1176–1181.

21 Chung, V., Liu, L., Bian, Z., *et al.* (2006) Efficacy and safety of herbal medicines for idiopathic Parkinson's disease: a systematic review. *Movement Disorders*, **21**, 1709–1715.

22 Bonuccelli, U. and Del Dotto, P. (2006) New pharmacologic horizons in the treatment of Parkinson Disease. *Neurology*, **67** (Suppl. 2), S30–S38.

23 Suchowersky, O., Gronseth, G., Perlmutter, J., Reich, S., Zesiewicz, T., and Weiner, W.J. (2006) Practice parameter: neuroprotective strategies and alternative therapies for Parkinson Disease (an evidence-based review). Report of the Quality Standards Subcommittee of the American Academy of Neurology. *Neurology*, **66**, 976–982.

24 Schleibs, R., Liebmann, A., Bhattacharya, SK, *et al.* (1997) Systemic administration of defined extracts from *Withania somnifera* (Indian ginseng) and *Shilajit* differentially affects cholinergic but not glutamatergic and GABAergic markers in the rat brain. *Neurochemistry International*, **30**, 181–190.

25 Nagashayana, N., Sankarankutty, P., Nampoothiri, M.R.V., *et al.* (2000) Association of L-DOPA with recovery following *Ayurveda* medication in Parkinson's disease. *Journal of the Neurological Sciences*, **176**, 124–127.

26 Chen, J.-F., Xu, K., Petzer, J.P., *et al.* (2001) Neuroprotection by caffeine and A2A adenosine receptor inactivation in a model of Parkinson's disease. *Journal of Neuroscience*, **21**:(10), 1–6.

27 Hernan, M.A., Takkouche, B., Caamano-Isorna, F., *et al.* (2002) A meta-analysis of coffee drinking, cigarette smoking, and the risk of Parkinson's Disease. *Annals of Neurology*, **52**, 276–284.

28 Ascherio, A., Zhang, S.M., Hernan, M.A., *et al.* (2001) Prospective study of caffeine consumption and risk of Parkinson's Disease in men and women. *Annals of Neurology*, **50**, 56–63.

29 Hancock, D.B., Martin, E.R., Stajich, J.M., *et al.* (2007) Smoking, caffeine, and nonsteroidal anti-inflammatory drugs in families with Parkinson Disease. *Archives of Neurology*, **64**, 576–580.

30 Durrant, K.L. (2002) Known and hidden sources of caffeine in drug, food, and natural products. *Journal of the American Pharmaceutical Association*, **42**, 525–537.

31 Kitagawa, M., Houzen, H., and Tashiro, K. (2007) Effects of caffeine on the freezing of gait in Parkinson's disease. *Movement Disorders*, **22** (5), 710–712.

32 Deleu, D., Jacob, P., Chand, P., *et al.* (2006) Effects of caffeine on levodopa pharmacokinetics and pharmacodynamics in Parkinson Disease. *Neurology*, **67**, 897–899.

33 Secades, J.J. and Frontera, G. (1995) CDP-choline: pharmacological and clinical review. *Methods and Findings in Experimental and Clinical Pharmacology*, **17** (Suppl. B), 1–54.

34 Adibhatla, R.M. and Hatcher, J.F. (2005) Cytidine 5′-diphosphocholine (CDP-choline) in stroke and other CNS disorders. *Neurochemical Research*, **30**, 15–23.

35 Manyam, B.V., Giacobinin, E., and Colliver, J.A. (1990) Cerebrospinal fluid choline levels are decreased in Parkinson's disease. *Annals of Neurology*, **27**, 682–685.

36 Grunewald, K.K. and Bailey, R.S. (1993) Commercially marketed supplements for bodybuilding athletes. *Sports Medicine*, **15**, 90–103.

37 Masso, M. and Urtasun, J.F. (1991) Citicoline in the treatment of Parkinson's disease. *Clinical Therapeutics*, **13**, 239–242.

38 Eberhardt, R., Birbamer, G., Gerstenbrand, F., *et al.* (1990) Citicoline in the treatment of Parkinson's disease. *Clinical Therapeutics*, **12**, 489–495.

39 Cubells, J.M. and Hernando, C. (1988) Clinical trial on the use of cytidine diphosphate choline in Parkinson's disease. *Clinical Therapeutics*, **10**, 664–671.

40 Angoli, A., Ruggieri, S., Denaro, A., *et al.* (1982) New strategies in the management of Parkinson's disease: a biological approach using a phospholipid precursors (CDP-choline). *Neuropsychobiology*, **8**, 289–296.

41 Dechent, P., Pouwels, P.J.W., and Frahm, J. (1999) Neither short-term nor long-term administration of oral choline alters metabolite concentrations in human brain. *Biological Psychiatry*, **46**, 406–411.

42 Shults, C.W., Flint Beal, M., Nakano, K., *et al.* (1998) Absorption, tolerability, and effects on mitochondrial activity of oral coenzyme Q10 in parkinsonian patients. *Neurology*, **50**, 793–795.

43 Storch, A., Jost, W.H., Vieregge, P., *et al.* (2007) Randomized, double-blind, placebo-controlled trial of symptomatic effects of coenzyme Q10 in Parkinson Disease. *Archives of Neurology*, **64**, 938–944.

44 Shults, C.W., Oakes, D., Kieburtz, K., *et al.* (2002) Effects of coenzyme Q10 in early Parkinson Disease. *Archives of Neurology*, **59**, 1541–1550.

45 Muller, T., Buttner, T., Gholipour, A.F., *et al.* (2003) Coenzyme Q10 supplementation provides mild symptomatic benefit in patients with Parkinson's disease. *Neurosciences Letters*, **341**, 201–204.

46 Shults, C.W., Flint Beal, M., Song, D., *et al.* (2004) Pilot trial of high dosages of coenzyme Q10 in patients with Parkinson's disease. *Experimental Neurology*, **188**, 491–494.

47 Horstink, M.W.I.M., and van Engelen, B.G. (2003) The effect of coenzyme Q10 therapy in Parkinson Disease could be symptomatic. *Archives of Neurology*, **60**, 1170–1172.

48 Strijks, E., Kremer, H.P.H., and Horstink, M.W.I.M. (1997) Q10 therapy in patients with idiopathic Parkinson's disease. *Molecular Aspects of Medicine*, **18** (Suppl.), S237–S240.

49 Harris, R.C., Soderlund, K., and Hultman, E. (1992) Elevation of creatine in resting and exercised muscle of normal subjects by creatine supplementation. *Clinical Sciences*, **83**, 367–374.

50 Mujika, I., Padilla, S., Ibanez, J., *et al.* (2000) Creatine supplementation and sprint performance in soccer players. *Medicine and Science in Sports and Exercise*, **32** (2), 518–525.

51 Haas, C.H., Collins, M.A., and Juncos, J.L. (2007) Resistance training with creatine monohydrate improves upper-body strength in patients with Parkinson Disease: a randomized trial. *Neurorehabilitation and Neural Repair*, **21** (2), 107–115.

52 Baker, S.K. and Tamopolsky, M.A. (2003) Targeting cellular energy production in neurological disorders. *Expert Opinion on Investigational Drugs*, **12**, 1655–1679.

53 Klivenyi, P., Gardian, G., Calingasan, N.Y., *et al.* (2003) Additive neuroprotective effects of creatine and a cyclooxygenase 2 inhibitor against dopamine depletion in the 1-methyl-4-phenyl-1,2,3,6-tetrahydropyridine (MPTP) mouse model of Parkinson's disease. *Journal of Molecular Neuroscience*, **21** (3), 191–198.

54 Bender, A., Koch, W., Elstner, M., Schombacher, Y., Bender, J., Moeschl, M., *et al.* (2006) Creatine supplementation in Parkinson Disease: a placebo-controlled randomized pilot trial. *Neurology*, **67**, 1262–1264.

55 Haas, C.J., Collins, M.A., and Juncos, J.L. (2007) Resistance training with creatine monohydrate improves upper-body strength in patients with Parkinson Disease: a randomized trial. *Neurorehabilitation and Neural Repair*, **21** (2), 1-7-115.

56 Bender, A., Samtleben, W., Elstner, M., and Klopstock, T. (2008) Long-term creatine supplementation is safe in aged patients with Parkinson Disease. *Nutrition Research*, **28**, 172–178.

57 NINDS PET-PD Investigators (2006) A randomized, double-blind, futility clinical trial of creatine and minocycline in early Parkinson Disease. *Neurology*, **66**, 664–671.

58 Rabey, J.M., Vered, Y., Shabtai, H., *et al.* (1992) Improvement of parkinsonian features correlate with high plasma levodopa values after broad bean (*Vicia faba*) consumption. *Journal of Neurology, Neurosurgery, and Psychiatry*, **55** (8), 725–727.

59 Rabey, J.M., Vered, Y., Shabtai, H., *et al.* (1993) Broad bean (*Vicia faba*) consumption and Parkinson's disease. *Advances in Neurology*, **60**, 681–684.

60 Apaydin, H., Ertan, S., and Ozekmekci, S. (2000) Broad bean (*Vicia faba*) – a natural source of L-dopa prolongs "on" periods in patients with Parkinson's disease who have "on-off" fluctuations. *Movement Disorders*, **15** (1), 164–166.

61 Pan, T., Fei, J., Zhou, X., *et al.* (2002) Inhibitory effects of green tea polyphenol on dopamine transporter *in vitro* and *in vivo*. *Annual Meeting of the American Academy of Neurology, 16 April, 2002, Denver, Colorado.*

62 Li, R., Huang, Y.-G., Fang, D., *et al.* (2004) Epigallocatechin gallate inhibits lipopolysaccharide-induced microglial activation and protects against inflammation-mediated dopaminergic neuronal injury. *Journal of Neuroscience Research*, **78**, 723–731.

63 Suganuma, M., Okabe, S., Oniyama, M., *et al.* (1998) Wide distribution of [³H] (–)-epigallocatechin gallate, a cancer-preventive tea polyphenol, in mouse tissue. *Carcinogenesis*, **19**, 1771–1776.

64 Manal, M., Mohsen, A.E., Kuhnle, G., *et al.* (2002) Uptake and metabolism of epicatechin and its access to the brain after oral ingestion. *Free Radical Biology and Medicine*, **33**, 1693–1702.

65 Ross, G.W., Abbott, R.D., Petrovitch, H., *et al.* (2000) Association of coffee and caffeine intake with the risk of Parkinson Disease. *Journal of the American Medical Association*, **283**, 2674–2679.

66 Tan, L.C., Koh, W.P., Yuan, J.M., *et al.* (2008) Differential effects of black versus green tea on risk of Parkinson's Disease in the Singapore Chinese Health Study. *American Journal of Epidemiology*, **167**, 553–560.

67 Preux, P.M., Condet, A., Anglade, C., *et al.* (2000) Parkinson's disease and environmental factors. Matched case-control study in the Limousin region, France. *Neuroepidemiology*, **19** (6), 333–337.

68 Checkoway, H., Powers, K., Smith-Weller, T., *et al.* (2002) Parkinson's disease risks associated with cigarette smoking, alcohol consumption, and caffeine intake. *American Journal of Epidemiology*, **155** (8), 732–738.

69 Morano, A., Jimenez, F.J., Molina, J.A., *et al.* (1994) Rick factors for Parkinson's disease: case-control study in the province of Caceres, Spain. *Acta Neurologica Scandinavica*, **89** (3), 164–170.

70 Antolin, I., Mayo, J.C., Sainz, R.M., *et al.* (2002) Protective effect of melatonin in a chronic experimental model of Parkinson's disease. *Brain Research*, **943** (2), 163–173.

71 Perry, T.L. and Young, R.S. (1986) Idiopathic Parkinson's disease, progressive supranuclear palsy and glutathione metabolism in the substantia nigra of patients. *Neuroscience Letters*, **67**, 269–274.

72 Saggu, H., Cooksey, J., Dexter, D., *et al.* (1989) A selective increase in particulate superoxide dismutase activity in Parkinsonian substantia nigra. *Journal of Neurochemistry*, **53**, 692–697.

73 Dexter, D.T., Wells, F.R., Lees, A.J., *et al.* (1989) Increased nigral iron content and alterations in other metal ions occurring in brain in Parkinson's disease. *Journal of Neurochemistry*, **52**, 1830–1836.

74 Bordet, R., Devos, D., Brique, S., *et al.* (2003) Study of circadian melatonin secretion pattern at different stages of Parkinson's disease. *Clinical Neuropharmacology*, **26** (2), 65–72.

75 Miller, E.R., Pastor-Barriuso, R., Dalal, D., *et al.* (2004) Meta-analysis: high-dosage vitamin E supplementation may increase all-cause mortality. *Annals of Internal Medicine*, **142**, 1–11.

76 Etminan, M., Gill, S.S., and Samii, A. (2005) Intake of vitamin E, vitamin C, and carotenoids and the risk of Parkinson's disease: a meta-analysis. *Lancet Neurology*, **4**, 362–365.

77 Zhang, S.M., Hernan, M.A., Chen, H., *et al.* (2002) Intakes of vitamins E and C, carotenoids, vitamin supplements, and PD risk. *Neurology*, **59**, 1161–1169.

78 The Parkinson Study Group (1993) Effects of tocopherol and deprenyl on the progression of disability in early Parkinson's disease. *New England Journal of Medicine*, **328**, 176–173.

79 Olanow, C.W. (2003) Dietary vitamin E and Parkinson's disease: something to chew on. *Lancet Neurology*, **2**, 74.

80 Weber, C.A. and Ernst, M.E. (2006) Antioxidants, supplements, and Parkinson's disease. *Annals of Pharmacotherapy*, **40**, 935–938.

A Patient's Story

Living with Parkinson's

Alison Wood

I was at home, reacting to an air quality problem in our school, when I first noticed the shaking in my left hand. I was 46 years old. Three years later in, 2003, I was diagnosed with Parkinson's. There was no history of the disease in my family, and the news was devastating.

Everything I had planned for my retirement – needlepoint, crocheting, photography, making jig-saw puzzles, traveling, handbell ringing, conducting, giving workshops, playing piano, and painting – would all be affected by the tremors in my hands.

In addition to problems with mobility, I read that Parkinson's sufferers can have trouble with speaking, smiling, writing and other forms of communication, which scared me. Communication has always been vital to my careers as a teacher and handbell conductor, but more importantly in my relationships with friends and family – all the things that I feel make life worth living.

Despite my diagnosis, I've chosen to do everything I can for as long as I can and fill my time with the things I love to do.

I went back to teaching, but only part-time, so I could deal with the increased fatigue, concentrate on getting the exercise, and deal with sleep problems.

I have always directed several handbell choirs at school and church, and accepted the job of Executive Director of the International Handbell Committee. I also sing in the Richard Eaton Singers, an auditioned choir of about 150 people, best known for singing with the Edmonton Symphony. Singing has always been important to me, and I began taking lessons after reading about some the studies of Professor Dr Harold Wiens, a music professor who is studying the benefits of singing in Parkinson's patients. Many people are astounded to find that my voice is presently much stronger than it was prior to Parkinson's disease.

Although I tried physiotherapists and chiropractors for help with the posture issues that have always been problematic and are exacerbated by Parkinson's, it is the Alexander Technique lessons that have been extremely helpful with this. I can now stand straighter than I have been able to do since my teens, have learned to walk with a normal gait, can get out of low cars, and have made steady improvement with other symptoms such as tremors as well. I hope to take "Yoga Breath" lessons in the future, so that I will have some strategies when breathing, becomes something I have to remember to do.

I find acupuncture treatments helpful, and want to resume Tai Chi and exercise programs that made such a difference in previous years. A few summers ago I brought out my needlepoint and crochet hooks for the first time in years, and am enjoying the challenge of overcoming the tremors to complete the project.

I do still have some fears about the future and what it will mean for my mobility and especially my independence, but I'm happy knowing that right now I'm doing the things I love, and I will have many great memories to cherish.

7
Can the Art of Medicine use Arts as Medicine?
A Personal Perspective

Joyce Pinckney

> "'Yes', he said thoughtfully, 'I do enjoy working with people who have
> Parkinson Disease. They are busy, productive, often talented–they are the
> movers and shakers!' I shot him a glance. Was he joking? But, no. He was
> serious, seemingly unaware of the aptness of his words."
>
> (Excerpt from a conversation I was having with Harold Wiens in 2004)

He may have been on to something. A number of prominent public figures are
known to have had Parkinson disease (PD), and yet have dealt effectively
with demanding jobs. After learning that I could be part of this group, I began
to research the disease, the lives of those who had it, and their hopes and expectations for the future. Many of these people are truly extraordinary people who are
rising above their disability, often exhibiting artistic, athletic, intellectual and
managerial skills. *Surviving Adversity* [1] is a good source of inspiration and encouragement filled with the kind of personalities we would all like to be. Uniformly,
they agree that a proactive attitude helps them deal with the disease more
effectively.

The following is a commentary reflecting my experiences as a person with PD.
It also provides a summary of results reported by some scientific reports; however,
it is not a systematic review of the scientific literature published on the topic.

Parkinson disease is not immediately life-threatening, though it is chronic,
progressive, and relentless. It mostly reduces the enjoyment of life. As there is no
doubt that the severity of symptoms is increased by stress and negative feelings,
a warm and encouraging approach by the healthcare professionals and therapists
is probably as important a positive factor as the activity itself.

Pleasure-producing activities allow people with PD to experience moments of
wellness and an alleviation of restraints. I have participated in, and benefited from,
the following adjunctive therapies:

- one on one physical therapy in a pool, involving strengthening and toning
  muscles
- speech therapy in group lessons
- massage therapy

Parkinson Disease – A Health Policy Perspective. Edited by Wayne Martin, Oksana Suchowersky,
Katharina Kovacs Burns, and Egon Jonsson
Copyright © 2010 WILEY-VCH Verlag GmbH & Co. KGaA, Weinheim
ISBN: 978-3-527-32779-9

- arts-related activities, such as playing and listening to music, teaching belly-dancing, taking singing lessons and performing in a chorus
- writing poetry, short stories, songs and music
- breathing exercises in private and group settings.

The activities that have made me feel the best are related to the arts.

7.1
Music Therapy–Let's Listen, Let's Play

Music is good medicine, as it stimulates the mind, spirit and the physical body. Music is not dangerous – it may be obtained easily from places as diverse as the airwaves and libraries and, more importantly, it is *free*. It begins to work immediately and has no adverse side effects. Participation in making music ourselves is even more effective than listening to the most expensive performance. Music touches the soul and enriches life.

We know that music affects us emotionally and physically. It can make us sway, tap our feet, clap our hands, cry, or rejoice. It can wake us up or put us to sleep, incite us to action, or help us to relax. Relaxation is a benefit to a person with PD who is experiencing too many tremors (part of the disease) or dyskinesias (writhing movements, the side effects of medications). Music calms me down and clears the clouds from my mind.

David Frey, a reporter for Associated Press, wrote an article [2] about a young woman who was coming regularly to a neonatal unit at a hospital. She would play her harp and sing lullabies. In a busy stressful intensive care unit with 150 premature babies, not only were the babies soothed and comforted, but parents and the staff members were also relaxed. The nurses stated that music was an antidote to the stress of caring for the babies and also masked any frightening mechanical sounds. In fact, the gentle melodies calmed everyone.

The results of a Japanese study conducted in 12-week-old rats with high blood pressure [3] showed that music could indeed lower blood pressure. (Can you picture the rats sitting around their speaker in a closed cage, listening to Mozart's Adagio from Divertimento No. 7 in D Major, K. 205, played repeatedly for 2 hours?) A comparison with a non-music control group showed that "music-loving" rats' blood pressures fell dramatically. The title of this study – *Music improves dopaminergic neurotransmission: demonstration based on the effect of music on blood pressure regulation* – may perhaps be confusing and distract us from the practical approach. Better to say that music improves the action of dopamine and lowers blood pressure. The research group that carried out the study admitted that it was unclear exactly how the brain function was changed. Listening to music raised calcium levels in the listener, which increased dopamine (of interest to people with Parkinson) and lowered the high blood pressure.

Losing track of our focus may be what we are doing by demanding more and more research, instead of simply using music with people who have PD. We know that music makes a difference in our own lives, so why do we hesitate to use it freely for people whose quality of life is jeopardized? Why not prescribe "participation in the arts" in addition to medications?

I got the idea that music might help alleviate the suffering and slow the progression of PD, perhaps because I had used the piano for comfort as a youngster, then later to work out my teenage angst or to ease my sorrows. When I finally received the diagnosis that I had PD and began to research the condition, it was no surprise to find my idea supported by studies performed worldwide. Now, being afflicted with PD, and having been an active teacher and performer of the Middle Eastern belly-dancing art, I often play dancing music when I am overly stiff and in pain – and suddenly I am moving with grace and ease.

Another source of information is the writing of Oliver Sacks whose book, *The Man Who Mistook his Wife for a Hat and Other Clinical Tales* [4], describes rare neurological conditions presented by his patients. I watched the movie *Awakenings* [5], which depicts Oliver Sacks' experience as the physician who conducted the first trials of L-dopa. The drug was used to awaken a group of people who had been victims of the 1920 influenza epidemic. They appeared to be paralyzed and did not speak or respond to questions, but were not really unconscious. It was more as if their minds were asleep in bodies that were awake but unable to move. When the new L-dopa was given to these people they became able to walk, talk, dance, play a musical instrument – in short, they were able to live again. Unfortunately, however, some serious side effects prevented the use of the drug until further testing was completed. Nonetheless, the drug had disclosed that these patients had been locked by Parkinsonian rigidity in their own bodies, as surely as David had been locked inside the uncarved piece of marble waiting for the genius of Michelangelo to release him.

Since then, Dr Sacks has written many books and articles about the strange and fascinating conditions of the human mind. Oliver Sacks' commentary "The Power of Music," in *Brain Magazine* [6] is both captivating and convincing. His books are case studies of his own experiences with patients; moreover, his writings not only contain compassion and hope but are also easy to read and appeal to the general public. Having them as a required reading for all medically oriented people might indeed revolutionize the practice of medicine [7].

7.2
Gait – Let's Make Tracks

Concetta Tomaino [8] maintains that certain types of music therapy stimulate the production of dopamine and serotonin, both of which are needed by PD patients, and has shown that the music choice makes a difference as to how well such stimulation occurs. The music chosen must appeal to the person and create an urge to move. De Bruin [9], from Lethbridge, Alberta, agrees that in order for music to improve the walking gait it should be familiar and appealing to the walker, and should be adjusted for their stride. The music therapist and patient can work together to find the best combination of rhythm and melody. This study also touches on the use of rhythm to help with walking, balance, and movement.

I know that music helps me; it is such a large part of my life, and I believe it has the power to slow down and control the progress of my PD. I also know that dancing or moving in time to music from the outside, or music from the inside (mind and memory) is used by many people with PD to help them move more naturally. One way of combating the freezing effect is to sing or encourage the patient to sing, to count consecutive numbers, or to provide a rhythmic beat.

In 1996, a gait training program for PD showed that people who trained with audio tapes with metronome pulse patterns and rhythmically accented instrumental music improved their gait, speed, stride length, and step cadence [10]. A diversity of studies[11–13] has shown that walking while listening to rhythmic drumbeats, as regular as a metronome (with or without music) can improve the stride, speed, and walking form (gait) of people with PD. This does not seem strange to me – it would be stranger if people were listening to one drummer and walking to another. De Bruin [9] suggested that such rhythms would significantly improve movement in patients, but the carry-over effect would depend on motivating the patients to continue practicing at home alone. That the improvement may not be sustained over time is not a surprise to me if the patients do not continue to practice the exercise when they have completed the course.

A study conducted in 1997 showed that the use of metronomes significantly reduced the number of steps, the time that the walking took, and also diminished the number of freezing episodes. Marching music was less effective, while tapping in time on the patient's shoulder made the symptoms worse [14]. Nowadays, digital metronomes are small, compact, inexpensive and easy to find in music stores. Perhaps every person with PD should have one handy.

Rhythmic counting may be helpful to some people, and I often find myself counting in my mind as I walk. I seem to have started at random, beginning with any number, usually in the two-digit range, and then reciting the numbers, apparently counting my steps. I have no memory of any thought starting this, or any reason for doing it, but once having noticed it I continue to march happily along, counting as I go.

Group activities such as music making, singing, dancing are inviting, and viewed as *fun* not *work* and as *art*, not *exercise*. This may be why dancing is so successful as an exercise, since it addresses being with people, the lure of music, the beat of beckoning drums, and maybe even elements of romance.

7.3
Voice – Let's Make a Joyful Noise

The aim for the management of PD is to obtain symptom control and remove the disabling effects. In 1998, a quality of life study [15] found that active therapy, such as improvising on an instrument or the use of voice, or playing rhythm instruments was more effective than passive therapy (listening to the music).

In 2004, I participated in a study group at the University of Alberta [16] which included five participants – three women and two men in varying stages of PD. We met three days per week for 1 hour of individual attention, and one day per week for 1 hour of communal time. We had vocal lessons which included breathing exercises, warm-up physical exercises of stretches and bending, and instruction in vocal sound production.

When the research group videotaped part of each lesson to chart the students' progress, the changes were quite obvious to see and hear. Each week, they measured our voice quality and strength using audio equipment (these data are available) [16].

It was a very positive experience – the leaders were unfailingly encouraging, and created an environment of laughter, approval, communication and cooperation. The social interaction was an added benefit, and the group bonded into a supportive family. The change over several weeks was obvious to us and to others. At the first meeting, one person in particular wore the "mask" of PD – a poker face – while his voice was scarcely audible and had no variation in pitch. But as we continued our meetings he regained volume and quality in his speaking, and his smile developed in front of our eyes. The singing and breathing exercises also reactivated his ability to communicate.

My voice gained power and clarity, and I learned to take a deep breath before beginning a sentence, so that I didn't trail off at the end and lose the punch line, or the final word. Prior to voice training, I had begun to choke and cough while eating, with the coughing often being quite intense, but as the voice training progressed I had fewer coughing spells. My friends and family also said that I was speaking louder, and was easier to hear. I noted that requests to repeat my comments were rarely necessary.

As well as learning new techniques to facilitate actual voice production, during the study [16] we were admonished to look at our listener, get closer if we weren't being heard, to take a deep breath, plan what we were trying to say and, if the words were jumbling up, to separate and say them carefully. We became very aware of *how* we were speaking; one husband requested that his wife finish her sentences in the same room that she started them! I observed that, ironically, every person with PD seemed to be married to someone who was going deaf!

One therapist remembered a patient who had come to her for speech therapy, and mentioned in passing that her dog had become deaf. However, as the therapy continued she was delighted to report that the dog's hearing seemed to have improved remarkably – in fact, he had completely recovered!

One fellow told us at the start of the study [16] that he was no longer able to sing, but once he had started the lessons he regained confidence and even performed a solo at the Christmas party, accompanying himself on the guitar. We were so pleased with the course that, by mutual consent, we extended the study a little longer in order to say our farewells with Seasons Greetings. At least three of us continued with the singing lessons or joined choirs to keep the joy of music in our lives.

Except for the videotapes, the hard data collected did not dramatically demonstrate the great improvement that we, as participants, knew we had experienced. In the article written by Harold Wiens [16], he concentrated on the qualitative but not the quantitative results. When we consider the perceived improvement in our quality of life, the subjective opinions of the participants would justify the use of vocal training as a viable treatment.

A study similar to that completed by Harold Wiens [15] was conducted by Haneishi [17, 18] at the University of Kansas, in which the articles described in detail the way in which the measurements of vocal production were obtained.

Although very few studies have concentrated on singing lessons, the *Lee Silverman Voice Technique* (speech pathology) with similarities to voice lessons, has been used in the treatment of PD.

Merrill (Tanner) Semple, a singer and speech-language pathologist in Edmonton, collaborated with Wiens in 2003, on a project, for which Harold Wiens stated [16]:

> "Our objective at that time was to examine specifically the effects of voice lessons on the speech intelligibility of individuals with Parkinson's ..." and "As we completed our study, we found that voice training did indeed have an effect on speech, but what surprised us was the feedback we received from participants, who indicated that their swallowing abilities and coughing reflexes had also strengthened during training sessions. These unexpected results encouraged us to broaden our focus, to expand the exercise regime we were using, and to see if voice training would also influence other symptoms of Parkinson's disease."

7.4
Art – Let's Create a Masterpiece

Although PD is generally associated with loss of function, some patients have experienced an unexpected gain, suddenly acquired a new artistic talent. In fact, many people afflicted with PD develop an expertise or interest in art forms such as poetry, painting, writing, music, sculpture, or photography.

It is indeed surprising how many people find their lives moving in a new direction – often artistic – as they begin to be affected by PD, and this was a common thread found in many stories [18], the proposal having been made in some studies that the resultant brain damage may spark the development of an artistic creativity. It might be that the medications used to treat PD may have side effects of augmenting creativity and productivity, or it could be that these traits surface to make up for the loss of other skills such as speed, dexterity, or fine motor skills. In other words, the body finds new opportunities for growth – when one avenue is closed, a new one opens up.

One such case involved a man who had been diagnosed with PD at the age of 40 years, and who started treatment with a dopamine agonist and levodopa at the age of 44 [19]. Although, subsequently, his symptoms improved and he had no side effects, except for an increase in libido, he had difficulty in adjusting his medication so as to obtain a balance between the dyskinesias and the symptoms. Within the first month of starting treatment he began writing poetry for the first time in his life, and went on to write ten poems within the first year. He continued writing with success, winning a prize in the annual contest of the International Association of Poets and publishing several poems in newspapers and magazines [19].

In 2005, I visited Seymour's Art Gallery in Deep Cove, British Columbia, which was hosting an event to showcase the various talents of Canadian people with PD. Although most of the artists lived in British Columbia, there were some from other provinces. I was astonished at the variety of media used, the excellent quality of the art, and the wide range of subject matter I saw, with self-portraits graphically depicting the ravages that PD had imposed on these artists. These photographs and sculptures had allowed us to see the world through their eyes.

Chatterjee [20] described a 68-year-old, right-handed graphic designer with PD who was alert, oriented, and without evidence of dementia. Although e spoke and understood well, he had a masked face, and a resting tremor in the right arm and left leg. His movements were slow, bilaterally and he had cogwheel rigidity, and his writing was small and tremulous. During the treatment of his depression he had begun to paint and draw—the lines of his paintings were regular and smooth, and he said that he felt completely in control when painting, even though he was frustratingly restricted in his everyday activities. His works were large, maybe 60 cm by 90 cm, full of color, and gradually became more abstract; he also began to use color pencil, which allowed more detail. He described himself as being "obsessed with art," with a "... sense of bursting forth and tearing back walls." He had an urgent need to create before "the time runs out" and had produced hundreds of paintings.

A female physician and artist with PD thinks her paintings were enhanced since her diagnosis [21]. She said her paintings were "... less precise but more vibrant and I have a need to express myself more. I let myself go sometimes painting with enraged fingers."

Available case studies and anecdotal reports have shown that PD did not adversely affect the artistic expression of established artists. One male patient who had always sketched occasionally began to produce vast quantities of art after receiving a dopamine agonist [22]. He developed inappropriate sexual behavior, with his art changing in subject matter to concentrate on the female form. He believed that the medication had positively affected his creativity and was unwilling to make any change, although the artistic critiques of his paintings were varied.

7.5
Dance – Let's Groove

Mark Morris Dance group [23], a modern dance company, in collaboration with the Brooklyn Parkinson's group, have developed dance classes for people with PD. They teach the classes in a large dance studio with live piano accompaniment, and in five years the group has grown from fewer than nine participants once monthly, to weekly classes of 20 to 30 people. Professional dancers teach the classes in traditional ballet format adapted for people who use a walker, cane, or wheelchair, people with tremors, freezing, retropulsion (being propelled backward), and people with difficulty getting out of a chair or walking backwards.

In response to the question, "why dance?"; dancing incorporates movement, rhythm, grace, self-knowledge, ego building, social interaction, and cooperation. It provides elements of physiotherapy, but it is more fun. Although it provides music therapy, and you think it is just music to dance to, it also teaches a much more intimate knowledge of how your body works and moves [23].

Interestingly enough, therapists are beginning to believe that dancing the "tango" is specifically appropriate for benefiting people with PD [24]. The act of turning (which is a very important part of the tango) is particularly difficult for patients with PD to accomplish without falling. This is because turning triggers something in the brain that makes people with PD freeze in the middle of the movement – they say they feel as if their feet are "glued to the floor." But, with the tango they have to practice turning in many different directions. The dance is impassioned, impressive and – one would think – impossible, but those people with PD who have tried it are convinced that, in particular, the Argentine Tango is terrific – it is better than walking to help with their balance.

The *Edmonton Journal* reprinted an article by Cynthia Billhartz Gregorian of the McClatchy News Service in St Louis, entitled "The tango may help prevent falls in Parkinson's patients"; here is an excerpt:

> "A retired engineer and his wife have been dancing the tango in their kitchen for more than a year. Dance has always been a part of their life, since they met at a dance studio. When he was at University he signed his whole fraternity up for dance classes, in response to complaints from the local ladies about their lack of skill, 'cutting a rug.' When Wilfried developed Parkinson's his loss of balance and frequent falls discouraged and interfered with their dancing. He saw a flyer stating that the University researchers were looking for Parkinson's patients to participate in a study involving the Tango. Despite his body's betrayals, Wilfried is a man with a twinkle in his eyes and a palpable joy for life. So this was right up his alley. He went home and announced in his German accent: 'We are going to do the tango.' What? The Tango? his wife asked in astonishment. 'I pictured all these moves where you lean into your partner. And I thought: 'Oh my god. Spare me''" [25]

They tell us it wasn't that bad, even though it's very precise footwork with lots of crossing over. Sometimes they get it and sometimes they don't, but who cares – they love every minute of it. The following quotation from Pamela Quinn, a professional dancer for 20 years before she was diagnosed with PD, describes how I, too, feel about my body:

> "For anyone, learning that you have a serious illness is a shock, but for a dancer having a condition that directly affects your ability to move is profoundly shattering [...]. Eventually I recognized that in addition to the medications I was taking (which are essential), the greatest resource I had was the understanding of the body that my life in dance had given me. Those of us who spend out lives working with the body are learning how to speak to the body: how to question it, coax it, finesse it, scold it, trick it if necessary – like a child for whom we have the utmost tenderness but whom we sometimes must guide. In a crisis of disease, this understanding has the potential to affect the course of our condition" [26].

I wrote the following poem in 1997, soon after I was diagnosed with Parkinson disease:

To Dance
"I used to walk on wings.
For one brief, shining moment
I was a star.
I had it all.
Romance, glamor, beauty, power, joy
I loved my body,
knew what it could do,
and it did everything I asked it to.
Swirling, twirling,
spinning without end.
Nothing made me dizzy.
I never feared to fall.
I used to walk on wings.
The gauzy veils aloft
on air and energy,
floating, teasing, framing, falling
draped about a dancing form,
creating living sculpture.
My body, an instrument:
the artist's brush, musician's horn
the potter's wheel, sculptor's file.
Through me, the music passed:
ethereal soundwaves fleeting, transient
touching briefly listener's ear,

transformed by dance
into a rainbow of color,
a palette of rhythm,
a virtual, visible painting of sound.
My body, conduit of art to earth.
A celebration of the joy of woman
the rites of femininity,
the power of sex.
A catalyst to resurrection
of an art form bridging centuries.
I used to walk on wings."

Joyce Pinckney, May 31, 1997

Inspired by the musical *Wings*, adapted by Arthur Perlman, from the play *Wings*, by Arthur Kopit.

7.6
Conclusion

If people with PD who use arts are happier or perceive themselves to be happier, if they are bringing pleasure to others by adding culture to the society, and if they are preventing their own depression and minimizing their symptoms, then what could be the harm in acting as if these therapies are successful?

In my opinion, the subjective views of the afflicted persons should hold as much weight as any objective measures of improvement. The kinds of improvement which we are seeing are difficult to measure using cups, liters, inches, feet, grams, pounds and other conventional units of measurement. We should take advantage of the wonderful response that people derive from participating in the arts. Moreover, while we are waiting to prove scientifically that this is an effective treatment, we should actively encourage the development of programs and the training of people to carry them out.

Such programs could include: singing lessons and vocal therapy with participation in choirs (I've heard of a Parkinson's singing group who call themselves the Tremble Clefs. What do you think of the "Movers and Shakers"), dance classes (people dancing with walkers, here's an opportunity for cane dancing), listening and responding to music (how about painting to music or joining a regular or percussion band), exercise groups which take into consideration people in wheelchairs or walkers (or exercise or therapy in swimming pools).

The possibilities are limited only by our hesitancy to think "outside the box."

References

1 Carley, G. (2007) *Surviving adversity – living with Parkinson's disease*. Available at: http://www.survivingadversity.com/index.html.

2 Frey, D. (2000) Harp sounds soothe newborns who are battling for survival. *Los Angeles Times*, April 29, p. A-25. Available at: http://articles.latimes.com/2000/apr/29/news/mn-24654.

3 Sutoo, D. and Akiyama, K. (2004) Music improves dopaminergic neurotransmission: demonstration based on the effect of music on blood pressure regulation. *Brain Research*, **1016** (2), 255–262.

4 Oliver, S. (1970) *The Man Who Mistook His Wife for a Hat*, Harper & Row, New York.

5 Marshall, P. (director) (1990) *Awakenings*. Columbia Pictures Corporation.

6 Sacks, O. (2006) The power of music. *Brain*, **129** (10), 2528–2532.

7 Sacks, O. (2007) *Musicophilia: Tales of Music and the Brain*, Knopf, New York.

8 Tomaino, C. (2000) Using music therapy with Parkinsonians. *Loss Grief Care*, **8** (3–4), 169–171.

9 de Bruin, N., Bonfield, S., Hu, B., Sucherowsky, O., Doan, J., and Brown, L. (2008) Walking while listening to music improves gait performance in Parkinson's disease. *Movement Disorders*, **23** (Suppl. 1), S220.

10 Thaut, M.H., McIntosh, G.C., Rice, R.R., Miller, R.A., Rathbun, J., and Brault, J.M. (1996) Rhythmic auditory stimulation in gait training for Parkinson's disease patients. *Movement Disorders*, **11** (2), 193–200.

11 Hayashi, A. (2005) Music therapy in Parkinson's disease: Improvement of parkinsonian gait and depression with rhythmic auditory stimulation. *Journal of Neurological Science*, **238**, S344.

12 Hayashi, A., Nagaoka, M., and Mizuno, Y. (2006) Music therapy in Parkinson's disease: improvement of parkinsonian gait and depression with rhythmic auditory stimulation. *Parkinsonism and Related Disorders*, **12**, S76.

13 Koss, A.M., Tramo, M.J., Flaherty, A.W., and Young, A.B. (2006) Effect of auditory stimulation with popular music on visuomotor integration and gait in Parkinson's disease. *Neurology*, **66** (5), A47.

14 Enzensberger, W., Oberlander, U., and Stecker, K. (1997) Metronome therapy in patients with Parkinson Disease. *Der Nervenarzt*, **68** (12), 972–977.

15 Pacchetti, C., Mancini, F., Aglieri, R., Fundaro, C., Martignoni, E., and Nappi, G. (2000) Active music therapy in Parkinson's disease: an integrative method for motor and emotional rehabilitation. *Psychosomatic Medicine*, **62** (3), 386–393.

16 Wiens, H., McNutt Campbell, M., and Wiens, J. (2008) Effects of voice training on speech intelligibility of individuals with Parkinson's disease. Proceedings of the Phenomenon of Singing International Symposium V; 2005: St. John's, NL: Faculty of Education, Memorial University, 2008.

17 Haneishi, E. (2001) Effects of a music therapy voice protocol on speech intelligibility, vocal acoustic measures, and mood of individuals with Parkinson's disease. *Journal of Music Therapy*, **38** (4), 273–290.

18 Haneishi, E. (2006) The effects of a music therapy voice protocol on selected perceptual and acoustic parameters of the speaking voice and psychological states of individuals with Parkinson's disease. PhD Thesis, University of Kansas.

19 Schrag, A. and Trimble, M. (2001) Poetic talent unmasked by treatment of Parkinson's disease. *Movement Disorders*, **16** (6), 1175.

20 Chatterjee, A., Hamilton, R.H., and Amorapanth, P.X. (2006) Art produced by a patient with Parkinson's disease. *Behavioural Neurology*, **17** (2), 105–108.

21 Pinker, S. (2002) Art movements. *Canadian Medical Association Journal*, **166** (2), 224.

22 Walker, R.H., Warwick, R., and Cercy, S.P. (2005) Augmentation of artistic productivity in Parkinson's disease. *Movement Disorders*, **21** (2), 285–286.

23 Westheimer, O. (2008) Why dance for Parkinson's disease. *Topics in Geriatric Rehabilitation*, **24** (2), 127–138.

24 Hackney, M.E., Kantorovich, S., Levin, R., and Earhart, G.M. (2007) Effects of tango on functional mobility in Parkinson's disease: a preliminary study. *Journal of Neurologic Physical Therapy*, **31** (4), 173–179.

25 Billhartz Gregorian, C. (2008) The tango may help prevent falls in Parkinson's patients. *Edmonton Journal*, **23**, G7.

26 Quinn, P. (2007) Struggling to move. *Dance Magazine*, **81** (12), 76.

Further Reading

1 Fox, M.J. (2002) *Lucky Man: A Memoir*, Hyperion, New York.

2 Levitin, D.J. (2006) *This Is Your Brain on Music: The Science of a Human Obsession*, Dutton, New York.

3 Green, B. and Gallwey, W.T. (1986) *The Inner Game of Music*, Doubleday, Garden City, New York.

4 Gaynor, M.L. (1999) *The Healing Power of Sound: Recovery from Life-Threatening Illness Using Sound, Voice, and Music*, Shambhala, Boston.

5 Ristad, B. (1982) *A Soprano on Her Head: Right-Side-Up Reflections on Life and Other Performances*, Real People Press, Boulder, CO.

6 Blanche, C. and Beattie, A. (2000) *The Power of Music: Harness the Creative Energy of Music to Heal the Body, Soothe the Mind, and Feed the Soul*, Lansdowne, Sydney.

7 Schnebly-Black, J. and Moore, S.F. (1999) *The Rhythm Inside: Connecting Body, Mind, and Spirit Through Music*, Sterling, New York.

8 Doidge, N. (2007) *The Brain That Changes Itself: Stories of Personal Triumph from the Frontiers of Brain Science*, Viking, New York.

9 Jourdain, R. (1997) *Music, the Brain, and Ecstasy: How Music Captures Our Imagination*. W. Morrow, New York.

A Patient's Story

Living with Parkinson's

Georg Kriegel

For most people, skiing 55 km of cross-country trail while carrying a 5.5 kg pack might seem a bit challenging, but for 66-year-old Georg Kriegel, who has had Parkinson's disease for three years, skiing the annual Birkebeiner in Edmonton is a matter of pride and tradition.

As an active individual for as long as he can remember, Georg has always loved the outdoors; cycling, running, mountain biking, downhill skiing, and even qualifying to compete in several Ironman triathlons. When his three daughters were young, Georg traded in his downhill skis for cross-country ones, and the winter activity quickly became a family affair. He joined the Edmonton Nordic ski club and has been going strong ever since, participating in as many as five cross-country events a year.

It wasn't until a few years ago, when he first mistook a slight lag in his left arm for a pinched nerve, that he began experiencing the early symptoms of Parkinson's.

> "My left ski pole started dragging in the snow–I had to think more about [my arm], it wasn't natural."

Even when walking, Georg notices his arm doesn't swing like it used to. Although he's given up running, Georg is still an avid skier. Since becoming a member of the Parkinson's Society of Alberta, he has participated in the movement disorder exercise program, and attends "maintenance" classes to keep his strength up.

The Canadian Birkebeiner is the largest Classical Cross-Country Ski Festival in North America. In 1985, fewer than 130 people took part in the very first Birkebeiner, but it has grown substantially over the years and reached a record high in 1999 with 2500 participants.

For Georg, the festival is the highlight of the ski season–even a nasty hamstring pull couldn't keep him from finishing the Birkie, so Parkinson's isn't going to stop him either.

Although the last three years have proven a bit more challenging–he's a little slower and his pole strides have been out of sync–Georg is determined to add his twentieth Birkie award to his collection.

"It's harder to keep up" he says, "... my times aren't what they used to be but as long as I finish, that's what matters. I don't have anything to prove to myself. Even if I only had one hand, I would still ski!"

8
The Costs of Parkinson Disease

Arto Ohinmaa

8.1
Introduction

Parkinson disease (PD) is a progressive chronic disease, and thus has significant impact on a patient's health status, health care utilization, and costs that are either directly or indirectly related to the condition. Although the majority of PD patients are elderly, a significant proportion of them are diagnosed before their normal retirement age [1]. Many of these patients either retire earlier or change to part time work, which causes significant losses in production. Parkinson disease is not only a physically disabling disease, but it is also connected to several mental health comorbidities such as psychiatric problems (e.g., anxiety, depression, cognitive problems, and fatigue), as well as musculoskeletal and pulmonary problems [2].

Economic studies that guide decision and policy making emerge basically from three areas:

- The economic burden or cost of illness studies that evaluate how much resources the different stakeholders are using for health care in different diseases.
- Economic evaluations of alternative treatments and programs; that is, comparing the costs and the benefits of different programs and choosing the alternatives that provide the best combinations of costs and outcomes (cost-effectiveness).
- Healthcare financing that deals with the questions of how much public money should be given to health care, how it should be distributed to different diseases and healthcare providers, and how much private money will be used.

In PD, all of these aspects of health economics are very important and are linked together. For example, the reorganization of homes and long-term care for severe elderly PD patients have positive and negative cost implications for different stakeholders, but it may also have substantial health implications for the PD patients and their caregivers.

The aim of this chapter is to review the international literature relating to the cost of PD by taking a societal perspective–that is, both direct and indirect costs

Parkinson Disease – A Health Policy Perspective. Edited by Wayne Martin, Oksana Suchowersky, Katharina Kovacs Burns, and Egon Jonsson
Copyright © 2010 WILEY-VCH Verlag GmbH & Co. KGaA, Weinheim
ISBN: 978-3-527-32779-9

are included, such as costs that have been paid by the public or private insurance system, patients and their family or caregivers, other sectors of the society (e.g., social services), and lost productivity of patients and caregivers. These types of study answer questions such as: How much resources are used or lost due to PD in society? The studies can be used to estimate the magnitude of the problem, as well as to estimate the economic impact of new effective and cost-effective PD treatments on the cost and outcomes in society.

8.2
Methods

8.2.1
Description of the Costs

The cost of illness studies may include both direct and indirect costs:

- *Direct costs* that are related to medical treatment may include physician visits, hospitalizations, diagnostic procedures, emergency care, drugs, and rehabilitation. Direct nonmedical costs may include transportation, social and other services, equipment, caregiving, and home health services.
- *Indirect costs* or productivity losses include lost working time due to sick leave, and long-term productivity losses due to early retirement or death.

Since the information from all direct and indirect cost components are not available in every study, the comparison of different cost of illness studies requires a close analysis of the cost components in each study.

The cost of illness studies reviewed here have been conducted in different countries, and in different years. This means that an accurate comparison of the studies would require inflating the costs in each study to the same year (e.g., 2005), and also to take into consideration the different purchasing powers of money in different countries. Many studies have either transformed the costs to $US or € values but, where possible, this chapter includes cost estimates in either of these two currencies or in Canadian $ so as to enable better comparisons. In order to compare the European studies, all costs have been discounted to €-values in the same year as was used to value the original costs. However, the study does not transfer costs to the same year (e.g., 2008), as that would have been time-consuming and the time horizon in the studies was from 1987 to 2004. Different studies in different countries have also included slightly different costs, which limits the comparability to some degree.

8.2.2
Literature Search

A comprehensive literature search was conducted in June 2008. All major data bases that indexes economic and PD related literature were included. The databases used in the search included the Cochrane Library, Medline, PubMed, CDR, Embase, Web of Science, PsycINFO, and Econlit databases. A large variation of economic terms and the term Parkinson disease (including its variants) were used to identify as many economic studies from PD as possible. The search was restricted to publications published since January 1998 until the search in June 2008. (The full search strategy is available from the author by request.)

8.2.2.1 Inclusion and Exclusion Criteria

The aim of the study was to examine the cost of illness/economic burden of PD for different stakeholders (societal perspective) in different countries. On order for a study to be included in the review, the following points were sought:

- An estimation of healthcare costs in a broad way, including direct medical costs (e.g., physician visits, hospitalizations, drug costs).
- The use of a PD population sample that represents the PD population well in the target area (e.g., survey to a sample of patients, patient claims, or registry data).
- An aggregation of the costs should be either means or medians, using some disease severity classification system [e.g., Hoen & Yahr (HY) stage], or if a random/consecutive sample of the patients was used, the mean/median in the whole PD population.
- The duration of the follow-up period should be clearly indicated to enable transformation of the costs to annual PD costs.

In addition, we were seeking the direct nonmedical costs such as transportation, social and other help, and equipment and lost productivity due to PD. Since different studies were reporting different combinations of the above-mentioned costs, the results showed the main categories separately. Finally, only those articles written in the English language were included.

Studies that were drug-related, or other clinical trials where the cost of PD was not estimated from a representative sample of PD patients and where the treatment protocol had some effects to the chosen healthcare services, were excluded. Studies that included both the pretreatment and treatment periods were assessed separately for inclusion and exclusion criteria. Studies were excluded that included only selected subgroups of the PD patients (e.g., dementia or falls and PD), while studies that included only part of the direct medical costs, such as the drug cost of PD, were excluded due to their narrow focus for this study.

8.2.3
Results

8.2.3.1 Literature Search Results

The search identified 521 abstracts that included economic and PD-related search terms. Those abstracts were first reviewed by a senior health economist (A.O.), after which studies that included economic data from the PD population were extracted to create a new database incorporating 137 studies. From this database of abstracts, a final set of 74 abstracts was selected using the above-mentioned selection criteria; these articles were then ordered for closer analysis by the same health economist.

A total of 22 studies was assessed to include detailed primary information from the cost of illness of PD; these articles are summarized in Table 8.1. In addition, five reports evaluated the economic burden of PD in different countries, providing primarily information about the magnitude of the PD cost on a country level. Twenty-five of the 27 articles were identified from the literature search, and two from the references in the reviewed article. The remainder of the articles ($n = 49$) were excluded from the detailed review as they did not provide sufficient information about the costs or patient population, they used other published studies to model total cost of PD in a country, or did not show details from the population average costs. However, a few studies from the excluded category were used to obtain information about certain special areas of the costs, such as lost productivity or drug costs of the PD patients.

8.2.3.2 Results from Global Economic Burden Studies

The first group of articles includes reports that have estimated the magnitude of PD-related costs compared to other brain-related diseases and gross domestic product (GDP) in their countries.

One of the most ambitious projects in this area is the study of "cost of disorders of the brain in Europe" [3]. Although the brain disorders' estimated burden of disease (expressed as lost Disability Adjusted Life Years; DALY) was 35% of total burden of all diseases, their cost of illness was not known. The study included 25 European Union countries and Iceland, Norway and Switzerland, and makes prevalence-based cost estimates [€ Purchasing Power Parity (PPP) 2004 values] – that is each prevalent case is multiplied by the average annual cost in the disease, age, and gender category. This provides comparable results to other healthcare expenditures in Europe [3].

The estimated European average cost of PD was €7577 per case per year (includes direct medical and nonmedical costs and productivity lost), varying between €11 138 in Germany and €2533 in Estonia. The PD case was estimated to be about as costly as schizophrenia, and about twice as expensive as depression cases, while the cost of stroke was estimated to be more than twofold higher and the cost of brain tumor patients about fivefold higher than for PD patients. The total cost of PD in Europe was €10.72 (€PPP billion), of which €4.58 billion was healthcare costs and €6.14 billion direct nonmedical costs (lost productivity not estimated). This represented 3.4% of healthcare costs and 8.5% of direct nonmedical costs for all brain disorders, and 21.5% and 30.3% of healthcare and direct nonmedical costs of neurological diseases [3]. In addition to the European cost of illness of brain diseases, the results also noted that several country-specific studies for brain diseases have been published, including PD estimates [3–6].

In 2007, the Canadian Brain and Nerve Health Coalition (CBANHC) published the details of a study for the burden of neurological diseases, disorders, and injuries in Canada. The study results showed that the total cost of the eleven

Table 8.1 Summary of cost of illness studies, their basic background variables and annual direct cost of services directed to Parkinson disease (PD) or to all conditions.

Country and year/ Reference	No. of patients	Age (mean ± SD)/ Median (years)	Mean duration of PD (years)	Data collection and costs included	Mean annual direct cost (year)	Comments
France (2006) [31]	971	–	11.5	Insurance registry data, direct medical costs	€6394 (1999 values)	Over 45-year-old PD medication patients with PD drug(s)
Germany (1998) [27]	40	60.3 ± 9.8	11.5	Survey of total costs	€11 986 (1995 values)	Drug treatment patient; equal size of HY stage groups
UK (2003) [10]	440	Median ≈ 75	≤4 41%	GP and patient surveys of total costs	€9554 (1998 values)	Random sample made to be representative for UK PD patients.
Canada (2003) [13]	15 306	Over 90% were aged >60	–	Six years' registry data; compares PD and control patients	Incremental $CAN 1691 (year missing)	Includes only physician visits and drug costs
Sweden (2002) [14]	127	30% <65	–	Medical records and survey, PD costs	€7700 (2000 values)	Random sample; PD cost survey details not shown (inclusion/ exclusion)
UK (2005) [15]	1859	Median 70–75	Median ≈ 0–4	Patient interview, total medical and social costs	£5630 (1996 values)	Randomized study (patients used PD drugs); the costs from controls on year 2
USA (2005) [32]	20016	73.6 ± 12.1	–	Claims data, control group, incremental (PD) costs	Incremental $US 10349 (2002 values)	Costs adjusted for differences in comorbidities between PD and non-PD groups

Study	N	Age	Duration	Methods	Cost	Comments
France (1999) [16]	294	68	9	Representative sample of PD patients surveyed to obtain total healthcare costs	€4710 (1996 values)	Random sample of general practitioners and all neurologists were used to get patients; includes only PD medication patients; excludes new patients (<1 year)
USA (2006) [17]	92	Median onset 70	0–10	Incremental medical cost of PD; medical records	Incremental median 1st yr $US 581; 10y $US 468 (year missing)	Includes patients from onset of PD (1987–1995) forward for 10 years (study ends 2004)
USA (2001) [18]	450 (in cost study)	72.4	–	Medical and pharmacy claims for PD cost only	$US 2161 (1995–1998 values?); 1st yr cost $US 3120	Population-based study in large healthcare plan, using patients with PD codes. Cost of all claims $US 8671.
Finland (2003) [21]	260	66.5 ± 10.6	4.3 ± 4.4	Consecutive patients in six centers, total costs collected using survey and patients records	€4900 (1998 values)	Study includes direct costs, informal care and early retirement that represent 41%, 16% and 43% of total burden of PD, respectively
United Kingdom (2007)[20]	175	70.8 ± 8.1	7.0 ± 6.4	Client Service Receipt Inventory used to survey patients total costs	£13 804 (2002/2003 values)	Includes direct costs, informal care and productivity losses; representative community sample; formal care represents 20% and informal care 80% of total costs.
USA (2006) [2]	717	78.3	–	From 1992–2000 national survey and personal healthcare data; total medical costs	Incremental cost of PD $US 7710 (2002 values)	Medicare Current Beneficiary Survey data includes healthcare and other services funded and out of pocket; over 65 years old population only

Table 8.1 *Continued*

Country and year/ Reference	No. of patients	Age (mean ± SD)/ Median (years)	Mean duration of PD (years)	Data collection and costs included	Mean annual direct cost (year)	Comments
USA (2006) [36]	735	76.2	–	1999 and 2000 Medicare beneficiaries; annual Medicare cost	$US 18 528 (PD incremental $US 7710) (2003 values)	Study compares annual Medicare costs in different functional limitation levels in PD and non-PD populations.
Italy (2002) [33]	253	–	–	Surveyed a sample from PD patients in a clinic, PD costs (not clearly stated)	€7018 (year not known)	Clinic included patients (N = 7500) from all Italy. Abstract that includes distribution of costs to different areas
USA (1997) [28]	43	73.7	–	National survey about health resource use and medical expenditure	$US 10168 (incremental $US 5648) (1987 values)	US National Medical Expenditure survey (NMES), non-institutionalized population, three matched controls for PD patients.
USA (2001) [23]	70	71.2 ± 8.4	5.5 ± 3.6	Sample of patients in North Carolina, interviewed, total costs	During 3rd yr good health group $US 6362: poor health 9591 (1997 values)	Three-year follow-up study (first year see below Whetten-Goldstein *et al.*). Third-year informal care was between $US 130–5057 and lost productivity $US 5556–11198 in good and poor health

Country (year) [ref]			Method	Cost	Notes
Germany (2005) [19]	145	67.3 ± 9.6		Patients from special clinics and GPs, patient diary used to collect PD-related costs	€4390 (informal care €17 560) (2000–2002 values)	Includes costs from different funders of the healthcare for PD in Germany, and the cost of lost productivity.
China (2006) [22]	190	67.9	6	Patient interview (Shanghai) including PD resource use and lost productivity	$US 917 (2004 values)	Consecutive series of all patients in one department. The economic burden of PD was very high (57% of mean annual income).
USA (1997) [24]	109	71.7	5.9	In-home interview, North Carolina	$US 5684 (1994 values) Informal care $US 5386, lost earnings $US 14 000	Comprehensive interview with standard questionnaires; includes societal, family and personal burden.
USA (2002) [25]	283/100 000	N/A	N/A	Cost model of direct cost of PD in USA using different databases and surveys	$US 8735 (1997 values)	Burden of PD in USA estimated to be $US 6.6 billion per year, excluding informal care and productivity loss.
Italy (2004) [34]	268	–	–	Surveyed a sample from PD patients in a clinic, PD costs (not clearly stated)	€5639 (year not known)	Clinic included patients (N = 7500) from all Italy. Includes both publicly funded and out of pocket (18.5%) expenses.

neurological conditions included in the study was about $8.8 billion, or 6.7% of the total cost of illness in Canada during 2000–2001 [35]. While these neurological conditions accounted for 2.4% of the total direct cost of illness, nine of them (including PD) accounted for 8.3% of the total indirect costs of illness in Canada during 2000–2001.

The CBANHC [35] based their PD calculations on the Parkinson Society of Canada's estimate of almost 100 000 PD cases in the country, affecting 1% of the population aged over 65 years, and 2% of the population aged 70 and above. Because of the increasing incidence by age, the number of PD cases is expected to increase in the future with the aging of the population. Based on the Public Health Agency of Canada (PHAC) calculations, the total cost of PD in 2000–2001 was $446.8 million; that is, about 5% of the total cost of the eleven neurological conditions. Of this figure, $201.9 million of the costs were direct, of which 44.2% were for hospital care, 6.6% for physician care, and 49.2% for drugs. Of the indirect costs ($244.9 million), 38.3% was associated with mortality costs, and 61.7% with morbidity costs (mainly early retirement). Based on the estimated number of PD patients in Canada, the average direct healthcare costs would be over $2000, and lost productivity over $2500 per year per case. The report also showed that the PD patients utilize more emergency, hospitalization, and complex continuing-care services than rest of the population.

8.2.3.3 PD Cost of Illness Studies

Since PD is a chronic progressive disease, healthcare utilization and costs are expected to increase with the both severity of the disease and the age of the population. In addition to the national burden of illness studies mentioned above, a further review identified 21 cost of illness-type studies that provided original cost data and were deemed to reflect the PD population's cost of illness in their country or region. In addition, several review studies were found that summarized results from other studies [7–12]. The 22 cost of illness studies found in the search, including their basic background variables and the average annual costs (linear transformation to one year if needed), are summarized in Table 8.1.

The data in Table 8.1 show that the cost of illness of PD varies between different countries, with the difference depending largely on what costs were included, and the time and place of the study. In general, the lowest cost estimates were in studies that measured incremental costs of PD; that is, estimating the additional cost of PD patients to their "healthy" comparators. Liebson et al. [17] found the incremental PD costs after onset to be $US581, while Guttman et al. [13] showed an incremental cost of $CAN 1691 for physician visits and drug treatment only. Most of the studies listed in Table 8.1 are between €5000 and €8000 or $US7000–9000. Random sample studies were all from Europe, and were in the same cost range as most of the other European studies [14–16, 26].

The higher end cost estimates were usually found in studies that were more inclusive of services (e.g., home care, special equipment), and these often included all healthcare costs (both PD and non-PD). The highest cost estimates were shown by McCrone et al. [20] (£13 804), Dodel et al. [27] (€11 986), and Rubenstein et al.

[21] ($US10 168) and all of them had some characteristics that can explain some of the cost differences. Although McCrone *et al.* [20] had relatively few patients in HY classes 4 and 5 (combined), a major proportion of the costs (80%) were estimated to come from informal care (mainly caregiver care at home) that was valued using social service costs in the United Kingdom. The study of Dodel *et al.* [27] included relatively severe PD patients due to equal numbers in each HY category, while Rubenstein *et al.* [28] reported the oldest data and thus may reflect a different structure of the services than the more recent studies.

Most of the studies that included some sort of severity scale indicated that the cost increased by the severity of the disease (Table 8.2). In order to make this type of comparison easier, Table 8.2 includes only European studies (all values converted to €) that utilized the HY scale as a severity indicator. This is one of the most frequently used indicators, and shows increasing severity usually on five-level scale [12]. Although the studies detailed in Table 8.2 show a relatively high variation in the mean total costs, they all show increasing cost pattern by severity (including Keranen *et al.* [21]). While the two studies from Germany [19, 27] showed relatively similar patterns of increasing costs by severity (considering that only one of them included non-PD costs), the two studies from the UK [10, 20] showed very different patterns by severity.

Tables 8.2 and 8.3 show the distribution of direct costs for different categories in the European and US studies, respectively, for studies where they were presented. In most European studies the drug costs were close to 20% of the direct costs, with the exception of the German studies which had much higher drug costs (30% and 45%). In the US studies, the drug costs varied between 7% [28] and 38% [23], where the first study used relatively old data when inpatient care was probably more common, and the second study acquired data from a more severe patient group where intensive drug treatment was more common. Both, inpatient and other formal care seemed to be largely substituting each other in different countries and systems. In most studies, these formed between 50% and 60% of all direct costs. Only the European studies provided any estimates for rehabilitation and physiotherapy costs; these were more than 10% of the direct health care costs. The physician and other outpatient care costs ranged from 1% in some European studies to 28% in the USA, and in general the physician-related costs in the USA were more than twofold those in Europe. However, this most likely reflects the differences in the way that physicians are compensated in the different systems (Tables 8.2 and 8.3).

Only a few studies provided cost estimates for the informal care that the patients' caregivers, friends, and family members provided. McCrone *et al.* [20], who valued informal care using social care tariffs, derived a more than ninefold higher estimate (€17 560) than Keranen *et al.* [21], and about a 3.5-fold higher estimate than in the USA [23, 24]. Transfer payments were provided only in a few studies, and these varied based on the healthcare system (Tables 8.2 and 8.3).

Lost productivity costs were between €5000 and €6000 in Europe, and between $US11 000 and $US14 000 in the USA (Tables 8.2 and 8.3). Early retirement was also studied by Martikainen *et al.* [1], who showed that only 16% of working aged

Table 8.2 Annual mean costs (€) in European Parkinson disease studies, by HY classification and in main cost categories.

Year of study/Reference	1998 [27][a]	1999 [16][b]	(2002)14][b]	2003 [21][a]	2003 [10][a]	2005 [19][b]	2007 [20][a]
Country	Germany	France	Sweden	Finland	UK	Germany	UK
Year of data/monetary value	1995/1995	1994–2005/1996	1996–2000/2000	1998–1999/1998	1998/1998	2000/2000–2002	2002–2003/2002–2003
Total mean direct cost (€)	11986[c]	4710	7700[e]	4900[d]	9554[f]	6760[g]	21953[h](4390)
HY I	3921	2720	1923	–	4736	3720	20184
HY II	6948	4596	3430	–	4886	3340	21807
HY III	11234	6422	13582	–	9857	6760	27573
HY IV	10117	10360	7088	–	16155	11860	25789
HY V	19787	10360	15216	–	29265	12220	25789
Proportion of direct costs (%)							
– Drugs	30	22	18	20	–	45	21
– Inpatient care	25	39	11	41	–	21	30
– Other formal/home care	27	11	59	21	–	6[g]	31
– Physician/outpatient	1	6	10	9	–	1	13
– Rehabilitation/physical therapy	15	17		9	–	12	5
– Other costs	2	5 (transport.)	2	–	–	15	–
Informal care				1890			17560
Indirect cost		6990	5652	5070		6360	
Transfer payment	6984					650	1380

a) Study includes PD-related costs and all or most of the other disease-related costs.
b) Study includes only PD-related costs.
c) German Mark changed to €, using 1998 exchange rate (€1 = DM 1.969; Eurostat).
d) Estimates of the HY scale values available in a figure in the article.
e) Used year 2000 exchange rates (€1 = Kr 9.255; Eurostat).
f) Used €-values directly from the publication.
g) Includes only Gesetzliche Krankenversicherung costs; in addition, Pflegeversicherung funded on average €2620 for nursing and €40 for special equipment.
h) Informal care valued using social service costs covers 80% of the total direct costs; £s changed to €s using 2002 exchange rate (€1 = £0.6288; Eurostat).
HY = Hoehn Yahr PD severity classification system.

Table 8.3 Distribution of the costs in the US Parkinson disease (PD) studies.

Study year/Reference	1997 [28]	1997 [24]	2001 [23]	2001 [18][c]	2002 [25]	2005 [32]	2006 [2][e]
Year of data/monetary value	1987/1987	1995/1994	1995–1997/1997	1995–1998/?	1994–1997/1997	1999–2002/2002	1992–2000/2002
Total mean direct cost (US$)	10168	5684[a]	9591[b]	2161 (PD) 8671 (all)	8735	10349	12586 (all costs)
Proportion of direct costs (%)							
– Drugs	7	19	38	27[c]	29	14	11
– Inpatient care	60	27	12	36[c]	17	15	25
– Other formal/home care	6	22	37	11[c]	48[d]	47	35
– Physician/outpatient	18	28	12	25[c]	5	24	23
– Rehabilitation/physical therapy	–	–	–	–	0.4	–	–
– Other costs	9	4	1	1[c]	–	–	6
Informal care (US$)	–	5386	5057	–	–	–	–
Indirect cost (US$)	–	14000	11198	–	–	–	–
Transfer payment (US$)	–	2089	–	–	–	–	–

a) Direct costs recalculated excluding compensated earnings and including family expenses.
b) Data from poor health category on third year (1997).
c) Littlefield et al. based on all health plan claims (no information from other costs).
d) Nursing home cost totals 43.7% of all costs (Wilson 22–28+32).
e) Noyes et al.[2] cost estimates represent Health Maintenance Organization (HMO) patient costs that were $4300 lower than Medicare FFS patient costs, but their distribution followed relatively closely the same pattern. Medicaid patients had much higher long-term care costs ($17 200). Leibson et al. (2006) [13] did not include details from different cost categories.

PD patients in Finland worked (12% full time, 4% part time). With regards to the 37% of patients who retired early due to PD, the median age for retirement was 53.4 years, and the median working time after diagnosis 1.7 years. In the study of Schrag and Banks [29] from the UK, the population that developed PD before the age of 65 years retired on average at age 55.8 years – that is, 4.9 years earlier than the remainder of the population. Survival analysis showed that 46% of the early-retired PD patients stopped working after 5 years of disease, and 82% after 10 years.

A study from China showed that the annual cost of PD was less than $US1000 [22], while another from India showed that in almost half of the PD patients their annual income was less than $US1450 per year, with patients using between 16% and 45% of their annual income to buy PD medications [30].

8.3
Discussion

The information provide in this chapter indicates that the cost of illness of PD is high when all direct costs, lost productivity and informal care at home was included. These costs will clearly increase by in terms of the patient age and severity of the PD. Based on the data sources studied, different annual costs of PD or total healthcare costs of PD patients became apparent. Those studies which used only claims-based data from one funding agency had somewhat lower cost estimates than did other studies in the same healthcare system. In the US, different beneficiaries have an impact on the observed healthcare costs in PD patients; in particular, HMOs and Medicare (fee-for-service) are less expensive than Medicaid [2].

One issue that influences the comparison of cost of illness studies is the inclusion and exclusion of non-PD-related costs. Studies such as those conducted by Gutman *et al.* [13], Liebson *et al.* [17], and Littlefield [18], which included only key PD-related costs or incremental costs, produced relatively low cost estimates (between $US600 and $US2260) for PD. However, other studies which provided incremental cost estimates, such as those of Noyes [2] and Rubenstein [28], derived several-fold higher cost estimates, of $US7700 and $US5600 (in year 1987 values), respectively. This can be explained mainly by the inclusion of other formal services such as long-term care, home care and other services that are not included in many medical benefits. The inclusion and exclusion of other formal care costs also explains some of the differences between the studies that included all healthcare expenditures.

From a societal perspective, the direct health and social care costs cover less than half of the total economic burden of the PD. Based on a UK and Finnish study [1], PD causes substantial early retirement and change to part time working for those individuals who develop the disease before the age of 65 years. Studies that have estimated the value of caregiving have also showed that its value may range from €2000 [21, 29] to €17 000 [20]. The magnitude of these estimates is largely dependent on the values used to calculate the monetary value of informal care. Those studies that use formal care costs for the informal care will derive substantially higher cost estimates.

It is difficult to estimate the quality of the economic studies in PD. Studies do not always provide details from where the values or the resource utilization, or even the year of the monetary values used in the study, were obtained. An even bigger problem is the inclusion and exclusion of those costs paid by the patients or by other insurance companies. In the claims-based studies, the missing or wrong diagnostic coding for PD-related costs can also substantially affect the estimated PD-related costs. Moreover, as categorization of the cost items is not standardized, this makes the comparison of the results from different studies relatively difficult. For example, physician payments and other outpatient costs are much higher in the US, whilst the rehabilitation/physiotherapy costs (which usually are about 10% or more) in the European studies are not reported in most US-based studies.

8.4
Summary and Conclusion

The economic burden of PD in western countries is substantial, and is expected to increase due to the aging of the population. Consequently, healthcare policies are required that are aimed at an early diagnosis and cost-effective treatments in order to slow the progression of the disease, and reduce the symptoms. Based on the European studies with data on HY categories (Table 8.2), a decrease of one category would mean about €3000 per patient per year (or about $CAN 4500) savings in total direct costs.

In Canada, if it were possible to slow the progression of PD so that one-quarter of the 100 000 PD patients would be one HY category milder, this would mean cost savings in the order of $CAN 112 million per year. Moreover, if the improvements in the productivity of the working-age PD population, a decreased need for caregiving, and the Health Related Quality of Life gains due to improved health status were also to be included, then the total societal savings would be substantially higher.

References

1 Martikainen, K.K., Luukkaala, T.H., and Marttila, R.J. (2006) Parkinson's disease and working capacity. *Movement Disorders*, **21** (12), 2187–2191.

2 Noyes, K., Liu, H., Li, Y., Holloway, R., and Dick, A.W. (2006) Economic burden associated with Parkinson's disease on elderly Medicare beneficiaries. *Movement Disorders*, **21** (3), 362–372.

3 Andlin-Sobocki, P., Jonsson, B., Wittchen, H.U., and Olesen, J. (2005) Cost of disorders of the brain in Europe. *European Journal of Neurology*, **12** (Suppl. 1), i–27.

4 McHugh, J.C. (2007) Cost of disorders of the brain in Ireland. *Irish Medical Journal*, **100**, 7.

5 Schoenen, J., Gianni, F., Schretlen, L., and Sobocki, P. (2006) Cost estimates of brain disorders in Belgium. *Acta Neurologica Belgica*, **106** (4), 208–214.

6 Sillanpaa, M., Andlin-Sobocki, P., and Lonnqvist, J. (2008) Costs of brain disorders in Finland. *Acta Neurologica Scandinavica*, **117** (3), 167–172.

7 Berchou, R. (2006) Economic and quality-of-life implications of Parkinson Disease and its treatment. *Formulary*, **41** (Suppl.), 39–44.

8 Dodel, R.C., Berger, K., and Oertel, W.G. (2001) Health-related quality of life and healthcare utilisation in patients with Parkinson's disease: impact of motor fluctuations and dyskinesias. *PharmacoEconomics*, **19** (10), 1013–1038.

9 Dowding, C.H., Shenton, C.L., and Salek, S.S. (2006) A review of the health-related quality of life and economic impact of Parkinson's disease. *Drugs and Aging*, **23** (9), 693–721.

10 Findley, L., Aujla, M., Bain, P.G., *et al.* (2003) Direct economic impact of Parkinson's disease: a research survey in the United Kingdom. *Movement Disorders*, **8** (10), 1939–1145.

11 Lindgren, P. (2003) Economic evidence in Parkinson's disease: A review. *European Journal of Health Economics*, **5** (Suppl. 1), S63–S66.

12 Lindgren, P., von Campenhausen, S., Spottke, E., Siebert, U., and Dodel, R. (2005) Cost of Parkinson's disease in Europe. *European Journal of Neurology*, **12** (Suppl. 1), 68–73.

13 Guttman, M., Slaughter, P.M., Theriault, M.E., *et al.* (2003) Burden of parkinsonism: a population-based study. *Movement Disorders*, **18** (3), 313–319.

14 Hagell, P., Nordling, S., Reimer, J., *et al.* (2002) Resource use and costs in a Swedish cohort of patients with Parkinson's disease. *Movement Disorders*, **17** (6), 1213–1220.

15 Hurwitz, B., *et al.* (2005) Scientific evaluation of community-based Parkinson's disease nurse specialists on patient outcomes and health care costs. *Journal of Evaluation in Clinical Practice*, **11** (2), 97–110.

16 LePen, C., Wait, S., Moutard-Martin, F., *et al.* (1999) Cost of illness and disease severity in a cohort of French patients with Parkinson's disease. *PharmacoEconomics*, **16** (1), 59–69.

17 Leibson, C.L., Long, K.H., Maraganore, D.M., *et al.* (2006) Direct medical costs associated with Parkinson's disease: a population-based study. *Movement Disorders*, **21** (11), 1864–1871.

18 Littlefield, R.S., Martin, S., and Heaton, A. (2001) Baseline cost of Parkinson Disease in a large health care plan. *Drug Benefit Trends*, **13**(12), 38–44.

19 Spottke, A.E., Reuter, M., Machat, O., *et al.* (2005) Cost of illness and its predictors for Parkinson's disease in Germany. *PharmacoEconomics*, **23** (8), 817–836.

20 McCrone, P., Allcock, L.M., and Burn, D.J. (2007) Predicting the cost of Parkinson's disease. *Movement Disorders*, **22** (6), 804–812.

21 Keranen, T., Kaakkola, S., Sotaniemi, K., *et al.* (2003) Economic burden and quality of life impairment increase with severity of PD. *Parkinsonism & Related Disorders*, **9** (3), 163–168.

22 Wang, G., Cheng, Q., Zheng, R., *et al.* (2006) Economic burden of Parkinson's disease in a developing country: a retrospective cost analysis in Shanghai, China. *Movement Disorders*, **21** (9), 1439–1443.

23 Schenkman, M., *et al.* (2001) Longitudinal evaluation of economic and physical impact of Parkinson's disease. *Parkinsonism and Related Disorders*, **8** (1), 41–50.

24 Whetten-Goldstein, K., Sloan, F., Kulas, E., *et al.* (1997) The burden of Parkinson's disease on society, family, and the individual. *Journal of the American Geriatrics Society*, **45** (7), 844–849.

25 Wilson, L., Huang, J., and Doshi, D. (2002) Health care burden, prevalence, and costs of Parkinson Disease. *Drug Benefit Trends*, **14** (5), 22–28, 32.

26 Findley, L.J. (2007) The economic impact of Parkinson's disease. *Parkinsonism and Related Disorders*, **13**(Suppl.), S8–S12.

27 Dodel, R.C., Singer, M., Kohne-Volland, R., *et al.* (1998) The economic impact of Parkinson's disease. An estimation based on a 3-month prospective analysis. *PharmacoEconomics*, **14** (3), 299–312.

28 Rubenstein, L.M., Chrischilles, E.A., and Voelker, M.D. (1997) The impact of Parkinson's disease on health status, health expenditures, and productivity. *PharmacoEconomics*, **12** (4), 486–498.

29 Schrag, A. and Banks, P. (2006) Time of loss of employment in Parkinson's disease. *Movement Disorders*, **21** (11), 1839–1843.

30 Ragothaman, M., Govindappa, S.T., Rattihalli, R., *et al.* (2006) Direct costs of managing Parkinson's disease in India: concerns in a developing country. *Movement Disorders*, **21** (10), 1755–1758.

31 Desboeuf, K., Grau, M., Riche, F., *et al.* (2006) Prevalence and costs of parkinsonian syndromes associated with orthostatic hypotension. *Thérapie*, **61** (2), 93–99.

32 Huse, D.M., Schulman, K., Orsini, L., *et al.* (2005) Burden of illness in Parkinson's disease. *Movement Disorders*, **20** (11), 1449–1454.

33 Pezzoli, G., Zecchinelli, A., Caprari, F., *et al.* (2002) Social costs of Parkinson's disease in Italy. *Movement Disorders*, **17** (Suppl. 5),130.

34 Zecchinelli, A., Caprari, F., Ponzi, P., Bonetti, A., and Pezzoli, G. (2004) Social costs of Parkinson disease in Italy. *Value in Health*, **7** (6) (Suppl.), 788.

35 Canadian Institute of Health Information. *The Burden of Neurological Disorders and Injuries in Canada*. Ottawa: CIHI, 2007.

A Daughter's Story

A Word from the Adult Daughter

Elda Pinckney

"I'm not leaving." I stand defiantly, next to my mother's hospital bed, only half-listening to the night nurse's "hospital policy" speech—the other half of my mind and heart is being torn apart by my mother's soft whispers of placation.

This is one of our few personality differences. My mom can get almost anyone to do almost anything for her, to bend rules, to overlook policies, just by being who she is. I, on the other hand, have inherited my father's tendency to move straight to the frustration stage.

> The nurse finally leaves, and I sit back down, relieved, and find another ice chip to gently place in my mother's parched mouth. She tries to talk about what's happening with the hospital, about what we're going to do. I simply say, "Mom, I am NOT leaving you. That's what's happening. End of story. They're gone, I think they got the -"

> "Miss ... ah ... Pinckney? I'm the supervisor on duty. May I speak to you in the hall?"

My mother has just finished an extremely invasive (non-Parkinson's-related) back surgery. She was in surgery for 8 hours or so, and I arrived late last night from Vancouver to stay with her in hospital. Dad's been great, but lacks the physical ability to stay up past about 9:30 pm, and so I volunteered to come and be with her overnight, for all seven to ten nights if necessary, never in a million years guessing that visiting hours would end at 11:00 pm, and include immediate family members.

The thing is, Mom's Parkinson's, although very well controlled by medication, has been exacerbated by the trauma of surgery. The nurses can't give her any more medication than they've been told to without a prescription, and so my mother is left even more unable to move than she would have been with just the surgery to contend with.

Unfortunately, my faith in this hospital has already been compromised. Apparently, nobody thought to give her even her regular doses of Parkinson's drugs while in surgery, the end result being that my father and I, as prepared as we could have been to see our invincible wife and mother rendered helpless by intense back surgery, found my mom—having not had her regular medication for hours—not only in intense pain, but completely rigid from Parkinson's.

The moment she saw us (and she could only whisper, which somehow made it all the more unbearable): "Bill, Elda—get my pills!! Please! The yellow ones! Quick!" Dad and I, barely managing to control our anger at the hospital, luckily had our own stash (which, of course, Mom had thought to tell us to pack), and gave her a dose of Sinimet, which would start working to loosen her muscles.

Needless to say, this did not inspire much confidence in the hospital staff, and now, 6 hours later, I was being told to leave her with them.

"Yes?"

"Miss Pinckney, I'm sorry, but visiting hours end at 11:00, and we simply can't allow you to stay overnight unless you're in a private room."

"Hmmm ... kind of like the private room we requested? Can we move to a private room now then?". (This is me, not making friends with the staff.)

"I'm sorry, but all of our private rooms are full right now. And visiting hours end at 11:00, so I'm afraid you'll have to leave."

"Yes, you mentioned that. So, would you like to sit next to my mother and feed her ice chips every 3 minutes until morning?"

"Miss Pinckney, obviously we don't have enough nurses to provide one for every patient. However, your mother can ring her buzzer if she needs anything and we will be there right away."

I take a deep breath, trying to be ... well, more like my mom.

"Riiiight. First of all, she needs something every 3 minutes—an ice chip. Second, she can't reach the buzzer because her Parkinson's disease is going crazy right now. Third, I pressed that goddamn button earlier tonight and it took 20 minutes for someone to get there! Oh! Hey! I have an idea! Why don't I just stay and give my mother the company and hydration she needs until tomorrow!".

"I'm sorry Miss Pinckney, but if we allowed you to stay, we would have to allow everyone else to stay too." (This is one of my all-time favorite ridiculous arguments, used by people in positions of power the world over.)

"Actually, you wouldn't. You could just allow me to stay with my mom, who can't move and who, a little while ago, when I told her to try to sleep, whispered to me that she thought, if she fell asleep, she would die."

My voice cracks. I'm losing it. I know the argument is pointless. I can't win against this kind of bureaucratic mumbo-jumbo. I also know, at this moment, that no matter what, I'm not leaving my mother alone.

"Miss Pinckney" (she's apparently dropped the "I'm sorry" at this point, which gives me a small measure of satisfaction), if you don't leave this hospital, we will have security escort you out."

This shocks my tears into submission, and I look her straight in the eye. "Really? I'd like to see you try."

I wipe my eyes, walk back into the room, and tell my mother, who has sat by my bedside countless times, not to worry. We have switched places, my mother and I, and I suddenly know, just as surely as she has for my entire life, that nothing could move me from her side.

****

Parkinson's sucks. It's a mean disease that takes away your strength, your movement, your expression, and your grace. My mother is a dancer, and her Parkinson's seems even more cruel because of this. The pills she takes, although they help immensely with regaining her movement, can't quite mimic the effect that actual dopamine has on her body, and make her move in an unnatural way.

I feel protective of her, of her self-esteem and her joy. Any of the changes that this disease imparts in her only make me more so.

It's like the hospital incident, except I can't just stand my ground and stop the Parkinson's from taking the reins. I wish I could. Like anyone who is forced to watch a loved one battle a disease—it makes us angry, but most of all, we're helpless to stop it, and that's the hardest part of all.

9

A Literature Summary on Parkinson Disease

Paula Corabian and Liz Dennett

9.1
Objective

This chapter provides a summary of the most recently published systematic reviews (SRs) and evidence-based clinical practice guidelines (CPGs) that have focused on the etiology, epidemiology, prevention, diagnosis, and/or management of Parkinson disease (PD).

This literature summary was conducted according to a predefined methodology that was formulated in consultation with the Parkinson Working Group. It does not represent a systematic review of the literature on this topic; thus, no firm conclusions are offered. In addition, the evidence was only summarized and no attempt was made to assess the veracity of the information contained within the included studies.

9.2
Methodology

9.2.1
Literature Search Strategy

The medical literature was searched to identify relevant SRs and CPGs on PD published between January 2006 and September 2008 (the full search strategy is available upon request from the authors). The date restriction was applied to ensure that the evidence collected was current and clinically relevant.

The search was conducted during September 2008, using key health information resources including PubMed/Medline, Embase, the Cochrane Library, and Center for Reviews and Dissemination (CRD) databases. The results were limited to humans and to the English language.

Although the bibliographies of articles retrieved in hard copy form were not searched systematically for relevant references that may have been missed in the

Parkinson Disease – A Health Policy Perspective. Edited by Wayne Martin, Oksana Suchowersky, Katharina Kovacs Burns, and Egon Jonsson
Copyright © 2010 WILEY-VCH Verlag GmbH & Co. KGaA, Weinheim
ISBN: 978-3-527-32779-9

database searches (pearling), any additional relevant references accidentally uncovered during the examination of these full-text articles were retrieved.

9.2.2
Study Selection

The initial and final study selection for both SRs and CPGs was conducted by one reviewer (P.C.) using selection criteria developed *a priori*. The initial study selection was based on titles and/or abstracts only. Articles were excluded that, on the basis of their abstract, clearly did not meet the inclusion criteria.

The final selection was based on full text articles. Copies of the full text of potentially relevant papers were retrieved and assessed for eligibility based on the selection criteria. In some cases, when the full text of the article was retrieved, a closer examination revealed that it did not meet the inclusion criteria specified by the protocol. Consequently, these papers were excluded (a list of the excluded papers and reasons for their exclusion is available upon request).

9.2.3
Inclusion Criteria

9.2.3.1 Types of Studies
For the purpose of this chapter, only published SRs and CPGs that were publicly available were included.

9.2.3.2 Systematic Reviews
The initial study selection considered citations of secondary research studies that mentioned in their titles/abstracts the following words: "review," "systematic review," "meta-analysis," "movement disorder," "neurodegenerative disease," "neurological disorders," "Parkinson," and/or "parkinsonism."

A SR is a critical assessment of existing evidence that addresses a focused clinical question, includes a comprehensive literature search, critically appraises the quality of studies, and reports results in a systematic manner. If the studies report comparable quantitative data and have a low degree of variation in their findings, a meta-analysis can be performed to derive a summary estimate of effect.

For the purpose of this chapter, the final selection considered only publicly available published reports of SRs that, by virtue of design and quality of reporting [1], were most likely to provide high level of evidence. Therefore, a secondary research study was deemed to be an SR if it met all of the following criteria (based on those set by Cook *et al.* [2]):

1) Focused clinical question
2) Explicit search strategy
3) Use of explicit, reproducible, and uniformly applied criteria for article selection

4) Critical appraisal of the included studies encompassing the use of a quality tool or checklist
5) Qualitative or quantitative data synthesis.

9.2.3.3 Clinical Practice Guidelines

The initial selection considered citations of articles that contained the words "guideline" or "recommendation" or "practice parameter" in its title and/or abstract or contained recommendations on preventing, diagnosing, prognosing progression of, and/or managing PD in the form of advice or instructions.

Evidence-based CPGs are recommendations for practice that are systematically developed by a multidisciplinary group of experts, and involve a comprehensive search of the literature and an evaluation of the quality of individual studies. In order for a CPG to be valid, the evidence supporting its recommendations must be cited and the recommendations graded so as to reflect the quality of the supporting evidence [3–7]. The search strategy, article/study selection, quality appraisal, and grading methods should be described explicitly, and be replicable by similarly skilled authors.

For the purpose of this chapter, the final selection considered only those publicly available published guidelines that, by virtue of design and quality of reporting [1], were most likely to provide valid recommendations (according to accepted methodology [3–8]).

Therefore, an article was deemed to be a CPG if it met all of the following criteria:

1) It was developed by a multidisciplinary team/group of experts using a transparent process that included a systematic review of the available literature and grading/rating of both the quality of the supporting evidence and the strength of the recommendation.
2) It provided details of the objectives, clinical question(s), and target population in the abstract, introduction, or methods section of the published guideline.
3) It clearly described the search strategy, the criteria for selecting the evidence, the study quality appraisal process, the grading/rating methods and the methods used for formulating the recommendations.
4) It provided an explicit link between the recommendations and the supporting evidence.

Any CPGs that were not evidence-based, such as consensus statements that contained recommendations based only on expert opinion without reference to any supporting evidence, were excluded.

Only CPGs formulated in countries with developed market economies were included, since the health status, cultural norms, access to healthcare, and the disease burden of individuals from countries with transitional or developing economies were likely to be too different from that of Canada so as to be clinically relevant. Countries deemed to have developed economies, as defined by the United Nations, were as follows: Australia, Canada, Japan, New Zealand, the United States of America, and Europe (except for Albania, Bulgaria, Czech Republic, Hungary, Poland, Romania, Slovakia, Bosnia and Herzegovina, Croatia, Slovenia, the former Yugoslav Republic of Macedonia, Yugoslavia, Estonia, Latvia, Lithuania, Belarus, the Republic of Moldova, the Russian Federation, and Ukraine) [9].

9.2.3.4 Target Population

Data were collected on adult patients (aged ≥18 years of age) with PD of any duration or stage.

The SRs were included if they reported results on etiology, epidemiology, pathology, screening, diagnosis, treatment, rehabilitation, prevention, prognosis of progression, management, and/or quality of life in PD.

Guidelines were included if they provided definitive recommendations for PD. Those that referred to parkinsonism, or (neuro)degenerative disorders, or movement disorders, or neurological disorders, or mental health disorders/ other comorbidities in and complications of PD but which provided specific recommendations for PD, were also included.

9.2.4
Study Methodology Appraisal

The included SRs/CPGs were not assessed with respect to any aspects of methodology and reporting using checklists specific for each particular study type.

9.2.5
Data Extraction

One reviewer (P.C.) extracted relevant data from the selected SRs/practice guidelines using standardized data extraction forms developed *a priori*.

9.3
Literature Search Findings

The literature search yielded 503 potentially relevant literature citations, following a review of which full text articles were retrieved for 166 reports of secondary research studies/guidelines. A closer examination of the retrieved full text articles revealed that 137 did not meet the selection criteria developed for this literature summary. Consequently, these were excluded either because they were available only in abstract format, *or* they did not meet all criteria for a SR/CPG, and they did not include PD cases or PD as a disorder, *and/or* they included PD among other (neuro)degenerative or neurological or movement disorders but did not report or provide separate results/recommendations for PD (a list of the excluded papers and reasons for their exclusion is available upon request).

9.4
Literature Summary

A closer examination of the 166 retrieved full text articles revealed that only 29 met the inclusion criteria developed for this review; these include 18 SRs [10–27] and 11 practice guidelines [1, 28–37].

For the purpose of this chapter, the main characteristics, findings, and conclusions from the published reports of the 18 selected SRs were summarized in tabular form (see Table 9.1). The methodological quality of these studies was not critically appraised, and no attempt was made to assess the validity of their findings.

Relevant data were also extracted from the selected practice guidelines; these are summarized in Table 9.2.

9.4.1
Available Systematic Reviews

Among the 18 selected SRs, one was focused on early features of PD [17], one on prognostic factors for progression of PD [26], 11 were focused on the therapy of early and late PD [10, 11, 16, 18–20, 23–25, 27, 38], four on comorbidities in and nonmotor complications of PD [12, 14, 22, 39], and one was focused on the quality of life in PD [13].

The following provides a brief summary of the key results from the 18 selected SRs on PD. More detailed information on each SR can be found in Table 9.1.

9.5
Early Features of PD

Ishihara and Brayne [17] reviewed the evidence for a relationship between PD and depression and other mental disorders. Although there were no prospective studies, a number of retrospective studies all indicated that a history of depression, mania and anxiety are associated with an increased risk of PD. More studies are needed to understand the cause and timing of this relationship.

9.5.1
Prognosis

In the area of prognosis, Post *et al.* [26] attempted to identify factors that predict changes in motor impairment, disability and in quality of life in PD, by reviewing studies that describe the course of the PD. Motor impairment may be negatively affected by lower baseline Unified Parkinson Disease Rating Scale Motor Examination (UPDRS-ME) scores, the presence of dementia, and a Schwab and England Disability Scale of less than 70%. There was also strong evidence that a higher age of onset and a higher Postural Instability and Gait Difference are prognostic

Table 9.1 Summary of relevant data extracted from selected systematic reviews.

Study	Objectives	Main findings[a] and conclusions[b]
Early features of PD		
Ishihara, L. and Brayne, C. [17] A systematic review of depression and mental illness preceding Parkinson's disease. *Acta Neurologica Scandinavica* 2006; **113** (4): 211–220.	To examine the association between PD and depression or other mental disorder (reviewed published literature relevant to the question "Do depression or other mental disorders precede the onset of PD?", and therefore indicate the possibility of a shared causal pathway	Main findings[a]: This SR included 10 CC studies, one NCC study and three cohort studies (of which one was prospective). Overall, evidence from five CC studies, one NCC study, and two cohort studies indicated that a history of depression is associated with an increased risk of PD. Anxiety and mania were positively associated with PD in retrospective cohort studies and only one examined anxiety levels. Conclusions[b]: This systematic review provides consistency in the finding that a diagnosis of depression is more common in PD patients before the onset of PD. However, no prospective studies examined depression. The reported findings suggest several possibilities for the relationship between PD and depression, anxiety, or other mental disorders. One hypothesis is that PD and mental disorders are caused by a general depletion of neurotransmitters; therefore, the time of disease onset would be relatively close. Another hypothesis could be that premorbid mental disorders are involved with underlying neurological changes that cause a higher susceptibility of the brain to PD. In this case, mental disorders might be apparent long before PD symptoms appear. Any conclusions made with respect to supporting the possible hypothesis depend on the selected time period of exposure. There is also the issue of what should be considered a sufficient lag time, as PD has an insidious onset and the length of the presymptomatic period is unknown. These issues should be addressed in future studies.
Prognosis		
Post, B., *et al.* [26] Prognostic factors for the progression of Parkinson's disease: a systematic review. *Movement Disorders* 2007; **22** (13): 1839–1851.	To summarize studies that describe the course of PD and to identify factors that predict change in motor impairment, disability, and QOL.	Main findings[a]: This SR included 27 cohort studies, of which 11 were considered to be of high methodological quality. Of these 11 studies, six described impairment, eight disability, and two QoL (more than one outcome measure possible in each study).

Table 9.1 *Continued*

Study	Objectives	Main findings[a] and conclusions[b]
		Limited evidence is found for lower UPDRS-ME at baseline, dementia and SE <70% as prognostic factors for future motor impairment. There is strong evidence for a higher age at onset and a higher PIGD-score; and limited evidence for higher bradykinesia-score, non-tremor-dominant subtype, symmetrical disease at baseline, and depression as prognostic factors for progression of disability. No evidence was found for predictors for future QoL in PD. Prognostic factors were identified for impairment and disability. Conclusions[b]: The literature on the prognosis in PD is not fulfilling the high methodological standards applied nowadays. There is a need for prospective cohorts of PD patients assembled at a common early point in the disease with long-term follow-up.

Therapy

Study	Objectives	Main findings[a] and conclusions[b]
Baker, W.L., *et al.* [10] Dopamine agonists in the treatment of early Parkinson's disease: A meta-analysis. *Parkinsonism and Related Disorders* 2008; **14** (4),287–294.	To perform a MA of RCTs of dopamine agonists (DA) as monotherapy, as well as adjunctive therapy for the early treatment of PD	Main findings[a]: This SR included 25 RCTs (total 5185 patients): 14 evaluated ergot DA (total 2656 patients) and 11 evaluated non-ergot DA (total 2529 patients). DA versus placebo (10 RCTs, 1781 patients): DA monotherapy showed superior efficacy but more frequent adverse events compared to placebo; in six RCTs, there was greater reduction in UPDRS ADL scores with DA than with placebo (WMD −1.64, 95% CI −2.65 to −0.62; P = 0016). In all 10 RCTs, there was greater reduction in UPDRS motor scores with DA than with placebo (WMD: 5.32, 95% CI −6.89 to −3.75; P<0.0001); in nine RCTs, DA was associated with significantly higher odds of withdrawal due to adverse events than placebo (OR = 2.49, 95% CI 1.69–3.65; P<0.0001) In four RCTs, DA was associated with nonsignificantly higher odds of dyskinesia than placebo (OR 2.20, 95% CI 0.78–6.14; P = 0.13) DA versus levodopa (10 RCTs, 2904 patients): DA demonstrated inferior efficacy to levodopa, but was associated with fewer motor complications. In RCTs assessing UPDRS ADL scores, DA had a significantly inferior response compared to levodopa (P < 0.0001). In six RCTs, patients receiving DA were significantly less likely to experience wearing-off than those receiving levodopa (OR 0.52, 95% CI 0.40–066; P < 0.0001). In nine RCTs, DA was associated with significantly higher odds of withdrawal due to adverse events than levodopa (OR = 2.46, 95% CI 1.44–4.20; P < 0.001). In four RCTs, DA was associated with significantly lower odds of dyskinesia than levodopa (OR 0.36, 95% CI 0.22–0.60; P < 0.0001).

Table 9.1 *Continued*

Study	Objectives	Main findings[a] and conclusions[b]
		<u>DA plus levodopa versus levodopa alone (six RCTs, 1202 patients)</u>: in three RCTs (606 patients), no statistically significant difference was seen between DA plus levodopa and levodopa alone in terms of wearing-off (OR = 0.44, 95% CI 0.17–1.44, $P = 0.09$. In four RCTs, DA plus levodopa was associated with significantly higher odds of withdrawals due to adverse events than levodopa alone (OR 4.0, 95% CI 1.5–10.64, $P = 0.0056$). In four RCTs, DA plus levodopa was associated with nonsignificantly lower odds of dyskinesia than levodopa alone (OR 0.4, 95% CI 0.16–1.01, $P = 0.053$)
		<u>Adverse events:</u> Upon MA of tolerability endpoints, the use of DAs was associated with significantly higher odds of experiencing side effects, such as hallucinations, somnolence, dizziness, and nausea, when compared to both placebo and levodopa ($P < 0.05$ for all).
		<u>Conclusions[b]:</u> "The use of DA is an effective treatment option for the treatment of early PD and appears especially useful among PD patients with wearing-off phenomenon or dyskinesias on levodopa; however, it may result in more adverse events and higher withdrawal rates"
Chung, V. *et al.* [11] Efficacy and safety of herbal medicines for idiopathic Parkinson's disease: a systematic review. *Movement Disorders* 2006; **21** (10): 1709–1715.	To assess the efficacy and safety of HMs, as a monotherapy or adjunct therapy, compared to placebo or conventional approaches for treatment of idiopathic PD	<u>Main findings[a]:</u> This SR included nine RCTs, each testing a different HM (551 patients in total). Three RCTs were relatively rigorous in design, whereas six had limited internal validity due to major flaws in design, including a lack of proper randomization; insufficient blinding; unclear inclusive criteria in terms of diagnostic criteria, baseline staging, and duration of disease; lack of proper sample size calculation; and insufficient data analysis.
		Three RCTs tested HMs as a monotherapy, five RCTs tested HMs as an adjunct therapy to conventional drugs, and one RCT simultaneously tested HMs as a monotherapy and as an adjunct therapy. All RCTs had a short-term duration.
		Imbalances in gender and ethnicity among the patients in the included trials were observed. No major adverse events emerged, and no specific pattern was detected from the trials describing such data. In addition to major methodological defects, heterogeneity in: (i) HM-tested; (ii) control treatment; and (iii) outcome measure hindered in-depth data analysis and synthesis.

Table 9.1 *Continued*

Study	Objectives	Main findings[a] and conclusions[b]
		Conclusions[b]: "Current evidence is insufficient to evaluate the efficacy and safety of various HMs. Further studies with improved trial design and reporting, with assessment on cost-effectiveness, quality of life, and qualitative data are warranted."
Dixon, L., *et al.* [25] Occupational therapy for patients with Parkinson's disease. [update of *Cochrane Database Systematic Reviews* 2001; (3): CD002813; PMID: 11687028]. *Cochrane Database of Systematic Reviews* 2007; (3): CD002813.	To compare the efficacy and effectiveness of occupational therapy with placebo or no interventions (control group) in patients with PD	Main findings[a]: This SR included two RCTs comparing occupational therapy with control group (84 patients in total). The two RCTs varied significantly in their methodology and used different interventions. Overall, their methodological quality and the standard of reporting was poor. Although both trials reported a positive effect from occupational therapy, all improvements were small. Conclusions[b]: "Considering the significant methodological flaws in the studies, the small number of patients examined, and the possibility of publication bias, there is insufficient evidence to support or refute the efficacy of occupational therapy in Parkinson's disease. There is now a consensus as to UK current and best practice in occupational therapy when treating people with Parkinson's disease. We now require large well-designed placebo-controlled RCTs to demonstrate occupational therapy's effectiveness in Parkinson's disease. Outcome measures with particular relevance to patients, carers, occupational therapists and physicians should be chosen and the patients monitored for at least six months to determine the duration of benefit. The trials should be reported using CONSORT guidelines."
Goodwin, V.A., *et al.* [15] The effectiveness of exercise interventions for people with Parkinson's disease: a systematic review and meta-analysis. *Movement Disorders* 2008; **23** (5): 631–640.	To systematically review RCTs reporting on the effectiveness of exercise interventions on outcomes (physical, psychological or social functioning, or QoL) for people with PD	Main findings[a]: This SR included 14 RCTs (495 patients in total), of which two were found to be of high methodological quality, 10 of moderate methodological quality, and two of low methodological quality. Evidence supported exercise as being beneficial with regards to physical functioning, (HR)QoL, strength, balance and gait speed for people with PD. There was insufficient evidence support or refute the value of exercise in reducing falls or depression. Conclusions[b]: "This review found evidence of the potential benefits of exercise for people with PD, although further good quality research is needed. Questions remain around the optimal content of exercise interventions (dosing, component exercises) at different stages of the disease."

Table 9.1 *Continued*

Study	Objectives	Main findings[a] and conclusions[b]
Hamer, M. and Chida, Y. [16] Physical activity and risk of neurodegenerative disease: a systematic review of prospective evidence. *Psychological Medicine* 2009: **39**; 3–11.	To quantify the association between physical activity and risk of neurodegenerative diseases using meta-analytical techniques	Main findings[a]: This SR included 16 prospective cohort studies in the overall analysis, which incorporated 163 797 nondemented participants at baseline with 3219 cases (488 PD cases) at follow-up. The two studies that examined risk of PD were considered to be high-quality studies. The pooled relative risk (RR) of overall dementia in the highest physical activity category compared with the lowest was 0.72 (95% CI 0.60–0.86, $P < 0.001$), for AD it was 0.55 (95% CI 0.36–0.84, $P = 0.006$), and for PD it was 0.82 (95% CI 0.57–1.18, $P = 0.28$). The results suggest that physical activity reduces the risk of dementia and AD by 28% and 45%, respectively. Physical activity was not associated with a significant reduction in risk of PD. There was significant heterogeneity for the association between physical activity and dementia [$\chi^2(13) = 46.66, P < 0.001$] and AD [$\chi^2(6) = 29.12, P < 0.001$] but not for PD [$\chi^2(2) = 3.09, P = 0.21$]

Conclusions[b]: "In conclusion, our results suggest that physical activity is protective against future risk of dementia and Alzheimer's disease. However, the optimal dose of physical activity for risk reduction remains to be accurately defined and this should be a focus of future research". |
| Kwakkel, G. [18] Impact of physical therapy for Parkinson's disease: A critical review of the literature. *Parkinsonism and Related Disorders* 2007; **13** (Suppl. 3): S478–S487. | To evaluate the efficacy of physical therapy (PT) in PD | Main findings[a]: This SR included 23 RCTs (all of moderate methodological quality). The RCTs reflected specific core areas of PT: transfer, posture, balance, reaching and grasping, gait, and physical condition. Most high-quality studies investigated the effects of exercise therapy, including the use of external rhythms to improve gait and gait-related activities.

Significant evidence was reported in favor of task-oriented exercise training to improve posture and balance control, gait and gait-related activities, and physical condition, suggesting that the PT effects are both task- and context-specific. The significant outcomes were closely related to the tasks specifically trained in the therapy, indicating that tasks that are trained tend not to generalize to activities that are not directly exercised in the PT program.

Despite the significant *P*-values for clinically meaningful outcomes, the size of changes remains unclear. The impact of the significant improvements in terms of strength, balance scores, gait and ADLs, as well as impact on patients' safety in terms of fall avoidance was unclear in all trials. |

Table 9.1 *Continued*

Study	Objectives	Main findings[a] and conclusions[b]
		Conclusions[b]: These results suggest that "... future programs should train meaningful tasks preferably in patients' home environment. In addition, the decline in treatment effects after an intervention has ended suggests the need for permanent treatment of patients with PD".

"Future studies should aim to develop responsive measurement instruments able to monitor meaningful changes in activities, as well as better understanding of insufficiently understood symptoms such as freezing, rigidity and bradykinesia and greater insight into neurophysiological mechanisms underlying training-induced changes in activities such as improved gait performance by rhythmic cueing." |
| Lam, Y.C., *et al.* [19] Efficacy and safety of acupuncture for idiopathic Parkinson's disease: a systematic review. *Journal of Alternative Complementary Medicine* 2008; **14** (6): 663–671. | To assess the efficacy and safety of acupuncture therapy (monotherapy or adjuvant therapy), compared with placebo, conventional interventions, or no treatment in treating patients with idiopathic PD (IPD) | Main findings[a]: This SR included 10 RCTs, with a total of 580 patients (60% males) who received acupuncture, placebo or conventional medications over periods varying from 2 weeks to 3 months. Each RCT used a different set of acupoints and manipulation of needles. No RCT reported the concealment of allocation, and only two mentioned the number of dropouts. Two used a nonblind method, while others did not mention their blinding methods. Nine RCTs were performed in China (*n* = 566 Chinese patients). Nine RCTs claimed a statistically significant positive effect from acupuncture as compared with their control; only one RCT indicated that there were no statistically significant differences for all variables measured. Only two studies described details about adverse events.

Conclusions[b]: "There is evidence indicating the potential effectiveness of acupuncture for treating IPD. The results were limited by the methodological flaws, unknowns in concealment of allocation, number of dropouts, and blinding methods in the studies. Large, well-designed, placebo-controlled RCTs with rigorous methods of randomization and adequately concealed allocation, as well as intention-to-treat data analysis are needed." |

Table 9.1 *Continued*

Study	Objectives	Main findings[a] and conclusions[b]
Lee, M.S., *et al.* [20] Effectiveness of acupuncture for Parkinson's disease: A systematic review. *Movement Disorders* 2008; **23** (11): 1505–1515.	To assess the clinical evidence for or against acupuncture as a treatment for PD	Main findings[a]: This SR included 11 RCTs, with a total 526 patients (52% males) who received needle acupuncture (with or without electrical stimulation), placebo, conventional drugs, or no treatment. Eight RCTs originated from China (387 patients), two from Korea (125 patients), and one from USA (14 patients). Six RCTs applied correct methods of randomization, only one RCT reported details on allocation concealment, three RCTs described patient blinding, and five RCTs described sufficient details of drop-outs and withdrawals.

Acupuncture versus placebo: MA of results from three RCTs (total of 139 patients) failed to show that acupuncture is superior in terms of UPDRS ($n = 96$, WMD, 5.7; 95% CI −2.8 to 14.2, $P = 0.19$, heterogeneity: $\tau^2 = 0$, $\chi^2 = 0.97$, $P = 0.62$, $I^2 = 0\%$); one RCT (14 patients) failed to show favorable results for electro-acupuncture for QoL and depression. In one RCT (55 patients), needle acupuncture was not superior to placebo for freezing of gait (FOG) and ADL, while individualized acupuncture showed favorable effects (not statistically significant) on FOG compared to placebo.

Acupuncture plus conventional drugs versus conventional drugs only: Six RCTs (290 patients) compared acupuncture plus conventional drugs on improvement of PD symptoms with drugs only. A MA of two of these RCTs suggested a positive effect of scalp acupuncture on UPDRS ($n = 106$, RR, 1.46, 95% CI = 1.15–1.87, $P = 0.002$; heterogeneity: $\tau^2 = 0.00$, $\chi^2 = 1.14$, $P = 0.29$, $I^2 = 12\%$). Two RCTs failed to show favorable effects of acupuncture plus levodopa compared to levodopa alone for severity of PD and for symptoms of PD, while reporting significantly fewer adverse events when compared with drug alone.

Acupuncture versus no treatment: A MA of two RCTs, which tested acupuncture versus no treatment, suggested beneficial effects of acupuncture on UPDRS ($n = 74$, WMD, 7.36, 95% CI = 5.58–9.14, $P < 0.001$; heterogeneity: $\tau^2 = 0.00$, $\chi^2 = 0.52$, $P = 0.0.47$, $I^2 = 0\%$). The results of the latter two types of RCTs fail to adequately control for nonspecific effects.

Table 9.1 *Continued*

Study	Objectives	Main findings[a] and conclusions[b]
		Conclusions[b]: "In conclusion, the evidence for the effectiveness of acupuncture for treating PD is not convincing. The number and quality of trials as well as their total sample size are too low to draw firm conclusions. Further rigorous trials are warranted but need to overcome the many limitations of the current evidence."
Stowe, R.L., *et al.* [23] Dopamine agonist therapy in early Parkinson's disease. *Cochrane Database of Systematic Reviews: Reviews* 2008; (2).	To quantify more reliably the benefits and risks of DAs compared to placebo or LD in early PD	Main findings[a]: This SR included 29 RCTs involving 5247 participants.
		Participants randomized to a DA were less likely to develop dyskinesia (OR 0.51, 95% CI 0.43–0.59; $P < 0.00001$), dystonia (OR 0.64, 95% CI 0.51–0.81; $P = 0.0002$) and motor fluctuations (OR 0.75, 95% CI 0.63–0.90; $P = 0.002$) than LD-treated participants.
		Various "non-motor" side effects, including edema (OR 3.68, 95% CI 2.62–5.18; $P < 0.00001$), somnolence (OR 1.49, 95% CI 1.12–2.00; $P = 0.007$), constipation (OR 1.59, 95% CI 1.11–2.28; $P = 0.01$), dizziness (OR 1.45, 95% CI 1.09–1.92; $P = 0.01$), hallucinations (OR 1.69, 95% CI 1.13–2.52; $P = 0.01$) and nausea (OR 1.32, 95% CI 1.05–1.66; $P = 0.02$) were all increased in DA-treated participants (compared with LD-treated participants).
		DA-treated participants were also significantly more likely to discontinue treatment due to adverse events (OR 2.49, 95% CI 2.08–2.98; $P<0.00001$). Symptomatic control of PD was better with LD than with DAs, but data were reported too inconsistently and incompletely to meta-analyze.
		There were no clear differences between types of DA, other than more hallucinations and somnolence with non-ergot-derived agonists. The reduction in dyskinesia does appear larger with nonergot agonists, but was correlated more closely with lower LD exposure in the agonist arm than type of agonist.
		Patients on a DA were more than twice as likely to discontinue treatment prematurely due to adverse events than control patients.
		Uncertainty still exists as to which class of drug is the most clinically and cost-effective in the treatment of early PD.

Table 9.1 Continued

Study	Objectives	Main findings[a] and conclusions[b]
		Conclusions[b]: "This 'umbrella' review is the first to assess dopamine agonists as a drug class and examines a more comprehensive range of outcomes than previous meta-analyses. It confirms the benefit of dopamine agonists in terms of reducing motor complications, as reported in several individual trials. However, the meta-analysis also provides conclusive evidence of a substantial increase in 'non-motor' side-effects among dopamine agonist-treated patients that has not been obvious from the publications of individual, usually commercially sponsored, trials. The non-motor side-effects appear at least as clinically important as the motor complications since patients randomised to a dopamine agonist were significantly more likely to withdraw from the trial due to adverse events than control patients.
		Unfortunately, the balance of risks and benefits remains unclear, as only one trial included overall quality of life and cost-effectiveness as outcome measures."
		"Larger, long-term comparative trials assessing patient-rated quality of life are needed to assess more reliably the balance of benefits and risks of dopamine agonists compared to levodopa."
van Hilten, J.J., et al. [24] Bromocriptine/levodopa combined versus levodopa alone for early Parkinson's disease. [update of Cochrane Database Systematic Reviews 2002; (2): CD003634; PMID: 12076493]. Cochrane Database of Systematic Reviews 2007; (4).	To determine the efficacy and safety of BR/ LD combination therapy in delaying the onset of motor complications associated with LD therapy in patients with PD	Main findings[a]: This SR included seven RCTs which randomized over 1100 patients to a LD or a BR/LD combination regimen. All studies failed adequately to describe randomization procedures. Only three were carried out according to a double-blind design. Differences were found between studies concerning participants' mean age, BR titration phase, maximum achieved daily dose of LD (62.5 to 1000 mg) and BR (5 to 50 mg), and the applied outcomes.
		This SR's results show no evidence of consistent differences between treatment groups in terms of occurrence and severity of motor complications, scores of impairment and disability, or occurrence of side effects.
		Conclusions[b]: This systematic review revealed no evidence to support or refute the use of early BR/LD combination therapy as a strategy to prevent or delay the onset of motor complications in the treatment of PD.

Table 9.1 *Continued*

Study	Objectives	Main findings[a] and conclusions[b]
van Hilten, J.J., et al. [27] Bromocriptine versus levodopa in early Parkinson's disease. [update of *Cochrane Database Systematic Reviews* 2000; (3): CD002258; PMID: 10908538]. *Cochrane Database of Systematic Reviews* 2008; (4): CD002258.	To assess the efficacy and safety of BR monotherapy for delaying the onset of motor complications associated with LD therapy in patients with PD	Main findings[a]: This SR included six RCTs with 850 participants. Methodological problems and incomparability of studies precluded the pooling of data in an attempt to perform meta-analysis. The occurrence of dyskinesias in three short trials was too low to draw any conclusion. The results of longer trials indicate a lower occurrence of dyskinesias in the BR tier. In five trials that evaluated dystonia, this motor complication occurred less frequently in the BR tier. However, for both dyskinesias and dystonia, a SS difference in favor of BR emerged only in the largest trial. There was a trend for wearing-off and on-off fluctuations to occur less frequently in the BR group. All trials evaluated participants at the impairment level, but only the largest trial reported a SS larger improvement for the LD tier during the first year of therapy. Concerning disability, evaluated by five trials, no SS differences were found. Overall, a statistically larger number of dropouts occurred in the BR group because of an inadequate therapeutic response or intolerable side effects. Conclusions[b]: Based on a qualitative review of the available data, the authors concluded "... that in the treatment of early Parkinson Disease, bromocriptine may be beneficial in delaying motor complications and dyskinesia with comparable effects on impairment and disability in those patients that tolerate the drug."

Comorbidities and/or complications

Study	Objectives	Main findings[a] and conclusions[b]
Coggrave, M., et al. [12] Management of faecal incontinence and constipation in adults with central neurological diseases. *Cochrane Database of Systematic Reviews* 2006; (2).	To determine the effects of management strategies for fecal incontinence and constipation in people with neurological diseases affecting the central nervous system	Main findings[a]: This SR included 10 RCTs (only one in people with PD). Most RCTs were small and of poor quality. One single-blind RCT, compared psyllium with placebo in seven people with PD. Psyllium was associated with increased stool frequency, but did not alter the colonic transit time. Eight weeks of psyllium was associated with a SS increased mean number of bowel motions (5.7 versus 3.5 mean stools per week, WMD -2.20, 95% CI -3.00 to -1.40) and mean stool weight (1300 versus 820 g per week, WMD -480.00, 95% CI -935.29 to -24.71). Mean colonic transit time was not altered (65 versus 58 h, WMD -7.00, 95% CI -24.67 to 10.67). Side effects were not reported.

Table 9.1 Continued

Study	Objectives	Main findings[a] and conclusions[b]
		Conclusions[b]:
		There is still little research on this condition, and it is not possible to draw any recommendations for bowel care in people with neurological diseases from the trials included in this review. Bowel management for these people must remain empirical until well-designed controlled trials with adequate numbers and clinically relevant outcome measures become available. It is widely accepted that the development of a bowel movement protocol/program should be based on a comprehensive, individualized, patient-centered assessment
Frieling, H., *et al.* [14] Treating dopamimetic psychosis in Parkinson's disease: structured review and meta-analysis. *European Neuropsychopharmacology* 2007; **17** (3): 165–171.	To evaluate which neuroleptic drugs can efficiently be used to treat DIP in PD	Main findings[a]: This SR included seven RCTs with a satisfactory allocation concealment and data reporting.
		Two RCTs compared low-dose clozapine versus placebo, with a significantly better outcome for clozapine regarding efficacy [significant improvement in psychotic symptoms with the BPRS in one RCT (WMD: −6.7, CI: −7.45 to −5.95)] and motor functioning [(significant improvement in UPDRS total and motor scores (UPDSR total: WMD: −2.39, CI: −3.58 to −1.20; UPDSR motor: WMD: −1.74, CI: −2.57 to −0.92)]. No significant difference in change of MMSE scores.
		One RCT compared clozapine versus quetiapine, showing equivalent efficacy and tolerability: no significant differences in terms of clinical efficacy (CGI: WMD: −0.20, CI: −0.57 to 0.17; BPRS: WMD: 0.10, CI: −1.00 to 1.20), motor functioning (UPDRS motor score: WMD: 2.70, CI: −3.58 to 8.98; AIMS: WMD: −0.60, CI −1.41 to 0.21), and in frequency of AE (RR: 0.40, CI: 0.09 to 1.83) between groups.
		In two placebo-controlled trials, quetiapine failed to show efficacy.
		In two other placebo-controlled trials olanzapine led to a significant worsening of Parkinson symptoms (UPDSR total, motor score and AD: SMD: 0.59, CI 0.40 to 0.78), did not improve psychotic symptoms [no significant difference in clinical efficacy assessed by CGI score (WMD: 0.13, CI: −0.27 to 0.53); using BPRS scores, a clear trend in favor of placebo was found only when sub-scores were analyzed (BPRS total: WMD: 0.71, CI: −1.73 to 3.15; BPRS positive and negative sub-scores and hallucination: SMD: 0.18, CI: −0.01 to 0.36); no differences were found concerning MMSE (WMD: −0.78, CI: −1.80 to 0.25) and caused significantly more extrapyramidal side effects.

Table 9.1 *Continued*

Study	Objectives	Main findings[a] and conclusions[b]
		Conclusions[b]:
		Only limited data exist on the best treatment strategy for DIP in PD. Based on randomized trial-derived evidence which is currently available, only clozapine can be fully recommended for the treatment of DIP in PD. Olanzapine should not be used in this indication. Further studies are needed to clarify the results for quetiapine and to evaluate newer antipsychotics or other drugs for this indication.
Maidment, I., *et al.* [39] Cholinesterase inhibitors for Parkinson's disease dementia. *Cochrane Database of Systematic Reviews* 2006; (1).	To assess the efficacy, safety, tolerability and health economic data relating to the use of cholinesterase inhibitors in PDD	**Main findings[a]:** This SR included one RCT (double-blind, placebo-controlled) involving 541 patients.
		Rivastigmine produced a 2.80 point ADAS-Cog improvement [WMD: −2.80, 95% CI: −4.26 to −1.34, $P = 0.0002$] and a 2.50 point ADCS-ADL improvement [95% CI: 0.43 to 4.57, $P = 0.02$] at 24 weeks relative to placebo. ADCS-CGIC found that using LOCF the change score from baseline to week 24 significantly favored rivastigmine [WMD: −0.50, 95% CI: −0.77 to −0.23, $P = 0.0004$].
		Clinically meaningful (moderate or marked) improvement occurred in 5.3% more patients on rivastigmine, and meaningful worsening occurred in 10.1% more patients on placebo.
		Significantly more patients on rivastigmine dropped out due to AE [62/362 versus 14/179, OR 2.44, 95% CI: 1.32 to 4.48, $P = 0.004$]; nausea [20/179 versus 105/362, OR 3.25, 95% CI: 1.94 to 5.45, $P<0.00001$]; tremor [7/179 versus 37/362, OR 2.80, 95% CI: 1.22 to 6.41, $P = 0.01$]; and vomiting [3/179 versus 60/362, OR 11.66, 95% CI: 3.60 to 37.72, $P<0.0001$] were significantly more common with rivastigmine. Significantly fewer patients died on rivastigmine than placebo [4/362 versus 7/179, OR 0.27, 95% CI: 0.08 to 0.95, $P = 0.04$].
		No reporting on the effect of rivastigmine in PDD on institutionalization rates, QoL measures for both patients and carers and health economic factors.

Table 9.1 Continued

Study	Objectives	Main findings[a] and conclusions[b]
		Conclusions[b]:
		"According to evidence from one RCT, rivastigmine appears to improve cognition and activities of daily living in patients with PDD. This results in clinically meaningful benefit in about 15% of cases. There is a need for more studies utilizing pragmatic measures, such as time to residential care facility and both patient and carer QoL assessments. Future trials should involve other cholinesterase inhibitors, utilize tools to analyze the data that limit any bias, and measure health economic factors. It is unlikely that relying solely on LOCF is sufficient. Publication of the observed case data in the largest trial would assist. Adverse events were associated with the cholinergic activity of rivastigmine, but may limit patient acceptability as evidenced by the high drop out rate in the active arm."
Reijnders, J.S., et al. [22] A systematic review of prevalence studies of depression in Parkinson's disease. *Movement Disorders* 2008; **23** (2): 183–189.	To calculate average prevalences of depressive disorders, taking into account the different settings and different diagnostic approaches of studies	Main findings[a]: This SR included 104 studies, of which 22 focused on the prevalence of depression in PD, and the remaining 82 had other primary objectives but also reported on prevalence of depression in the study sample (16 population-based studies, three studies in general practices, 71 studies in outpatient settings, five studies in hospital inpatient settings, two studies in nursing homes, and seven other studies). Only 51 articles fulfilled the quality criteria, and 15 from the same database were not included in the meta-analysis. In the remaining 36 articles, the weighted prevalence of major depressive disorder was 17% of PD patients, that of minor depression 22%, and dysthymia 13%. Clinically significant depressive symptoms, irrespective of the presence of a DSM-defined depressive disorder, were present in 35%. In studies using a (semi) structured interview to establish DSM criteria, the reported prevalence of major depressive disorder was 19%, while in studies using DSM criteria without a structured interview, the reported prevalence of major depressive disorder was 7%. Population studies report lower prevalence rates for both major depressive disorder and the clinically significant depressive symptoms than studies in other settings. Conclusions[b]: This systematic review suggests that the average prevalence of major depressive disorder in PD is substantial, but lower than generally assumed.

Table 9.1 *Continued*

Study	Objectives	Main findings[a] and conclusions[b]

Quality of Life

| Den Oudsten, B.L., et al. [13] Quality of life and related concepts in Parkinson's disease: a systematic review. *Movement Disorders* 2007; **22** (11): 1528–1537. | To review the conceptual and methodological quality of QoL studies among patients with PD and to identify factors associated with poor (HR)QoL | Main findings[a]:

This SR included 61 studies (of moderate methodological quality), of which 39 were cross-sectional studies.

The term "QoL" was often used inappropriately in the included 61 studies. In fact, almost all studies in this review actually assessed HS instead of QoL. The functioning of patients with PD on physical, social, and emotional domains is affected by PD. Their HS seems to be lower when compared to healthy persons or patients with other chronic diseases. Besides a declined functioning in the physical domain, patients also experience a diminished social and emotional functioning.

Conclusions[b]:

HS is conceived as a valuable construct. However, QoL is also an important factor in health care. Attention towards QoL is needed in order to draw valid conclusions regarding a person's subjective experience of well-being in a broad sense. In order to accomplish this, future studies should apply the QoL concept with more rigor, should use an adequate operational definition, and should employ sound measures. |

AD, Alzheimer's disease; A DAS-Cog, Alzheimer's Disease Assessment Scale–Cognitive subscale; ADCS–ADL, Alzheimer's Disease Cooperative Study–Activities of Daily Living; ADL, Activities of Daily Living; AE, adverse events/adverse side effects; AIMS, Abnormal Involuntary Movement Scale; ANCDS, Academy of Neurologic Communication Disorders and Sciences; BPRS, Brief Psychiatric Rating Scale; BR, bromocriptine; CC, case-control; CGI-S, Clinical Global Impression Severity Scale; ChEIs, cholinesterase inhibitors; CI, confidence interval; DA, dopamine agonist; DIP, drug-induced psychosis; DSM, Diagnostic and Statistic Manual for Mental Disorders; FOG, freezing of gait; GI, gastrointestinal; HM, herbal medicine; (HR)QoL, health-related quality of life; HS, health status; IPD, idiopathic Parkinson disease; LD, levodopa; LOCF, Last observation carried forward; LT, long-term; MA, meta-analysis; MMSE, Mini Mental Status Examination; mo, month(s); NCC, nested case-control; non-RCT, non-randomized controlled trial; OL, open-label study; OR, Odds ratio; QoL, quality of life; *P*, *P*-value; PD, Parkinson disease; PDD, Parkinson disease dementia/dementia with Parkinson disease; PIGD, postural instability and gait disorder; PRS, primary research study; RCT, randomized controlled trial; RR, relative risk; SE, Schwab and England Disability scale; SMD, Standardized Mean Difference; SR, systematic review; SS, statistically significant; UPDRS, Unified Parkinson's disease Rating Scale; UPDRS-ME, Unified Parkinson's disease Rating Scale Motor Examination; WMD, weighted mean difference.

a) Main findings regarding PD and/or PD complications and/or comorbidities in PD.

b) Conclusions summarize statements by the author(s) and/or quote statements directly from the published report.

Table 9.2 Summary of relevant data extracted from selected practice guidelines.

Item	Synopsis of recommendations[a]
Diagnosing PD	PD should be diagnosed clinically [1]. The UK Parkinson's Disease Society Brain Bank Criteria may be useful.
	People with suspected PD should be referred quickly and untreated to a specialist with expertise in differential diagnosis [1].
	Determining the presence of the following clinical features in early stages of disease should be considered to distinguish PD from other parkinsonian syndromes: (i) falls at presentation and early in the disease course; (ii) poor response to levodopa; (iii) symmetry at onset; (iv) rapid progression; (v) lack of tremor; and (vi) dysautonomia [30].
	Acute levodopa and apomorphine challenge tests should not be used in differential diagnosis of parkinsonian syndromes [1]. Levodopa and apomorphine challenge tests should be considered for confirmation when the diagnosis of PD is in doubt [30].
	Objective smell testing should not be used in differential diagnosis of parkinsonian syndromes, except in the context of clinical trials [1]. Olfaction testing should be considered to differentiate PD from PSP and CBD, but not PD from MSA [30].
	GH stimulation with clonidine, electro-oculography, and SPECT scanning may not be useful in differentiating PD from other parkinsonian syndromes [30].
	^{123}I-FP-CIT SPECT is recommended for people with tremor where essential tremor cannot be clinically differentiated from parkinsonism [1].
	PET should not be used in differential diagnosis of parkinsonian syndromes, except in the context of clinical trials [1].
	Structural MRI should not be used in differential diagnosis of PD [1].
	MRV should not be used in differential diagnosis of parkinsonian syndromes, except in the context of clinical trials [1].
	MRS should not be used in the differential diagnosis of parkinsonian syndromes [1].
Prognosis of new-onset PD	Older age at onset and rigidity/hypokinesia as an initial symptom should be used to predict a more rapid rate of motor progression [30].
	The presence of associated comorbidities (stroke, auditory deficits, and visual impairments), PIGD, and male gender may be used to predict a faster rate of motor progression [30].
	Tremor as a presenting symptom may be used to predict a more benign course and a longer therapeutic benefit to levodopa [30].
	Older age at onset and initial hypokinesia/rigidity should be used to predict an earlier development of cognitive decline and dementia [30].
	Older age at onset, dementia, and decreased dopamine responsiveness may be used to predict earlier nursing home placement as well as decreased survival [30].

Table 9.2 *Continued*

Item	Synopsis of recommendations[a]
Neuroprotection	For patients with PD, treatment with vitamin E should not be considered for neuroprotection [1, 36].
	Coenzyme Q10, DAs, and MAO-B inhibitors should not be used as neuroprotective therapies for people with PD, except in the context of clinical trials [1].
	Levodopa may be considered for the initial treatment of PD, as it does not accelerate disease progression and is safe (*although there is no long-term evidence to recommend levodopa for neuroprotection*) [36].
Management of early PD	*Initial pharmacotherapy*
	Levodopa is established as the most effective symptomatic antiparkinsonian drug, and may be used for early PD [1, 32]. After a few years of treatment, levodopa is frequently associated with the development of motor complications [1, 32].
	DAs may be used as a symptomatic treatment for early PD [1, 30]:
	– Pramipexole and ropinirole are effective as monotherapy in early PD, with a lower risk of motor complications than levodopa [32].
	– Bromocriptine is probably effective in managing patients with early PD [32].
	– The benefit of DAs in preventing motor complications, when compared with levodopa, must be balanced with the smaller effect on symptoms and the greater incidence of hallucinations, somnolence, and leg edema [32] Patients must be informed of these risks [32].
	MAO-B inhibitors may be used as a symptomatic treatment for early PD [1, 30]. Selegiline or rasagiline are established as effective symptomatic therapies [32]. The symptomatic effect is more modest than that of levodopa and (probably) DAs, but they are easy to administer (one dose, once daily, no titration) [32].
	Amantadine or anticholinergics may be used for symptomatic therapy in early PD [1, 30]. The symptomatic effect is smaller than that of levodopa [32]. As anticholinergics are poorly tolerated in the elderly, their use is mainly restricted to young people with early PD and severe tremor, but they should not be drugs of first choice due to a limited efficacy and the propensity to cause neuropsychiatric side effects [1, 30].
	Modified-release levodopa preparations should not be used to delay the onset of motor complications in early PD [1]. The early use of CR levodopa formulations is not effective in the prevention of motor complications [32].
	Adjustment of initial pharmacotherapy
	For patients with persistent or emerging disabling tremor, the use of clozapine is not advised for routine because of safety concerns [32].
	Surgical therapy

Table 9.2 *Continued*

Item	Synopsis of recommendations[a]
Management of late PD	*Pharmacotherapy* Motor fluctuations Modified-release levodopa preparations may be used to reduce motor complications in people with later PD, but should not be drugs of first choice [1]. DAs may be used to reduce motor fluctuations in later PD [1, 30, 35]. – Oral DAs are efficacious in reducing the "off" time in patients experiencing wearing-off [32]. Currently, no DA has proven better than another, but switching from one DA to another can be helpful in some patients [32]. – Pergolide[b], pramipexole, and ropinirole should be considered to reduce "off" time [35]. – Pergolide[b] should be used with caution; it will need to be monitored because of its association with valvulopathy [35]. – Apomorphine, and cabergoline may be considered to reduce "off" time [35]. – Intermittent apomorphine (subcutaneous) injections may be used to reduce "off" time in PD with severe motor complications [1]. – Sustained-release carbidopa/levodopa and bromocriptine may be disregarded to reduce "off" time [35]. – Ropinirole may be chosen over bromocriptine for reducing "off" time [35]. Otherwise, there is insufficient evidence to recommend one medication over another [35]. If oral therapy fails, the following strategies can be recommended: – Alternative delivery routes such as: oral dispersible levodopa, which might be useful for delayed on [32]; or – Alternative formulations of levodopa such as levodopa/carbidopa enteric gel administered through PEG, which can also be considered to stabilize patients with refractory motor fluctuations [32]. COMT and MAO-B inhibitors may be used to reduce motor fluctuations in people with later PD [1, 30, 35]. – Entacapone and rasagiline should be offered to reduce "off" time [35]. – There is no difference between entacapone and rasagiline (both are established as effective in reducing "off" time) [32]. – Tolcapone should be considered to reduce "off" time [35]. Tolcapone should be used with caution and require monitoring because of its association with hepatotoxicity [35]. – Selegiline may be considered to reduce "off" time [35]. – Rasagiline should not be added to selegiline (cardiovascular safety issues) [32]. Dyskinesia Amantadine may be considered to reduce dyskinesia in late PD [1]. Amantadine is established as effective for reducing peak-dose dyskinesia [32]. The use of other antiglutaminergic drugs is investigational [32]. Reducing the individual levodopa dose size is possibly effective in reducing peak-dose dyskinesia, at the risk of increasing "off" time [32]. The latter can be compensated for by increasing the number of daily doses of levodopa, or increasing the doses of a DA.

Table 9.2 *Continued*

Item	Synopsis of recommendations[a]
	Adding clozapine is established as effective for reducing peak-dose dyskinesia, with doses ranging between 12.5 and 75 mg per day up to 200 mg per day [32].
	Adding quetiapine is possibly effective in reducing peak-dose dyskinesia.
	Surgical therapy
	DBS of the STN may be considered to improve motor function and reduce "off" time, dyskinesia, and medication usage [32, 35].
	Preoperative response to levodopa should be considered as a factor predictive of outcome after DBS of the STN [35].
	Age and duration of PD may be considered as factors predictive of outcomes after DBS of STN [35].
Non-motor features of PD	*Mental health problems*
	<u>Dementia</u>
	The MMSE and the CAMCog should be considered as screening tools for dementia in patients with PD [28].
	The diagnosis of dementia remains clinical. There is good evidence to retain the diagnostic criteria currently in use [29].
	At present, the separation of DLB from PDD is based on the dominant clinical presenting feature of each syndrome, and relies on the duration of this feature: long duration of parkinsonian "motor" syndrome preceding dementia for PDD versus early/initial dementia accompanied by extrapyramidal symptoms for DLB [29].
	Adding therapy with ChEIs can be considered for PDD [28, 34, 37]: – Rivastigmine is established as effective and should be considered for the treatment of dementia in PD or DLB [34, 37] – Donepezil should be considered for the treatment of dementia in PD [28]. – Adding donepezil or galantamine is possibly effective as a treatment for PDD [38]. – Patients who discontinued treatment with ChEIs, should be closely monitored in order to assess withdrawal effects or worsening, in which case the treatment should be restarted [34].
	There is insufficient evidence for the use of memantine in PDD [34].
	The discontinuation of *anticholinergics* as potential aggravators is probably effective for treatment of PDD [37].
	The discontinuation of amantadine, tricyclic antidepressants, tolterodine and oxybutynin, and benzodiazepines, as potential aggravators is possibly effective for PDD treatment [37].
	<u>Depression</u>
	The BDI-I and HDRS should be considered for depression screening in PD [28].
	MADRS may be considered for screening of depression in PD [28].

Table 9.2 *Continued*

Item	Synopsis of recommendations[a)]
	Amitriptyline may be considered in the treatment of depression associated with PD (it is not necessarily the first choice) [28].

Psychosis

Clozapine is effective for treatment of psychosis/psychotic symptoms in PD, and should be considered [1, 28, 37]. Clozapine use is associated with serious adverse events (such as agranulocytosis that may be fatal), and its use requires monitoring [1, 28, 37].

Quetiapine may be considered for psychosis in PD [28].

Olanzapine is established as harmful and is not recommended (should not be routinely used) for psychosis in PD [28, 37].

Risperidone is possibly harmful and is not recommended for psychosis in PD [37].

Rivastigmine is probably effective for treatment of psychosis in PD (cognitive improvements are only modest, while tremor worsened in some patients) [37].

Donepezil is possibly effective for treatment of psychosis in PD (cognitive improvements are only modest while tremor worsened in some patients) [37].

Autonomic dysfunction/disturbance

For treatment of orthostatic hypotension add midodrine (established as effective) [37].

For gastrointestinal motility problems in PD add domperidone (probably effective) [37].

To treat erectile dysfunction add sildenafil (established as effective) [37].

Falls

An increased risk of falls is probable among patients with PD [31]. A history of falling in the past year strongly predicts the likelihood of future falls [31].

All of the patients with any fall risk factors should be asked about falls during the past year [31].

After a comprehensive standard neurologic examination, including an evaluation of cognition and vision, if further assessment of the extent of fall risk is needed, other screening measures to be considered include the Get-Up-And-Go Test or Timed Up-and-Go Test, an assessment of ability to stand unassisted from a sitting position, and the Tinetti Mobility Scale [31].

Item	Synopsis of recommendations
Alternative therapy and other health care interventions	*Physical therapy*

Physiotherapy should be available for people with PD; particular consideration should be given to: gait re-education, improvement of balance and flexibility; enhancement of aerobic capacity; improvement of movement initiation; improvement of functional independence, including mobility and ADL; provision of advice regarding safety in the home environment [1].

For patients with PD, exercise therapy may be considered to improve function [36].

Physical therapy, especially exercise and cueing strategies, are probably effective as adjunctive therapy in PD (*long-term benefits remain to be proven*) [32].

Table 9.2 *Continued*

Item	Synopsis of recommendations[a]
	It is plausible that [33]:

- the gait is improved by applying visual or auditory cues, which have been trained during active gait training;
- applying cognitive movement strategies improves the performance of transfers;
- balance training (where patients are taught to use visual and vestibular feedback), combined with lower-limb strength training, is effective in improving balance in patients with PD, and more effective than balance exercises alone;
- an exercise program aimed at improving range of motion combined with activity-related (e.g., gait or balance) exercises, improves ADL functioning;
- a strength-training program increases muscle power.

The Alexander Technique may be offered to benefit people with PD by helping them to make lifestyle adjustments that affect both the physical nature of the condition and the person's attitudes to having PD [1].

Specialist nurse interventions

People with PD should have regular access to: clinical monitoring and medication adjustment; a continuing point of contact for support, including home visits, when appropriate; a reliable source of information about clinical and social matters of concern to patients and their carers, which may be provided by a PD nurse specialist [1].

Speech and language therapy

For patients with PD complicated by dysarthria, speech therapy may be considered as an adjunctive therapy to improve speech (volume, vocal loudness and pitch range) [1, 32, 36].

Vitamin therapy

For patients with PD, vitamin E (2000 units) should not be considered for symptomatic treatment [36].

ADL, Activities of Daily Living; BDI-I, Beck Depression Inventory-I; CAMCog, Cambridge Cognitive Examination; CBD, corticobasal degeneration; ChEI, cholinesterase inhibitor; COMT inhibitor, catechol-*O*-methyltransferase inhibitor; CR, controlled-release; DA, dopamine agonist; DBS, deep brain stimulation; DLB, dementia with Lewis bodies; ECT, electroconvulsive therapy; EMG, electromyography; ESR, erythrocyte sedimentation rate; FDG PET, ^{18}F fluorodeoxyglucose positron emission tomography; GH, growth hormone; HDRS, Hamilton Depression Rating Scale; MADRS, Montgomery Asberg Depression Rating Scale; MAO-B inhibitor, monoamine oxidase isoenzyme B inhibitor; MAS, multiple system atrophy; MMSE, Mini-Mental State Examination; MRI, magnetic resonance imaging; MRS, magnetic resonance spectroscopy; MRV, magnetic resonance volumetry; PDD, Parkinson disease dementia; PEG, percutaneous gastrostomy; PET, positron emission tomography; PIGD, postural instability/gait difficulty: PPRS, Parkinson Psychosis Rating Scale; PSP, progressive supranuclear palsy; REM, rapid eye movement; RLS, restless legs syndrome; SPECT, single photon emission computed tomography; SSRI, selective serotonin reuptake inhibitor; STN, subthalamic nucleus.

a) Summarized are only recommendations specifically developed for or related to PD that are supported by controlled or comparative data.

b) Note from the National Guideline Clearinghouse (NGC) (www.guideline.gov): On March 29, 2007, Permax (pergolide) was withdrawn from the market in the US and worldwide, due to safety concerns of an increased risk of cardiovascular events. See the US Food and Drug Administration (FDA) Web site for more information.

factors for a more rapid progression of disability and, less conclusively, that a higher bradykinesia score, nontremor dominant subtype, symmetrical disease at baseline and depression may also predict a rapid progression of disability. However, none of the factors examined proved to be a good predictor of future quality of life in PD. Post *et al.* suggested that prospective cohorts of PD patients need to be assembled early on in the disease, and subsequently followed in long-term studies to better understand the prognosis of the disease.

9.5.2
Therapy

The bulk of systematic reviews about PD evaluate various treatments. Recently, four systematic reviews have been produced on the effectiveness of dopamine agonists in the treatment of PD; two of these have included the full class of dopamine agonists, and two examined the drug bromocriptine specifically. Baker *et al.* [10] synthesized the results of 25 randomized clinical trials (RCTs) with more than 5000 patients. Dopamine agonists, when compared to placebo, reduced the patients' motor impairment and improved their ability to perform activities of daily living, but also caused significantly more adverse events. When dopamine agonists were compared to levodopa, they were found to have a lower efficacy but produced fewer motor complications. The dopamine agonists had less of a wearing-off effect (i.e., the drug's potency decreasing over time) when compared to levodopa, but a higher percentage of the dopamine agonist-treated patients withdrew from the study because of adverse events. When dopamine agonists were assessed as a combined therapy with levodopa compared to levodopa alone, the combination was not significantly more effective, and there was a higher rate of adverse events in the combined therapy group. Thus, the authors concluded that dopamine agonists were an effective treatment option for the treatment of early PD, and particularly among PD patients who experience a wearing-off phenomenon or who have involuntary movements while using levodopa. Unfortunately, however, the dopamine agonists seemed to result in a greater number of adverse events and higher withdrawal rates.

Stowe *et al.* [23] also conducted a large systematic review (29 RCTs) on the effectiveness of dopamine agonists, and arrived at many of the same conclusions as Baker *et al.* [10] (this was not surprising as 16 of the RCTs were common to both systematic reviews). While motor impairment was reduced by the dopamine agonists, nonmotor side effects such as edema, somnolence, constipation, dizziness, hallucinations, and nausea were all more frequent than in dopamine agonist-treated patients than in those receiving levodopa. Moreover, the former group were more than twice as likely to discontinue treatment than levodopa patients.

Van Hilten *et al.*'s first systematic review [24] on the use of bromocriptine in early PD compared a bromocriptine/levodopa combined therapy to levodopa alone. Seven RCTs incorporating 1100 patients failed to show ant consistent difference between them, in terms of occurrence and severity of motor complications, scores of impairment and disability, or the occurrence of side effects. Van Hilten *et al.*'s other systematic review [27] compared bromocriptine as a monotherapy against levodopa. For this, although six RCTs were located with 850 patients, a meta-analysis was not possible as there were methodological problems and incomparable outcome indicators. In the larger and longer trials, there was evidence that bromocriptine improved motor impairments such as dyskinesias and dystonia. As in the other trials, a significantly greater number of bromocriptine-treated patients withdrew from the studies because of adverse effects, or because they felt that the bromocriptine was of no help to them. Like Baker *et al.* [10] and Stowe *et al.* [23], Van Hilten *et al.* [24] concluded that there was a role for the use of dopamine agonists in improving motor impairments in early PD, but only in those patients who could tolerate the drug.

Chung *et al.* [11] examined the effectiveness and safety of herbal medicines for PD, but concluded that the heterogeneity and methodological flaws of the included RCTs were such that no conclusions could be made.

Methodological flaws, a small study size, and the possibility of publication bias also prevented Dixon *et al.* [25] from making any conclusions in their systematic review regarding the effectiveness of occupational therapy in PD.

Kwakkel *et al.*'s systematic review [18] on the impact of physical therapy on PD included 23 RCTs of moderate methodological quality. The results of these studies suggested that physical therapy involving specific task-oriented exercise training was successful at producing the desired outcome such as improving posture, balance control, gait and gait-related activities, and physical condition, but did not result in any generalized improvement (e.g., exercises for gait only improved gait). There was also a decline in treatment effect after an intervention–that is, the improvements were not permanent. Hence, physical therapy in PD must be ongoing in order to be helpful.

Goodwin *et al.* [15] examined the effectiveness of exercise interventions for treating people with PD, by analyzing the data from 14 RCTs that included a total of 495 patients. The results supported the proposal that exercise was helpful for improving physical functioning, quality of life, strength, balance and walking speed for people with PD. Nonetheless, good quality research is still required to determine the optimal type and level of physical exercise for PD patients throughout the progression of their disease.

When Hamer and Chida [16] examined the relationship between levels of physical activity and neurodegenerative diseases, they located two high-quality prospective cohort studies which determined that a person's level of physical activity did not significantly alter the risk of PD.

Two recent systematic reviews have been published on the use of acupuncture in PD. Lam *et al.* [19] combined 10 RCTs with 580 patients, and Lee *et al.* [20] combined 11 RCTs with 526 patients (at least five but more likely six of these RCTs were common to both systematic reviews). In the study of Lam *et al.* [19], nine of the 10 RCTs contained a significant positive treatment effect; however, this result may have contained a bias because there was a limited reporting of proper concealment, blinding methods and numbers of adverse events and dropouts.

Lee *et al.* [20] compared acupuncture versus placebo, acupuncture plus conventional drugs versus conventional drugs, and acupuncture versus no treatments. For acupuncture versus placebo, a meta-analysis of three trials (with a total of 139 patients) was unable to demonstrate any superiority of acupuncture over the placebo. However, individualized acupuncture did result in a non-statistically significant gain in the freezing of gait when compared to placebo. Although seven other RCTs all showed positive results, the fact that they were not placebo-controlled suggested that any benefit might have been due to either nonspecific or placebo effects of the acupuncture. Lee *et al.* [20] concluded that the evidence relating to acupuncture was not convincing, and that larger, more rigorous trials would be needed to provide any conclusive evidence.

9.5.3
Comorbidities and Complications

Coggrave *et al.* [12] investigated the management of fecal incontinence and constipation in adults with central neurological diseases. Of the ten RCTs located, only a very small study of seven patients included PD patients, in which psyllium was compared to placebo. Although an eight-week treatment with psyllium caused an increase in the patients' stool frequency and stool weight (but not in colonic transfer time), the small number of patients enrolled limited the value of the findings.

The treatment of dopamimetic psychosis in PD is an important issue, for which Frieling *et al.* [14] completed a systematic review using seven good-quality RCTs. In two of the RCTs, low-dose clozapine was compared to placebo, and in both cases clozapine significantly improved both psychotic symptoms and motor functioning. An additional RCT in which clozapine was compared to quetiapine showed both drugs to have similar efficacies, motor function and frequencies of adverse events, but in two placebo-controlled trials quetiapine failed to show any efficacy. In two trials of olanzapine versus placebo, the former caused a significant worsening of Parkinson syndrome and did not improve psychotic symptoms. Thus, only clozapine could be recommended in PD patients, while olanzapine was contraindicated.

Maidment *et al.* [39] examined cholinesterase inhibitors for dementia in PD, but could identify only one valid RCT, albeit a large, good-quality trial that included 541 patients to evaluate rivastigmine versus placebo. Although 15% of patients receiving rivastigmine experienced a clinically meaningful improvement in cognition and activities of daily living, there was a significantly higher number of adverse events such as nausea, tremor and vomiting, and a larger number of rivastigmine-treated patients withdrew than did those receiving the placebo.

The prevalence of depression in PD has long been observed. Indeed, Reijinders *et al.* [22] calculated the prevalence of major depressive disorder at 17% and minor depression at 22%, using a weighted mean of the data from 36 studies among a variety of settings. The authors concluded that, although this rate was high, it appeared lower than was previously assumed.

9.5.4
Quality of Life

In an attempt to understand the well-being of patients with PD, den Oudsten *et al.* [13] reviewed the evidence from studies on quality of life (QoL) in PD. Although a total of 61 studies of moderate methodological quality was identified, only two of these truly assessed QoL, while the remainder assessed the patients' health status. Typically, patients with PD have a lower health status compared to healthy people or those with other chronic diseases. PD patients will experience diminished physical, social, and emotional functioning. Further research must be conducted in an effort to measure the QoL in PD patients, in order to understand their subjective experience of well-being.

9.6
Available Clinical Practice Guidelines

Six of all the selected CPGs were developed by multidisciplinary groups in North America [28–31, 35, 36], and five in Europe [1, 32–34, 37]. The selected CPGs used various rating/grading systems and provided different recommendation grades/levels for several items.

For the purpose of this chapter, from all selected CPGs only those recommendations supported by controlled or comparison data were extracted and summarized (see Table 9.2, in which a synopsis of these recommendations is provided). Good practice points or recommendations based only on clinical experience, expert opinion, formal consensus, and/or evidence from nonanalytical, descriptive studies (such as uncontrolled studies, case series, and case reports) are not summarized in Table 9.2.

References

1 National Institute for Health and Clinical Excellence (2006) *Parkinson's Disease: Diagnosis and Management in Primary and Secondary Care*, National Institute for Health and Clinical Excellence (NICE), London, p. 45.

2 Cook, D.J., Mulrow, C.D., and Haynes, R.B. (1997) Systematic reviews: synthesis of best evidence for clinical decisions. *Annals of Internal Medicine*, **126**, 376–380.

3 Wilson, M.C., Hayward, R.S., Tunis, S.R., Bass, E.B., and Guyatt, G. (1995) Users' guides to the medical Literature. VIII. How to use clinical practice guidelines. B. what are the recommendations and will they help you in caring for your patients? The evidence-based Medicaine Working Group. *Journal of the American Medical Association*, **274** (20), 1630–1632.

4 The AGREE Collaboration (2008) Appraisal of Guidelines for Research and Evaluation (AGREE) Instrument. Available at: http://www.agreecollaboration.org/instrument (accessed 3 October 2008).

5 National Institute for Health and Clinical Excellence (2008) *The Guidelines Manual*, National Institute for Health and Clinical Excellence, London. Available at: www.nice.org.uk (accessed 3 October 2008).

6 Veldhuijzen, W., Ram, P., Vander, W.T., Wassink, M., and Van, D.V. (2007) Much variety and little evidence: a description of guidelines for doctor-patient communication. *Medical Education*, **41** (2), 138–145.

7 World Health Organization (2003) *Guidelines for WHO Guidelines, Global Programme on Evidence for Health Policy*. World Health Organization, Geneva, Switzerland.

8 Aggressive Research Intelligence Facility. ARIF Critical Appraisal Checklist. Available at: http://www.arif. bham.ca.uk/critical-appraisal-checklist. shtml (accessed 7 October 2009)

9 United Nations Public Administration Network (1995) *List of Country Groupings and Sub-Groupings for the Analytical Studies of the United Nations World Economic Survey and other UN Reports* (ed. United Nations Public Administration Network), United National Public Administration Network.

10 Baker, W.L., Silver, D., White, C.M., Kluger, J., Aberle, J., Patel, A.A., *et al.* (2009) Dopamine agonists in the treatment of early Parkinson's disease: a meta-analysis. *Parkinsonism and Related Disorders*, **15** (4), 287–294.

11 Chung, V., Liu, L., Bian, Z., Zhao, Z., Leuk Fong, W., Kum, W.F., *et al.* (2006) Efficacy and safety of herbal medicines for idiopathic Parkinson's disease: a systematic review. *Movement Disorders*, **21** (10), 1709–1715.

12 Coggrave, M., Wiesel, P.H., and Norton, C. (2006) Management of faecal incontinence and constipation in adults with central neurological diseases. *Cochrane Database of Systematic Reviews*, Issue 2, Article no. CD002115.

13 Den Oudsten, B.L., Van Heck, G.L., and De Vries, J. (2007) Quality of life and related concepts in Parkinson's disease: a systematic review. *Movement Disorders*, **22** (11), 1528–1537.

14 Frieling, H., Hillemacher, T., Ziegenbein, M., Neundorfer, B., and Bleich, S. (2007) Treating dopamimetic psychosis in Parkinson's disease: structured review and meta-analysis. *European Neuropsychopharmacology*, **17** (3), 165–171.

15 Goodwin, V.A., Richards, S.H., Taylor, R.S., Taylor, A.H., and Campbell, J.L. (2008) The effectiveness of exercise interventions for people with Parkinson's disease: a systematic review and meta-analysis. *Movement Disorders*, **23** (5), 631–640.

16 Hamer, M. and Chida, Y. (2009) Physical activity and risk of neurodegenerative disease: a systematic review of prospective evidence. *Psychological Medicine*, **39** (1), 3–11.

17 Ishihara, L. and Brayne, C. (2006) A systematic review of depression and mental illness preceding Parkinson's disease. *Acta Neurologica Scandinavica*, **113** (4), 211–220.

18 Kwakkel, G. (2007) Impact of physical therapy for Parkinson's disease: a critical review of the literature. *Parkinsonism and Related Disorders*, **13** (Suppl. 3), S478–S487.

19 Lam, Y.C., Kum, W.F., Durairajan, S.S., Lu, J.H., Man, S.C., Xu, M., *et al.* (2008) Efficacy and safety of acupuncture for idiopathic Parkinson's disease: a systematic review. *Journal of Alternative and Complementary Medicine*, **14** (6), 663–671.

20 Lee, M.S., Shin, B.C., Kong, J.C., and Ernst, E. (2008) Effectiveness of acupuncture for Parkinson's disease: a systematic review. *Movement Disorders*, **23** (11), 1505–1515.

21 Ballard, C., Lane, R., Barone, P., Ferrara, R., and Tekin, S. (2006) Cardiac safety of rivastigmine in Lewy body and Parkinson's disease dementias. *International Journal of Clinical Practice*, **60** (6), 639–645.

22 Reijnders, J.S., Ehrt, U., Weber, W.E., Aarsland, D., and Leentjens, A.F. (2008) A systematic review of prevalence studies of depression in Parkinson's disease. *Movement Disorders*, **23** (2), 183–189.

23 Stowe, R.L., Ives, N.J., Clarke, C., van Hilten, J., Ferreira, J., Hawker, R.J., *et al.* (2008) Dopamine agonist therapy in early Parkinson's disease. *Cochrane Database of Systematic Reviews*, Issue 2, Article no. CD006564.

24 van-Hilten, J.J., Ramaker, C.C., Stowe, R.L., and Ives, N.J. (2007) Bromocriptine/levodopa combined versus levodopa alone for early Parkinson's disease. *Cochrane Database of Systematic Reviews*, Issue 4, Article no. CD003634.

25 Dixon, L., Duncan, D.C., Johnson, P., Kirkby, L., O'Connell, H., Taylor, H.J., and Deane, K. (2007) Occupational therapy for patients with Parkinson's disease. *Cochrane Database System Reviews*, Issue 3, Article no. CD002813.

26 Post, B., Merkus, M.P., de Haan, R.J., and Speelman, J.D., CARPA Study Group (2007) Prognostic factors for the progression of Parkinson's disease: a systematic review. *Movement Disorders*, **22** (13), 1839–1851.

27 van Hilten, J.J., Ramaker, C.C., Stowe, R., and Ives, N. (2007) Bromocriptine versus levodopa in early Parkinson's disease. *Cochrane Database Systematic Reviews*, Issue 4, Article no. CD002258.

28 Miyasaki, J.M., Shannon, K., Voon, V., Ravina, B., Kleiner-Fisman, G., Anderson, K., *et al.* (2006) Practice Parameter: evaluation and treatment of depression, psychosis, and dementia in Parkinson Disease (an evidence-based review): report of the Quality Standards Subcommittee of the American Academy of Neurology. *Neurology*, **66** (7), 996–1002.

29 Robillard, A. (2007) Clinical diagnosis of dementia. *Alzheimer's and Dementia*, **3** (4), 292–298.

30 Suchowersky, O., Reich, S., Perlmutter, J., Zesiewicz, T., Gronseth, G., Weiner, W.J., *et al.* (2006) Practice Parameter: diagnosis and prognosis of new onset Parkinson Disease (an evidence-based review): report of the Quality Standards Subcommittee of the American Academy of Neurology. *Neurology*, **66** (7), 968–975.

31 Thurman, D.J., Stevens, J.A., Rao, J.K., and Standards, Q. (2008) Subcommittee of the American Academy of Neurology. Practice parameter: assessing patients in a neurology practice for risk of falls (an evidence-based review): report of the Quality Standards Subcommittee of the American Academy of Neurology. *Neurology*, **70** (6), 473–479.

32 Horstink, M., Tolosa, E., Bonuccelli, U., Deuschl, G., Friedman, A., Kanovsky, P., *et al.* (2006) Review of the therapeutic management of Parkinson's disease. Report of a joint task force of the European Federation of Neurological Societies and the Movement Disorder Society-European Section. Park I: early (uncomplicated) Parkinson's disease. *European Journal of Neurology*, **13** (11), 1170–1185.

33 Keus, S.H., Bloem, B.R., Hendriks, E.J., Bredero-Cohen, A.B., and Munneke, M., and the Practice Recommendations Development Group (2007) Evidence-based analysis of physical therapy in Parkinson's disease with recommendations for practice and research. *Movement Disorders*, **22** (4), 451–460.

34 Waldemar, G. (2007) Recommendations for the diagnosis and management of Alzheimer's disease and other disorders associated with dementia: EFNS guideline. *European Journal of Neurology*, **14** (1), e1–e26.

35 Pahwa, R., Factor, S.A., Lyons, K.E., Ondo, W.G., Gronseth, G., Bronte-Stewart, H., *et al.* (2006) Practice Parameter: treatment of Parkinson Disease with motor fluctuations and dyskinesia (an evidence-based review): report of the Quality Standards Subcommittee of the American Academy of Neurology. *Neurology*, **66** (7), 983–995.

36 Suchowersky, O., Gronseth, G., Perlmutter, J., Reich, S., Zesiewicz, T., Weiner, W.J., *et al.* (2006) Practice Parameter: neuroprotective strategies and alternative therapies for Parkinson Disease (an evidence-based review): report of the Quality Standards Subcommittee of the American Academy of Neurology. *Neurology*, **66** (7), 976–982.

37 Horstink, M., Tolosa, E., Bonuccelli, U., Deuschl, G., Friedman, A., Kanovsky, P., *et al.* (2006) Review of the therapeutic management of Parkinson's disease. Report of a joint task force of the European Federation of Neurological Societies (EFNS) and the Movement

Disorder Society-European Section (MDS-ES). Part II: late (complicated) Parkinson's disease. *European Journal of Neurology*, **13** (11), 1186–1202.

38 Adams, C.E., Rathbone, J., Thornley, B., Clarke, M., Borrill, J., Wahlbeck, K., *et al.* (2005) Chlorpromazine for schizophrenia: a Cochrane systematic review of 50 years of randomised controlled trials (Brief record). *BMC Medicine*, **3**, 15.

39 Maidment, I., Fox, C., and Boustani, M. (2006) Cholinesterase inhibitors for Parkinson's disease dementia. *Cochrane Database Systematic Reviews*, (1), 004747.

A Patient's Story

Parkinson's Story

Gunnar Henriksson

When I was diagnosed with Parkinson's disease in the spring of 2004 I thought life was over. I thought I would be in a wheelchair in two years, and dead in four. And I thought this way in spite of what my neurologist told me. I'll never forget the feeling of despair, of wondering, "Is this all there is?"

But when I met with the counselor at the Parkinson's Society she assured me this wasn't the case, and that people often lived for 10 or 20 or more years with Parkinson's. She then took me down to the movement disorder clinic at the General Hospital, where I met the physiotherapist. When she found out that I lifted weights, the physiotherapist encouraged me to do some leg work every time I went to the gym, to keep my legs strong – because when they're gone, I would be in trouble.

So, I did as I was told and over the next couple of years my legs got stronger, until eventually I was lifting weights that I hadn't lifted for 20 years. In November 2006, I was having lunch with Dennis, a friend of mine who happens to be a professional powerlifting coach. We were talking about weightlifting, and he asked me if I had ever seen the Alberta Powerlifting website. I said no, but later that evening I checked it out.

I discovered that there were separate categories for older lifters. Masters 1 for the 40- to 49-year-olds, Masters 2 for 50- to 59-year-olds, Masters 3 for 60- to 69-year olds, and Masters 4 for those aged 70 and over. Out of curiosity, when I checked out the 125 kg weight class for the 50-year-olds I discovered that the squat record was 175 kg (385 lb). At the time, as I was squatting about 320 lb, I wondered if Dennis could coach me and help me take a run at the squat record?

I approached Denis with the idea, and then took two months to convince him I was serious! When he began coaching me in February 2007 we started off on a four days a week training regimen – on Tuesday we did squats and bench press, on Thursday the bench press and deadlift, on Saturday squats and bench press, and on Sunday the bench press and deadlift. I had never trained so consistently before, and certainly never four days a week.

Right around the same time I approached Ray Williams, the executive director of the Parkinson's society, and told him what I was doing. I asked him how I could inspire others with Parkinson's, or those who might be diagnosed with Parkinson's in the future, to not give in to the disease and just quit living. How could I encourage them to strive for new goals and successes, in spite of Parkinson's? How could I show them that there is a life after Parkinson's? How could I give them hope? Ray's answer to me was just to carry on with what I was doing, and they would report my story in their newspaper – which they did in March 2007.

In June 2007, at the provincial championships, I was fortunate enough to set a new squat record, which led to the Parkinson's society doing a follow-up story on me in the October edition of the paper. And added to that, in September 2007 I appeared on Global TV and on CTV, promoting the Super walk charity event.

Over the months, many people have approached me in the gym, asking if I'm "that guy on TV." In fact, the whole thing has taken on a new life – I've been told by many people from all walks of life, that I inspire them and give them hope. So many people have told me how proud they are of me – I'm flattered and humbled. I'm just a guy who happens to be good at lifting weights, and I wanted to encourage people with Parkinson's not to quit. I never realized so much more would come of this.

I'm very fortunate that all I have at the moment is the tremors or shaking, although once in a while I get severe cramps. There are people with Parkinson's who can't walk without a walker, or can't even walk at all. Some people also have difficulty swallowing and eating, and others with Parkinson's can't drive anymore, and many of them can't work. And sadly, quite often when Parkinson's is diagnosed they lose their spouse too.

For me, the hardest part about having Parkinson's is knowing what's coming up as the condition progresses, and worrying about how am I going to survive. But I refuse to quit, and I'll try to keep improving at my sport for as long as I can.

So, where do we go from here? I can squat 445 lb now, and plan to do 600 lb, I can bench press 365 lb, and plan to do 500 lb, and I can deadlift 445 lb, and plan to do 600 lb. That's assuming that I have the time!

People often ask me why I do all this. Why do you put yourself through the pain that you do? But my coach sent me an e-mail explaining it all – pain is temporary, pride is forever! I'm very proud of what I can lift, and I like telling people at the gym that if I can do this with Parkinson's at my age, think of what you could when you are younger and healthy?

Over the years I have met some of the most wonderful people because of Parkinson's, and I am so grateful. The folk I have met through weightlifting have welcomed me into their sport and have helped me, coached me, and encouraged me. And the people I've met from the Parkinson's society are the kindest and sweetest you could ever meet. I'm very fortunate that I came down with Parkinson's and have met the people I have because of it. Yes, life is a challenge – but it's what you make of it that counts.

10
Highlights of Current Research in Parkinson Disease

Wayne Martin and Bin Hu

Whilst a tremendous amount of information has been learned about the causes, pathophysiology, and treatment of Parkinson disease (PD) since its original description in 1817 (much of which is summarized elsewhere in this book), there remain many "unknowns." A great deal of research activity is currently under way in many centers worldwide, with the general objective of extending knowledge related to the basic mechanisms that underlie the development and progression of PD, the short-term goal of improving treatment and lessening disability, and the long-term goal of altering the course of the disease process itself, ultimately to achieve a cure. A PubMed search of the term "Parkinson's" yields more than 15 000 citations published during the past five years. The aim of this chapter is not to discuss the entire spectrum of current research activities, but rather to review some recent developments and emerging trends pertaining to PD and its management, with specific reference to current research in the province of Alberta.

10.1
Overview of Research Policy

Traditionally, research activities in PD fall into two main streams: basic and clinical. Fundamental theoretical or experimental investigations designed primarily to advance scientific knowledge are usually categorized as "basic research." In contrast, clinical research may involve a particular person or group of people (e.g., patients with PD), and include studies of the mechanisms of human disease, of clinical trials of new treatments, the development of new technologies related to disease management, of epidemiological and behavioral studies, and of the outcomes and health services research. One major objective of clinical research is to improve the understanding and treatment of specific disease processes. During recent years, much emphasis has been placed on translational research [1, 2] which, in a nutshell, is by itself not a new genre. Rather, it is a framework or mechanism that can be utilized to facilitate interactions between basic and clinical research, and to streamline the process that translates discovery into application. The need for such a framework is both obvious and overdue. Life science in

Parkinson Disease – A Health Policy Perspective. Edited by Wayne Martin, Oksana Suchowersky,
Katharina Kovacs Burns, and Egon Jonsson
Copyright © 2010 WILEY-VCH Verlag GmbH & Co. KGaA, Weinheim
ISBN: 978-3-527-32779-9

general – and health research in particular – is transdisciplinary in nature, and often involves a lengthy process of iteration and trial by error. It is becoming increasingly difficult to bring a new procedure, technique or drug from the laboratory to clinical use, as the process is extremely complex, time-consuming, and expensive. A translational research approach could be expected to help alleviate some of these problems by encouraging basic and clinical scientists to form partnerships, to share resources, and to engage in collaborative efforts. It is hoped that this will create a path of minimum resistance through which not only the quality of research will itself be significantly enhanced, but the entire process of discovery, innovation, and application will become more coherent, focused, and affordable. It is noteworthy that the push for "translational research" is taking place on both sides of the Canada/US border, and has received strong endorsements from many granting agencies, including the Michael J Fox Foundation (which to date has distributed US$129 million), the National Institutes of Health, and the Morris K. Udall Parkinson Disease Center of Excellence Programs in the US. In Canada, the Canadian Institutes of Health Research (CIHR) has funded two translational research teams in PD. The first team, headquartered at the University of Calgary and led by Professor Bin Hu, is investigating sensory-motor cueing and the non-pharmaceutical management of PD. The second team is located at the University of British Columbia (headed by Professor Jon Stoessl), and is focused on functional brain imaging. In addition, NeuroScience Canada supports a PD research team led by Louise Trudeau and David Park at the University of Ottawa to study the mechanism of dopaminergic cell death. It is believed that, given its financial health, entrepreneurial culture and desire to reduce escalating cost of healthcare delivery, the province of Alberta should play a significant role in PD research.

10.1.1
Basic Research

In the past, PD has been considered to be one of the best understood neurodegenerative disorders, thus promoting the speculation that a cure would be in sight within the decade. Unfortunately, however, it has become increasingly clear that the underlying etiology and pathological changes of PD are significantly more complex than originally anticipated, with both genetic and environmental factors now known to play roles in the development of the disease.

10.1.2
Genetic Predisposition

Overall, less than 10% of PD cases have a strict familial etiology, whereas the majority are sporadic. Some 13 genetic loci (denoted PARK1 to 13) have been identified so far for PD, five of which have clear genetic products that can be causatively linked to the disease [3–5]. A prominent example of this is the PARK1 gene which encodes α-synuclein. Three missense mutations in α-synuclein gene are associated with autosomal dominant PD. It has been shown that α-synuclein normally functions as an unfolded presynaptic protein [6–8]. Certain truncated forms of the protein can form dense neurotoxic aggregates or inclusions in neuronal somata and/or neurites, causing cell death [8, 9]. Indeed, α-synuclein is a major component of Lewy body inclusions, which are found in dopaminergic nigrostriatal neurons and other brain regions in PD patients (including sporadic cases) [10]. The level of α-synuclein in the cerebrospinal fluid of PD patients is also significantly reduced, which suggests that it may serve as a biomarker of disease progression [11]. However, recent studies of α-synuclein neurotoxicity in animals have yielded conflicting results, it has been shown that an accumulation of misfolded proteins *per se* may either be toxic or neuroprotective [10, 12–15]. Clearly, further research is required to establish the existence of any causal relationship between α-synuclein, neuronal death, and the appearance of behavioral abnormalities. The characterization of other mutations is also providing increasing evidence as to the etiology and pathogenesis of PD. In spite of the growth in this area, analysis for genetic mutations is available only for research purposes and should not be used for confirmation of diagnosis of PD.

10.1.3
Environmental Factors

There is strong epidemiological and genomic data supporting an environmental etiology of idiopathic PD. For example, elevated levels of iron in the substantia nigra (SN) have been associated with sporadic PD [16–18]. In mice, a combined environmental paraquat and neonatal iron exposure can result in an age-related degeneration of the nigrostriatal dopaminergic neurons, though this can be partially rescued by the administration of antioxidants [19]. In a recent study of industrial emissions of manganese in the cities of Toronto and Hamilton, Finkelstein and Jerrett have shown that exposure to ambient manganese was associated with an earlier age of diagnosis of PD in a cohort of 110 000 subjects [20]. Hence, a diminishing environmental exposure to certain toxic heavy metals and compounds such as paraquat may prove to be an important area of research in disease prevention. On a cautionary note, however, research teams interested in pursuing environmental toxicity in PD must consider any potential legal implications (especially in the US), as research into this subject has already led to high-profile lawsuits and broad media attention [21].

10.1.4
Mechanism of Disease Progression

The results of recent pathological and genetic studies have made it clear that PD is not a homogeneous disease entity affecting only dopaminergic system. Rather, extensive neuropathological examinations have demonstrated the presence of neurodegenerative inclusions in the noradrenergic neurons of the locus coeruleus, in the cholinergic neurons of the nucleus basalis of Meynert, as well as in nerve cells in the dorsal motor nucleus of the vagus, the pedunculopontine nucleus, olfactory region, cerebral cortex, spinal cord, and peripheral autonomic nervous system [22]. Some of the degeneration in nondopaminergic regions may precede the development of a dopaminergic pathology [22]. These findings support clinical data showing that many PD symptoms do not respond to levodopa treatment. For example, gait disturbances – such as freezing of gait and falling – are common and potentially disabling features in advanced patients with PD. Nevertheless, gait and postural instability typically shows a minimal – if any – response to levodopa. Furthermore, certain non-motor symptoms, including sleep disturbances, impaired olfaction, and constipation, often precede the onset of the classic motor features of PD [23–25]. Indeed, the Sydney multicenter study has found that, after 15 years of treatment, the disabilities of PD patients are primarily related to levodopa-unresponsive symptoms [23]. Therefore, future basic research should perhaps invest more efforts towards understanding the non-dopamine-related mechanisms of disease progression.

10.2
Clinical Research

10.2.1
Neuroimaging

10.2.1.1 Functional Brain Imaging

Generally, PD is diagnosed on the basis of its characteristic clinical features, since routine imaging procedures do not demonstrate any significant abnormalities. However, extensive investigations have been conducted with several types of functional brain imaging, utilizing positron emission tomography (PET) and single photon emission computed tomography (SPECT). The application of these techniques can allow for the quantitation of processes that are specific to the dopaminergic pathway, and are impaired in patients with PD [26]. While definite PD-related abnormalities can often be detected, these techniques remain primarily in the research environment, and have not seen widespread application in the diagnosis or management of patients, in part because their diagnostic accuracy is not significantly greater than a clinical examination and because, in the absence of any treatments that alter disease progression, there may be little to be gained with an early confirmation of the diagnosis. However, once effective neuroprotective treatments have been developed, an early diagnosis will become very important. Nonetheless, at present these techniques are extremely useful within a research setting, in order to study features such as disease progression and compensatory mechanisms [27–29].

In clinical trials with new medications in PD, it is common to demonstrate a substantial symptomatic benefit even in the placebo-treated group. An interesting application of PET has resulted in an improved understanding of the physiological basis for this placebo response, with the demonstration that the expectation of a symptomatic benefit alone can result in dopamine release in the brain [30, 31]. This serves to emphasize the importance of including appropriate placebo-treated groups when evaluating potential new treatments for PD.

10.2.1.2 Structural Imaging

Although, conventional magnetic resonance imaging (MRI) shows no convincing abnormalities in PD, more advanced MRI techniques have been useful in elucidating some of the associated structural changes that occur in the brain. The present authors' group at the University of Alberta has utilized a technique to estimate regional iron content in the midbrain in patients with PD, to show that iron accumulation in the lateral substantia nigra correlates with the severity of the motor symptomatology in the early disease [16]. This provides a tool that may be of value in assessing disease progression since, unlike clinical assessments, the MRI abnormalities will not be affected by medications that provide symptomatic benefit. MRI has also been utilized to measure tissue volumes in PD, and has shown that patients with PD who are developing dementia have evidence of atrophy affecting the hippocampus [32]. It has also been shown that the right amygdala is atrophic in PD, while data have been acquired suggesting that this abnormality may occur very early during the course of the disease [33]. These observations attest to the multisystem nature of PD, and provide further support for the impression that non-dopaminergic mechanisms are an important part of the disease process.

10.2.2
Treatment

10.2.2.1 Cell Therapy

In recent years, the transplantation of cells to the brain has been pursued as a potential symptomatic treatment for PD, based on the rationale that cells producing dopamine or growth factors may be effective at replacing the dysfunctional nigral dopaminergic input that underlies many of the motor features of the disease, as recently reviewed by Bjorklund *et al.* [34] and Laguna Goya *et al.* [35]. Initial attempts at cell replacement therapy used an autologous transplantation of the patient's own adrenal medulla as a source of dopaminergic neurons. After some initial enthusiasm [36], however, this procedure has been abandoned because of the minimal clinical improvements and significant morbidity and mortality associated with the procedure [37].

Extensive preclinical experimentation in animal models of PD has demonstrated that the implantation of tissue derived from the fetal midbrain can be effective at ameliorating the motor symptoms associated with dopamine depletion [34]. Subsequently, clinical trials have shown that the transplantation of fetal midbrain tissue into the striatum of individuals with PD can be associated with the long-term survival of implanted neurons, with the development of functional connections with striatal neurons, and with clinical benefit in some patients. However, there are major problems associated with this method of treatment, including the observations that clinical efficacy varies substantially among individuals, and that a significant number of treated patients have developed graft-induced dyskinesias [38, 39].

More recently, there has been widespread excitement regarding the potential for *stem cells* to reverse the motor symptomatology of PD. Stem cells can potentially provide a renewable source of dopamine-producing midbrain neurons, alleviating many of the ethical and practical concerns associated with the use of human fetal tissue, while introducing other ethical and political issues [34]. Although extensive experimentation has shown that a variety of human stem cells can provide a source of dopaminergic or growth factor-producing neurons, many unanswered questions currently stand between the theoretical advantages of this type of treatment and its clinical implementation as a routine procedure. One important issue is that the uncontrolled proliferation of transplanted undifferentiated embryonal stem cells may potentially lead to tumor (teratoma) formation [40].

An additional concern with any type of cell-based therapy directed at dopaminergic motor mechanisms, is that it is becoming increasingly clear that PD is a multisystem disorder affecting more than the dopaminergic neuronal systems. Non-dopaminergic motor and other clinical features are a major source of disability, particularly in patients with more advanced PD. Dopamine replacement alone, whether by medication, fetal transplantation, or stem cell-derived implants, would not be expected to have any significant impact on disability related to non-dopaminergic mechanisms [24].

10.2.2.2 Neural Growth Factors

Over the past decade, evidence has accumulated that the adult human brain has the potential to generate its own neurons, and is therefore much more plastic than was previously thought. Several growth factors have been identified that may play roles in promoting the regrowth of dysfunctional nigral neurons and/or nigrostriatal connections, with glial cell line-derived neurotrophic factor (GDNF) having received particular attention [41]. However, in spite of some promising findings in animal studies and open-label studies in humans, a large-scale double-blind, placebo-controlled study of GDNF infused directly into the putamen did not improve motor symptoms in patients with PD [42]. Issues related to this negative study, and to the future of trophic factor therapy in PD, have recently been reviewed [43].

10.2.2.3 Gene Therapy

The rationale underlying a gene therapy approach is that cells can be induced to produce specific substances by introducing an appropriate gene directly into the affected cells [44]. Potential approaches in PD include the insertion of a gene involved in dopamine production in nigrostriatal neurons in an attempt to normalize levels of the enzyme amino acid decarboxylase (AADC), which is deficient in PD [45], or of a gene involved in growth factor production (such as neurturin, a growth factor that is closely related to GDNF) to stimulate the proliferation of affected neurons [46]. Another approach currently being explored involves the insertion of a gene involved in the production of γ-aminobutyric acid (GABA), the major inhibitory neurotransmitter in the brain. This is based on the hypothesis that the reestablishment of normal brain activity within motor circuits might reverse the motor features of PD [47]. While pilot studies utilizing these approaches have been completed, much additional research is required, first to refine the techniques used to deliver the gene to relevant cells, and subsequently to evaluate the efficacy and safety of the procedure. The potential risks and design issues to be considered in clinical trials of gene therapy have recently been reviewed [48]. Issues related to the multisystem nature of PD, as described previously, are as important in considering the potential impact of gene therapy and other neurotrophic factor delivery systems as they are in considering cell-based therapies.

10.2.2.4 Deep Brain Stimulation

Deep brain stimulation (DBS) is associated with significant improvements of motor complications and the patients' quality of life in advanced PD [49–51]. Recently, high-frequency stimulation of the subthalamic nucleus (STN) has become the surgical therapy of choice, although there is no evidence that DBS offers any neuroprotective effect that may retard disease progression [49, 52]. Some controversy persists, however, regarding the ideal target location for DBS, and a clinical trial is currently under way examining the relative merits of an STN versus globus pallidus interna target [53, 54]. The potential neuropsychological disturbances caused by STN-DBS have been examined in several recent clinical studies, and cognitive complications have been recognized as rare; however, suicides have been reported following DBS for movement disorders [55, 56]. An international multicenter retrospective survey has shown the suicide rates during the first postoperative year following STN-DBS (263 in 100 000 patients per year; 0.26%) to be higher than the World Health Organization suicide rate [56]. It is possible that STN-DBS may also cause a unique form of impulsivity, which is unaffected by the dopaminergic medication status [57, 58].

Whether DBS in the pedunculopontine nucleus (PPN) can provide a better relief of gait disturbances and akinesia than STN-DBS has been examined in two recent studies [59, 60]. Subsequently, PPN-DBS was found to be particularly effective on gait and posture, whilst combined STN and PPN-DBS provided an additive improvement when compared to single-target stimulation [60]. Previous studies in animals have identified PPN as a major region involved in locomotion control and sleep regulation [61]. For example, it has been shown in the cat, that the depletion of monoamines with reserpine can lead to the activation of PPN cholinergic neurons, which in turn triggers an abnormally long episode of rapid eye movement (REM) sleep during the daytime and the appearance of eye movement-related activities in the visual thalamus [62, 63]. Such abnormal neural activity is proposed to contribute to visual hallucinations, which are common in PD patients and those with dementia with Lewy bodies [64, 65]. Therefore, the PPN may be an important site for the DBS treatment of sleep- and locomotion-related symptoms.

10.2.3
Translational Research in Alberta

During the past three years, the Hotchkiss Brain Institute and its Movement Disorders and Therapeutic Brain Stimulation Program at the University of Calgary, together with Behavioral Neuroscience Center at the University of Lethbridge, have embarked on a series of translational research projects.

10.2.3.1 Parkinson Disease Rehabilitation

Although PD patients with advanced disease struggle with slowness in movement and stooped posture, it is known that many of them can move normally for a short time period when provided with visual or auditory cues [66–68]. Some can even dance to music with perfect steps, and sing eloquently with joy. Although sensorimotor cueing as a rehabilitation training tool has been formally incorporated the practice guidelines in Europe and USA, the subject is poorly understood. A research team consisting of neurophysiologists, neurologists, neurosurgeons, engineers and physiotherapists was assembled in 2006 at the Universities of Calgary and Lethbridge. The ultimate goal of the research is to test the hypothesis that sound and music can activate alternative sensorimotor pathways, bypassing the dysfunctional basal ganglia. For example, as mentioned above, the PPN can form an important extrastriatal pathway for gait initiation and locomotion regulation [61]. It is also well known that the PPN is a brain site that is highly sensitive to sound stimuli [63, 69, 70]. Hence, auditory or music-based rehabilitation training aimed at the plasticity modulation of these extrastriatal pathways may allow a sustainable reestablishment of certain basic motor function in PD patients. Research conducted by Ian Whishaw has shown that familiar ultrasonic sounds can activate movement in rats, even when they are severely Parkinsonian and cataleptic, supporting the alternative cueing pathway hypothesis [71]. Consistent with these animal studies, Kiss has observed that metronome tones or music elicited no significant auditory responses in the basal ganglia in PD patients [72]. Hu further showed that single neurons in the association auditory cortex, which provide attention and cueing signals, can form widespread and direct connections to various sensorimotor pathways [73]. Clinical trials conducted by Suchowersky and Brown have shown that patients who completed a two- to three-month exercise program while walking to music, experienced noticeable improvements in their gait and balance.

10.2.3.2 Cellular Mechanism of Deep Brain Stimulation

Although DBS has been adopted as an effective treatment of late-stage PD, its mechanism of action remains elusive. Through a series of complementary studies in rats and humans, it was possible to show that the neural basis of DBS therapy involves rapid neurotransmitter depletion at the axonal terminals, leading to a functional deafferentation [74–78]. Furthermore, the cellular effect of DBS can vary significantly, according to which axons are stimulated. For example, myelinated axons can conduct high-frequency DBS pulses to remote sites, away from the stimulated structure, where they can deplete transmitter release and cause functional deafferentation. In contrast, only low-frequency stimulation pulses are conducted along unmyelinated fibers, thereby promoting transmitter release at the target [74]. The notion of functional deafferentation also provides an explanation for many DBS-related phenomena. For example, the reduced excitability of nigral dopaminergic neurons during high-frequency STN stimulation and the enhanced activities of the thalamus and cortex proposed for low-frequency PPN stimulation can both be readily explained based on the deafferentation and axonal filtering mechanisms mentioned above.

10.2.3.3 New Technologies and Medical Devices for Managing Gait Disorder

Recent advances in microchip technology have led to a new generation of miniature sensing devices that are particularly suitable for gait and mobility assessment, and rehabilitation training in clinical settings. The GaitMeter™, a prototype device developed by Dr. Hu and his colleagues [79–82], utilizes a miniature triaxial accelerator and gyroscope and system-on-the-chip technology to acquire high-frequency gait and mobility data during long-distance natural walking. The device, which is controlled by a wearable personal digital assistant (PDA), is equipped with high-speed wireless and video connectivity, and can provide real time feedback. It is currently being tested in pilot trials. A personal Gait Trainer™ is the second line of device under development; this utilizes precise kinematic data collected during a gait cycle and feedback capability to trigger an auditory remainder, either to alert the patient about a potential fall, or to facilitate stepping.

10.2.4
Future Research in Parkinson's Disease

Despite this broad spectrum of ongoing research activity, many questions remain unanswered. Although numerous genetic and environmental influences related to the development of PD have been identified, the complex interaction between these factors remains largely unexplored. It is probable that different combinations of these factors are operative in different patients and different families. Indeed, it may well be that PD does not have a single cause in all cases.

Although it is well established that PD is a progressive disorder, the mechanisms responsible for such inexorable progression have yet to be fully elucidated. Both, mitochondrial dysfunction and increased oxidative stress may play critical roles in the pathogenesis of PD in some individuals. Mitochondrial dysfunction has not been identified, however, in all individuals with PD, indicating that other factors are also involved. It is necessary to identify these additional factors as a preliminary step to developing individualized neuroprotective strategies for altering disease progression. Establishing an effective therapeutic strategy to alter the natural history of the disease is a high priority for the research teams and, of course, for the patients and their families.

The potential effects of symptomatic treatments such as levodopa and dopamine agonists on the natural history of PD have been studied extensively. Although as yet there is no convincing evidence that these treatments have a deleterious effect on disease progression, it is less clear whether they may be beneficial in terms of slowing progression. Independently from any potential effect on progression, it is clear that dopaminergic treatments are frequently associated with motor complications such as fluctuations and dyskinesias. It is important to establish an effective means of decreasing the prevalence of these complications, and to lessen the associated disability when these complications do occur. Similarly, it is necessary to establish effective means of dealing with the non-motor complications of treatment, such as the excessive daytime somnolence and impulse control disorders (e.g., pathologic gambling, hypersexuality, binge eating, and compulsive shopping) that may be associated with some of these medications.

In the past, PD has been considered to be a disorder primarily of dopaminergic neurons, with motor dysfunction being the major clinical abnormality. It is becoming increasingly clear, however, that other (non-dopaminergic) neuronal systems are also involved and that disability, particularly in those with more advanced disease, is related in large part to non-motor symptoms. The effective implementation of disease-altering treatments will need to address not only the dopaminergic but also the non-dopaminergic aspects of the disease. Dementia is a particularly important source of disability in patients with more advanced PD. New treatments are desperately needed to lessen the morbidity associated with this non-dopaminergic aspect of brain functioning.

Research into how best to provide the health services required by individuals with PD is an important prerequisite to achieving the goals of decreasing disease-related morbidity and, through effective knowledge transfer, of bringing advances derived from basic and clinical research to the bedside. While the nature of health service needs may change with disease progression, all affected individuals require access to multidisciplinary care from individuals with expertise in medical, surgical, nursing, rehabilitation, dietary, and psychological aspects of this complex disorder. Patients with advanced disease, many of whom are living in long-term care facilities, present a particular challenge as their predominant problems may not be responsive to traditional dopaminergic or surgical treatments.

References

1 Horig, H., Marincola, E., and Marincola, F.M. (2005) Obstacles and opportunities in translational research. *Nature Medicine*, **11**, 705–708.

2 Horig, H. and Pullman, W. (2004) From bench to clinic and back: perspective on the 1st IQPC Translational Research conference. *Journal of Translational Medicine*, **2**, 44.

3 Dawson, T.M. (2007) Unraveling the role of defective genes in Parkinson's disease. *Parkinsonism and Related Disorders*, **13** (Suppl. 3), S248–S249.

4 Cookson, M.R. (2005) The biochemistry of Parkinson's disease. *Annual Review of Biochemistry*, **74**, 29–52.

5 von Bohlen und Halbach, O., Schober, A., and Krieglstein, K. (2004) Genes, proteins, and neurotoxins involved in Parkinson's disease. *Progress in Neurobiology*, **73**, 151–177.

6 Thomas, B. and Beal, M.F. (2007) Parkinson's disease. *Human Molecular Genetics*, **16**, R183–R194.

7 Abeliovich, A., Schmitz, A., Fariñas, I., *et al.* (2000) Mice lacking [alpha]-synuclein display functional deficits in the nigrostriatal dopamine system. *Neuron*, **25**, 239–252.

8 Yavich, L., Tanila, H., Vepsäläinen, S., and Jäkälä, P. (2004) Role of α-synuclein in presynaptic dopamine recruitment. *Journal of Neuroscience*, **24**, 11165–11170.

9 Spillantini, M.G., Crowther, R.A., Jakes, R, Hasegawa, M., and Goedert, M. (1998) Alpha-synuclein in filamentous

inclusions of Lewy bodies from Parkinson's disease and dementia with Lewy bodies. *Proceedings of the National Academy of Sciences of the United States of America*, **95**, 6469–6473.

10 Periquet, M., Fulga, T., Myllykangas, L., Schlossmacher, M.G., and Feany, M.B. (2007) Aggregated alpha-synuclein mediates dopaminergic neurotoxicity *in vivo*. *Journal of Neuroscience*, **27**, 3338–3346.

11 Tokuda, T., Salem, S.A., Allsop, D., *et al.* (2006) Decreased alpha-synuclein in cerebrospinal fluid of aged individuals and subjects with Parkinson's disease. *Biochemical and Biophysical Research Communications*, **349**, 162–166.

12 Bodner, R.A., Outeiro, T.F., Altmann, S., *et al.* (2006) Pharmacological promotion of inclusion formation: a therapeutic approach for Huntington's and Parkinson's diseases. *Proceedings of the National Academy of Sciences of the United States of America*, **103**, 4246–4251.

13 Lo Bianco, C., Schneider, B.L., Bauer, M., *et al.* (2004) Lentiviral vector delivery of parkin prevents dopaminergic degeneration in an alpha-synuclein rat model of Parkinson's disease. *Proceedings of the National Academy of Sciences of the United States of America*, **101**, 17510–17515.

14 Chandra, S., Gallardo, G., Fernández-Chácon, R., Schlüter, O.M., and Südhof, T.C. (2005) Alpha-synuclein cooperates with CSPalpha in preventing neurodegeneration. *Cell*, **123**, 383–396.

15 Manning-Bog, A.B., McCormack, A.L., Purisai, M.G., Bolin, L.M., and DiMonte, D.A. (2003) Alpha -synuclein overexpression protects against paraquat-induced neurodegeneration. *Journal of Neuroscience*, **23**, 3095–3099.

16 Martin, W.R.W., Wieler, M., and Gee, M. (2008) Midbrain iron content in early Parkinson disease: a potential biomarker of disease status. *Neurology*, **70**, 1411–1417.

17 Griffiths, P.D., Dobson, B.R., Jones, G.R., and Clarke, D.T. (1999) Iron in the basal ganglia in Parkinson's disease: an *in vitro* study using extended X-ray absorption fine structure and cryo-electron microscopy. *Brain*, **122**, 667–673.

18 Sofic, E., Paulus, W., Jellinger, K., Riederer, P., and Youdim, M.B. (1991) Selective increase of iron in substantia-nigra zona compacta of parkinsonian brains. *Journal of Neurochemistry*, **56**, 978–982.

19 Peng, J., Peng, L., Stevenson, F.F., Doctrow, S.R., and Andersen, J.K. (2007) Iron and paraquat as synergistic environmental risk factors in sporadic Parkinson's disease accelerate age-related neurodegeneration. *Journal of Neuroscience*, **27**, 6914–6922.

20 Finkelstein, M.M. and Jerrett, M. (2007) A study of the relationships between Parkinson's disease and markers of traffic-derived and environmental manganese air pollution in two Canadian cities. *Environmental Research*, **104**, 420–432.

21 Racette, B.A., Bradley, A., Wrisberg, C.A., and Perlmutter, J.S. (2006) The impact of litigation on neurologic research. *Neurology*, **67**, 2124–2128.

22 Braak, H., Tredici, K.D., Rüb, U., de Vos, R.A.I., Jansen Steur, E.N.H., and Braak, E. (2003) Staging of brain pathology related to sporadic Parkinson's disease. *Neurobiological Aging*, **24**, 197–211.

23 Hely, M.A., Morris, J.G., Reid, W.G., and Trafficante, R. (2005) Sydney multicenter study of Parkinson's disease: non-l-dopa-responsive problems dominate at 15 years. *Movement Disorders*, **20**, 190–199.

24 Lang, A.E. and Obeso, J.A. (2004) Challenges in Parkinson's disease: restoration of the nigrostriatal dopamine system is not enough. *Lancet Neurology*, **3**, 309–316.

25 Nomoto, M. and Nagai, M. (2006) Pharmacological consideration of the symptoms resistant to dopaminergic therapy. *Parkinsonism and Related Disorders*, **12** (Suppl. 2), S83–S87.

26 Ravina, B., Eidelberg, D., Ahlskop, J.E., *et al.* (2005) The role of radiotracer imaging in Parkinson disease. *Neurology*, **64**, 208–215.

27 Adams, J.R., van Netten, H., Schulzer, M., *et al.* (2005) PET in LRRK2 mutations: comparison to sporadic

Parkinson's disease and evidence for presymptomatic compensation. *Brain*, **128**, 2777–2785.

28 Sossi, V., de la Fuente-Fernández, R., Schulzer, M., Troiano, A.R., Ruth, T.J., and Stoessl, A.J. (2007) Dopamine transporter relation to dopamine turnover in Parkinson's disease: a positron emission tomography study. *Annals of Neurology*, **62**, 468–474.

29 Martin, W.R., Wieler, M., Stoessl, A.J., and Schulzer, M. (2008) Dihydrotetrabenazine positron emission tomography imaging in early, untreated Parkinson's disease. *Annals of Neurology*, 63, 388–394.

30 de la Fuente-Fernández, R., Ruth, T.J., Sossi, V., Schulzer, M., Calne, D.B., and Stoessl, A.J. (2001) Expectation and dopamine release: mechanism of the placebo effect in Parkinson's disease. *Science*, **293**, 1164–1166.

31 de la Fuente-Fernández, R., Schulzer, M., and Stoessl, A.J. (2004) Placebo mechanisms and reward circuitry: clues from Parkinson's disease. *Biological Psychiatry*, **56**, 67–71.

32 Bouchard, T.P., Malykhin, N., Martin, W.R., *et al.* (2008) Age and demential-associated atrophy predominates in the hippocampal head and amygdale in Parkinson's disease. *Neurobiology and Aging*, **29**, 1027–1039.

33 Martin, W.R., Wieler, M., Gee, M., and Camcioli, R.M. (2009) Temporal lobe changes in early, untreated Parkinson's disease. *Movement Disorders*, **24**, 1949–1954.

34 Björklund, A., Dunnett, S.B., Brundin, P., *et al.* (2003) Neural transplantation for the treatment of Parkinson's disease. *Lancet Neurology*, **2**, 437–445.

35 Laguna Goya, R., Tyers, P., and Barker, R.A. (2008) The search for a curative cell therapy in Parkinson's disease. *Journal of Neurological Science*, **265**, 32–42.

36 Madrazo, I., Drucker-Colín, R., Díaz, V., Martínez-Mata, J., Torres, C., and Becerril, J.J. (1987) Open microsurgical autograft of adrenal medulla to the right caudate nucleus in two patients with intractable Parkinson's disease. *New England Journal of Medicine*, **316**, 831–834.

37 Goetz, C.G., Stebbins, G.T., III, Klawans, H.L., *et al.* (1991) United Parkinson Foundation Neurotransplantation Registry on adrenal medullary transplants: presurgical, and 1- and 2-year follow-up. *Neurology*, **41**, 1719–1722.

38 Freed, C.R., Greene, P.E., Breeze, R.E., *et al.* (2001) Transplantation of embryonic dopamine neurons for severe Parkinson's disease. *New England Journal of Medicine*, **344**, 710–719.

39 Olanow, C.W., Goetz, C.G., Kordower, J.H., *et al.* (2003) A double-blind controlled trial of bilateral fetal nigral transplantation in Parkinson's disease. *Annals of Neurology*, **54**, 403–414.

40 Roy, N.S., Cleren, C., Singh, S.K., Yang, L., Beal, M.F., and Goldman, S.A. (2006) Functional engraftment of human ES cell-derived dopaminergic neurons enriched by coculture with telomerase-immortalized midbrain astrocytes. *Nature Medicine*, **12**, 1259–1268.

41 Deierborg, T., Soulet, D., Roybon, L., Hall, V., and Brundin, P. (2008) Emerging restorative treatments for Parkinson's disease. *Progress in Neurobiology*, **85**, 407–432.

42 Lang, A.E., Gill, S., Patel, *et al.* (2006) Randomized controlled trial of intraputamenal glial cell line-derived neurotrophic factor infusion in Parkinson Disease. *Annals of Neurology*, **59**, 459–466.

43 Sherer, T.B., Fiske, B.K., Svendsen, C.N., Lang, A.E., and Langston, J.W. (2006) Crossroads in GDNF therapy for Parkinson's disease. *Movement Disorders*, **21**, 136–141.

44 Fiandaca, M., Forsayeth, J., and Bankiewicz, K. (2008) Current status of gene therapy trials for Parkinson's disease. *Experimental Neurology*, **209**, 51–57.

45 Eberling, J.L., Jagust, W.J., Christine, C.W., *et al.* (2008) Results from a phase I safety trial of hAADC gene therapy for Parkinson Disease. *Neurology*, **70**, 1980–1983.

46 Gasmi, M., Brandon, E.P., Herzog, C.D., *et al.* (2007) AAV2-medicated delivery of human neurturin to the rate nigristriatal system: long-term efficacy and

tolerability of CERE-120 for Parkinson's disease. *Neurobiology of Disease*, **27**, 67–76.

47 Kaplitt, M.G., Feigin, A., Tang, C., *et al.* (2007) Safety and tolerability of gene therapy with an adeno-associated virus (AAV) borne GAD gene for Parkinson's disease: an open label, phase 1 trial. *Lancet*, **369**, 2097–2105.

48 Lewis, T.B. and Standaert, D.G. (2008) Design of clinical trials of gene therapy in Parkinson disease. *Experimental Neurology*, **209**, 41–47.

49 Wichmann, T. and Delong, M.R. (2006) Deep brain stimulation for neurologic and neuropsychiatric disorders. *Neuron*, **52**, 197–204.

50 Perlmutter, J.S. and Mink, J.W. (2006) Deep brain stimulation. *Annual Review of Neuroscience*, **29**, 229–257.

51 Kleiner-Fisman, G., Fisman, D.N., Zamir, O., *et al.* (2003) Long-term follow up of bilateral deep brain stimulation of the subthalamic nucleus in patients with advanced Parkinson disease. *Journal of Neurosurgery*, **99**, 489–495.

52 Charles, P.D., Gill, C.E., Davis, T.L., Konrad, P.E., and Benabid, A.L. (2008) Is deep brain stimulation neuroprotective if applied early in the course of PD? *Nature Clinical Practice. Neurology*, **4**, 424–426.

53 Deogaonkar, M., Walter, B.L. , Boulis, N., and Starr, P. (2007) Clinical problem solving: finding the target. *Neurosurgery*, **61**, 815–825.

54 Melinda, P., Gary, M.A., and William, J.M., Jr. (2005) Deep brain stimulation for the treatment of Parkinson's disease: overview and impact on gait and mobility. *NeuroRehabilitation*, **20**, 223–232.

55 Appleby, B.A., Duggan, B.S., Regenberg, A., and Rabins, P.V. (2007) Psychiatric and neuropsychiatric adverse events associated with deep brain stimulation: a meta-analysis of ten years' experience. *Movement Disorders*, **22**, 1722–1728.

56 Voon, V., Krack, P., Lang, A.E., *et al.* (2008) A multicentre study on suicide outcomes following subthalamic stimulation for Parkinson's disease. *Brain*, **131**, 2720–2728.

57 Welberg, L. (2007) Neurological disorders: stimulating side effects. *Nature Reviews. Neuroscience*, **8**, 913.

58 Frank, M.J., Samanta, J., Moustafa, A.A., and Sherman, S.J. (2007) Hold your horses: impulsivity, deep brain stimulation, and medication in parkinsonism. *Science*, **318**, 1309–1312.

59 Plaha, P. and Gill, S.S. (2005) Bilateral deep brain stimulation of the peduncu-lopontine nucleus for Parkinson's disease. *NeuroReport*, **28**, 1883–1887.

60 Stefani, A., Lozano, A.M., Peppe, A., *et al.* (2007) Bilateral deep brain stimulation of the pedunculopontine and subthalamic nuclei in severe Parkinson's disease. *Brain*, **130**, 1596–1607.

61 Pahapill, P.A. and Lozano, A.M. (2000) The pedunculopontine nucleus and Parkinson's disease. *Brain*, **123**, 1767–1783.

62 Hu, B., Bouhassira, D., Steride, M., and Deschenes, M. (1988) The blockage of ponto-geniculo-occipital waves in the cat lateral geniculate nucleus by nicotinic antagonists. *Brain Research*, **473**, 394–397.

63 Hu, B., Steriade, M., and Deschenes, M. (1989) The cellular mechanism of thalamic ponto-geniculo-occipital waves. *Neuroscience*, **31**, 25–35.

64 Manford, M. and Andermann, F. (1998) Complex visual hallucinations. Clinical and neurobiological insights. *Brain*, **121**, 1819–1840.

65 Arnulf, I., Bonnet, A.M., Damier, P., *et al.* (2000) Hallucinations, REM sleep, and Parkinson's disease: a medical hypothesis. *Neurology*, **55**, 281–288.

66 Rubinstein, T.C., *et al.* (2002) The power of cueing to circumvent dopamine deficits: a review of physical therapy treatment of gait disturbances in Parkinson's disease. *Movement Disorders*, **17**, 1148–1160.

67 Nieuwboer, A. (2008) Cueing for freezing of gait in patients with Parkinson's disease: a rehabilitation perspective. *Movement Disorders*, **23** (Suppl. 2), S475–S481.

68 Lim, I., van Wegen, E., de Goede, G., *et al.* (2005) Effects of external rhythmical cueing on gait in patients with

Parkinson's disease: a systematic review. *Clinical Rehabilitation*, **19**, 695–713.

69 Reese, N.B., Garcia-Rill, E., and Skinner, R.D. (1995) The pedunculopontine nucleus–auditory input, arousal and pathophysiology. *Progress in Neurobiology*, **47**, 105–133.

70 Garcia-Rill, E., Homma, Y., and Skinner, R.D. (2004) Arousal mechanisms related to posture and locomotion: 1. Descending modulation. *Progress in Brain Research*, **143**, 283–290.

71 Clark, C.A., Sacrey, A.R., and Whishaw, I.Q. (2007) Activation following familiar sound: an animal model of music-induced improvement in Parkinson's disease. *Society for Neuroscience Annual Meeting Abstract*, **589**, 5/T9.

72 Heming, E.A., Britvina, T., Bonfeld, S.P., Sanden, A., Hu, B., and Kiss, Z.H. (2008) Auditory stimuli and movement modulate local field potential synchronization in the human basal ganglia. *Society for Neuroscience Annual Meeting Abstract*, **578**, 17/QQ19.

73 Chomiak, T., Peters, S., and Hu, B. (2008) Functional architecture and spike timing properties of corticofugal projections from rat ventral temporal cortex. *Journal of Neurophysiology*, **100**, 327–335.

74 Chomiak, T. and Hu, B. (2007) Axonal and somatic filtering of antidromically evoked cortical excitation by simulated deep brain stimulation in rat brain. *Journal of Physiology*, **579**, 403–412.

75 Kiss, Z.H., Mooney, D.M., Renaud, L., and Hu, B. (2002) Neuronal response to local electrical stimulation in rat thalamus: physiological implications for mechanisms of deep brain stimulation. *Neuroscience*, **113**, 137–143.

76 Iremonger, K., Anderson, T.R., Hu, B., and Kiss, Z.H. (2006) Cellular mechanisms preventing sustained activation of cortex during subcortical high frequency stimulation. *Journal of Neurophysiology*, **96**, 613–621.

77 Anderson, T., Hu, B., Pittman, Q., and Kiss, Z.H. (2004) Mechanisms of deep brain stimulation: an intracellular study in rat thalamus. *Journal of Physiology*, **559**, 301–313.

78 Anderson, T.R., Hu, B., Iremonger, K., and Kiss, Z.H. (2006) Selective attenuation of afferent synaptic transmission as a mechanism of thalamic deep brain stimulation-induced tremor arrest. *Journal of Neuroscience*, **26**, 841–850.

79 Hu, B., Melville Jones, G., Fletcher, W.A., Haffenden, A., and Block, E.W. (2007) Automated Timed Up and Go test and dynamic podographs. *Society for Neuroscience Annual Meeting Abstract*, **80**, 3/JJ7.

80 Block, E.W., Melville Jones, G., Fletcher, W.A., and Hu, B. (2007) NeuroExplore I: a wireless high speed sensing system for human kinematic recordings. *Society for Neuroscience Annual Meeting Abstract*, **80**, 1/JJ5.

81 Block, E., Melville Jones, G., Fletcher, W.A., and Hu, B. (2008) Neuroexplore I: a wireless high speed sensing system for human kinematic recordings. *2nd International Congress on Gait and Mental Function, Amsterdam*.

82 Block, E., Melville Jones, G., Block, E.W., Fletcher, W.A., Hu, B, and Horak, F. (2008) Locomotor expression of cognitive intent to walk round a known circular trajectory. *2nd International Congress on Gait and Mental Function, Amsterdam*.

Part II
The Case of Alberta, Canada

Parkinson Disease – A Health Policy Perspective. Edited by Wayne Martin, Oksana Suchowersky,
Katharina Kovacs Burns, and Egon Jonsson
Copyright © 2010 WILEY-VCH Verlag GmbH & Co. KGaA, Weinheim
ISBN: 978-3-527-32779-9

A Patient's Story

"I Have Parkinson's" – Three Words that Have Forever Changed My Life

Cindy Exton

That was seven years ago, when I was aged 42. My reaction? Totally devastated. All phases of grieving, images of my "new" future haunted me. How could this be happening to me? My initial symptom was a slight stiffness in my right hand, but we thought it was just a pinched nerve. After an MRI and many months of uncertainty, I was informed by a Movement Disorder Specialist that I had Young Onset Parkinson's Disease, and that was the day my life changed forever. I have a progressive debilitating brain disease for which there is no known cause or cure. I will never forget that day, sitting in my car in the parking lot at Foothills Hospital, feeling like I had just been kicked in the stomach, crying, and wishing I would wake up from this nightmare. Only it was not a nightmare, it was real.

Parkinson's is not just "shaking"; it is not just taking medication – it is real life, day-to-day coping with the changes and the losses. Everything is affected – family, relationships, career, lifestyle, self. Besides the physical implications, the innermost concept of self and self worth is impaired, and needs to be healed. But with the support of my family and friends I came to realize that PD does not define who I am, and with that came acceptance.

"Life is too short" means so much more. My focus has shifted to "today," not yesterday, and not tomorrow. I drive my Mustang convertible top-down, music-up, as often as I can. I stop to enjoy the view, it's amazing really how much I have to be thankful for.

Volunteer work at the Parkinson's Society has uncovered a passion I didn't know I had, and I know I am making a difference there. The best coping mechanism I have found is to get involved, to participate, contribute, educate, as Parkinson's is often misunderstood. It amazes me really how much one person can achieve if they really want to. As a board member, I challenge, debate, initiate, and support ideas that may help those with PD. I want to be an example of hope; I want to be seen, I want to be heard, I want to fight back while I still can. I want the world to see Parkinson's. I want my kids to learn that through adversity, that we still have choices.

My future ... thoughts of hope, uncertainty and fear. I'm afraid to look down that road, but everyday life gives you no choice. I am still the same person – mom, daughter, sister, auntie, friend, volunteer. This will never change, and for that I am thankful.

We need to find a cure, with proper funding and research, so that my future and the futures of the thousands of people living with PD, can be one to be looked forward to, without the fear.

11

The Incidence and Prevalence of Parkinson Disease in Alberta

Lawrence W. Svenson and Nikolaos W. Yiannakoulias

11.1
Introduction

Parkinson disease (PD) is a progressive neurological disorder with an onset typically occurring in later life. It is characterized by bradykinesia, resting tremor, rigidity, and impaired postural reflexes brought on as a result of degeneration of dopamine-containing neurons in the basal ganglia.

Parkinson disease was first described in 1817 by James Parkinson, an English physician and geologist, in a monograph entitled *An Essay on the Shaking Palsy* [1]. The vivid description of this disorder was based on Parkinson's experience with six patients, one of whom he was able to follow to death, and two he noticed on the streets of London; the fourth patient he saw for only three weeks, a fifth patient he saw "at a distance", and the sixth suffered a stroke. At the time when Parkinson was making his observations, the neurological examination had yet to be formally developed and, as a result, the muscular rigidity appeared to go unnoticed by Parkinson as he focused his attention on the tremor. He was, however, able to distinguish it from tremor due to alcoholism, caffeine, and senility [50].

The entity described by Parkinson was often confused with other conditions, but gradually became better recognized as a separate entity. Charcot and Vulpian [2–5] together published a three-part treatise in 1861 and 1862 which gave Parkinson credit as the first to have described this condition in sufficient detail; they then gave the condition its current name, *Parkinson disease*. Charcot, over the next few years, further elaborated on the description first provided by Parkinson when, during his famous Tuesday lectures, Charcot described the muscular rigidity, stooped posture, thermal paresthesias, and micrographia [6].

11.1.1
Onset and Progression

Parkinson disease can be considered an aging-related disorder with onset typically occurring in mid- to late-life. Idiopathic forms of PD are generally uncommon under the age of 50 years. Diamond *et al.* [51] studied the age of onset and

Parkinson Disease – A Health Policy Perspective. Edited by Wayne Martin, Oksana Suchowersky, Katharina Kovacs Burns, and Egon Jonsson
Copyright © 2010 WILEY-VCH Verlag GmbH & Co. KGaA, Weinheim
ISBN: 978-3-527-32779-9

progression among 47 men and 23 women with idiopathic Parkinson disease (IPD), and found no difference in the age of onset or duration of illness. Thus, it was concluded that PD may reduce the life expectancy of women to the same level as men.

Guttman *et al.* [52] identified a cohort of individuals with PD using administrative health data from Ontario. Thus, a total of 15 304 cases was identified as having parkinsonism as of 1993. To allow for a comparison of the relative risk of mortality, a control group was created in which two controls were selected for each case of parkinsonism. The controls were selected to have the same age and gender as the cases. When both the cases and controls were followed for six years and the mortality assessed, the odds of dying were increased more than two-fold (OR = 2.5, 95% CI: 2.4, 2.6) for PD cases over controls. At the end of the follow-up, 50.8% of PD cases had died, compared to 29.1% of the controls. A similar result was found in Italy by D'Amelio *et al.* [53], where cases with PD had a two-fold increased risk of death.

11.1.2
Male:Female Ratio

While many studies have reported a higher prevalence of PD among males [7–12], a few have found no significant difference [13–16]. In general, male:female ratios vary widely from about 1.2 to 3.7, with men having the higher prevalence. In Alberta, Svenson *et al.* [9] reported a higher prevalence among males, with a male:female ratio of 1.2:1.

11.1.3
Etiology

In 1983, Langston *et al.* [17] described the presence of a Parkinson-like syndrome among four young illicit drug users in California. Upon investigation, it was determined that during the manufacture of "synthetic heroin" the sample had been contaminated with 1-methyl-4-phenyl-1,2,3,6-tetrahydropyridine (MPTP). The latter compound breaks down in the body to 1-methyl-4-phenylpyridinium (MPP$^+$), which selectively destroys dopamine-containing neurons in the basal ganglia. This spawned research into the potential of environmental factors that may have similar characteristics as MPTP, as being causal in the development of PD.

Although a number of potential risk factors have been described, no clear causal mechanism has been fully described. The etiology of PD would appear to be related to a complex interaction between genetic predisposition and environmental exposures.

11.1.4
Risk Factors

A number of studies have been conducted to determine risk factors for PD, but no consistent factor or set of factors has been identified in such a way as to provide the needed evidence to reduce risk. Factors that appear to reduce the risk of PD include smoking, coffee consumption, and vitamin E, whereas factors that appear to be associated with an increased risk of developing PD include surrogate measures such as rural living, farming, and well-water consumption, pesticide exposure, welding, exposure to heavy metals (iron, manganese, copper, lead, amalgam, aluminum, zinc), a family history, and genetics. Monogenetic causes do not appear to have a role in the pathogenesis of PD, although a genetic predisposition may exist.

11.1.5
Incidence and Prevalence

A number of reports have described the incidence and prevalence of PD at several locations (see Table 11.1). Unfortunately, many methods and many different time frames have been used to ascertain cases, which means that any direct comparisons are not only difficult but must also be made with caution. Prevalence is a function of the duration of an illness; if the mortality and/or out-migration are lower than the incidence rate, then the prevalence will *increase* naturally. But prevalence will only be *decreased* if mortality and/or out-migration are in excess of newly diagnosed cases. Given this relationship, it is generally best to compare studies that not only use similar methods, but also have similar time periods. Otherwise, any observed differences in prevalence across multiple locations may be misinterpreted as geographic variations when in fact they may be more related to differing time periods of observation.

Whilst, internationally, there is great variation in the prevalence estimates of PD, there are also consistencies, despite the variations in reported incidences and prevalences. Generally, PD is rare before the age of 60 years, with prevalence estimates of around 300 per 100 000 population, but this increases with rising age by approximately 1% of the population over the age of 60 years [18].

Von Campenhausen *et al.* [19] reviewed 39 articles describing the incidence and prevalence of PD in a number of European countries over a four-decade period. They noted a wide variation in both incidence and prevalence across Europe, with prevalence estimates ranging from 65.6 per 100 000 to 12 500 per 100 000, and incidence estimates ranging from 5 to 346 per 100 000 population. The highest prevalence estimate was in a study conducted by Evers and Obladen [20], but this was restricted to the residents of a nursing home.

In most industrialized nations, the prevalence of PD is approximately 300 per 100 000 population [21, 22]. In Alberta, Svenson *et al.* [9] deduced values of 248.9 and 239.8 per 100 000 population for males and females, respectively.

11.1.6
Clusters

The clustering of disease events can offer an opportunity to better understand potential factors that may increase risk [49]. When Wastensson and coworkers [23] investigated a potential PD cluster among workers at a paper mill, based on the

Table 11.1 A summary of PD prevalence studies.

Location	Time period	Rate per 100000 population			M:F ratio	Reference
		Male	Female	Total		
North America						
Canada						
Alberta	1984–1989	248.9	239.8		1.03:1	Svenson et al. 1993 [9]
British Columbia	1996–1998	120 (1996)	99 (1996)	109 (1996)	1.21:1 (1996)	Lai et al., 2003 [30]
		129 (1997)	112 (1997)	120 (1997)	1.15:1 (1997)	
		134 (1998)	116 (1998)	125 (1998)	1.16:1 (1998)	
United States						
Nebraska	1999	406 (age 60–70)	298 (age 60–70)		1.36 (age 60–70)	Strickland and Bertoni 2004 [31]
		1794 (age 70–80)	991 (age 70–80)		1.81 (age 70–80)	
		4248 (Age >80)	2069 (age >80)		2.05 (age >80)	
Europe						
Estonia	1996	171 (urban)	157 (urban)	160 (urban)	1.09:1 (urban)	Taba and Asser, 2002 [32]
		128 (rural)	145(rural	139 (rural)	0.88:1 (rural)	
Faroe Islands	2005			206.7 (Idiopathic PD)		Wermuth et al. 2008 [33]
				227.4 (Parkinsonism)		
				561 (age ≥45)		
Greenland	2000			187.5		Wermuth et al., 2002 [34]
United Kingdom				257 (age ≥65)		Taylor et al., 2006 [35]
				285 (age ≥75)		
United Kingdom						
North Tyneside	2001			148		Porter et al., 2006 [36]
Spain						
Bidasoa	1999	1300 (age ≥65)	1600 (age ≥65)	1500 (age ≥65)	0.81:1	Bergareche et al., 2004 [37]
Italy						
L'Aquila district	2001	227.4	231.1	229.3	0.98:1	Totaro et al., 2005 [38]
South America						
Bolivia	1994	248	323	286	0.77:1	Nicoletti et al., 1993 [39]

Table 11.1 *Continued*

Location	Time period	Rate per 100 000 population			M:F ratio	Reference
		Male	Female	Total		
Brazil Columbia Antioquia	2001	33	53		0.62:1	Barbosa et al., 2006 [6]
	1996–2000			30.7		Saacutenchez et al. 2004 [40]
				176.4 (age >50)		
Asia						
China						
– Beijing	1997–1998	205 (age ≥65)	117 (age ≥65)	161 (age ≥65)	1.75:1	Zhang et al., 2005 [41]
– Shanghai	1997–1998	139 (age ≥65)	204 (age ≥65)	174 (age ≥65)	0.68:1	Zhang et al., 2005 [41]
– Xian	1997–1998	174 (age ≥65)	137 (age ≥65)	155 (age ≥65)	1.27:1	Zhang et al., 2005 [41]
Kinmen	1992			119		Wang et al., 1994 [42]
South Korea	1999–2001	498	271	374	1.84:1	Seo et al., 2007 [43]
Australasia						
Australia	1992–2004			104		Mehta et al., 2007 [44]
				362 for age >50 years		
– Bankstown, Sydney	1998–1999			776		Chan et al., 2005 [45]
– Randwick, Sydney	1998–1999			775		Chan et al., 2005 [45]
– Queensland				145		Peters et al., 2006 [46]
New Zealand	1990			110.4		Caradoc-Davies et al., 1992 [47]
Africa						
Nigeria	1982			10		Okubadejo et al., 2006 [48]
Libya	1982			31.4		Okubadejo et al., 2006 [48]
Tunisia	1985			43		Okubadejo et al., 2006 [48]
Ethiopia	1986			7		Okubadejo et al., 2006 [48]
Togo	1989			20		Okubadejo et al., 2006 [48]
	1995			20		Okubadejo et al., 2006 [48]

prevalence of PD reported in a Swedish community they calculated the expected number of cases to be 0.9. But their investigation determined that there were five cases, giving a relative risk of 5.6 (95% CI: 1.8, 13), and that there was a 1 in 500 chance of having a relative risk measure this high due to chance alone. It was concluded that a cluster of cases did exist, and that exposure to diphenyl may be a possible explanation.

Kumar *et al.* [24] examined three separate clusters of PD in Canada. The first cluster included four individuals who worked together, among a staff of 125 people. Upon investigation, the members of the staff were found to have worked in a poorly ventilated area with high concentrations of carbon dioxide. The second cluster involved four individuals from the same college, two of whom reported intermittent exposure to organic solvents such as benzene and toluene. The classroom used by these four individuals was also found to have been built over a filled-in waste dump. The third cluster involved three cases among a staff of seven at a garment-manufacturing factory, but no history of toxin exposure was found among these three. Across the three clusters investigated, the latency period between potential exposure and disease outcome ranged from 9.5 to 15.7 years. Kumar *et al.* have suggested that there might be a possible role for environmental factors such as viral infection and/or toxin exposure.

A number of steps are involved when investigating reported clusters of disease, one of which includes estimating the number of *expected* cases of disease among the target population. This makes the selection of a reference population very important, as it must bear relevance to the group under study; otherwise, it may be possible to identify elevations or reductions in risk that are not associated with the disease process, but rather with the appropriateness of the reference chosen. Obtaining accurate and consistent surveillance information on the incidence and prevalence of PD is also necessary if any investigation of potential clusters is to be properly undertaken.

11.1.7
Purpose

An understanding of the epidemiology of PD is important for the development of etiologic hypotheses, improved planning, and for policy decisions. By using data obtained from the Alberta Health Care Insurance Plan (AHCIP) administrative health data, it is possible to describe the incidence and prevalence of PD in the province of Alberta. This is done by using administrative health records, and the data acquired will form the basis for developing an on-going surveillance system to monitor the distribution of cases in both space and time.

11.2
Methods

The province of Alberta maintains a publicly funded, universally available health-care system. As part of the administration of this system, all residents of the province are required to register with AHCIP such that, once registered, a unique lifetime identifier – known as the "personal health number" – is assigned. This number is collected for each interaction with physicians, emergency departments, and hospital in- and out-patient services, allowing for linkage across data sources to create a longitudinal medical record. The AHCIP registry excludes members of the Canadian military, Royal Canadian Mounted Police, and federal inmates. Any dependents of these groups are, however, registered with the AHCIP registry. Consequently, over 99% of the population is registered with the AHCIP.

The majority of physicians submit claims for reimbursement from the AHCIP for services provided. As part of the claims submission, the physician can provide up to three diagnostic codes, coded using the 9th Revision of the International Classification of Diseases-Clinical Modification (ICD-9-CM) at the four-digit level. The patient's personal health number is also required, and the database includes information on the location and type of service, as well as physician specialty and amount paid for services.

11.2.1
Data

A fee-for-service claims data (henceforth referred to as "claims") is used as a basis for identifying PD cases in Alberta between 1995 and 2005. Cases of PD are defined as persons with two or more claims records in which PD (ICD-9-CM 332.x) is the primary diagnosis, or one or more claims records in which PD is the primary diagnosis made by a physician with a neurology specialty.

The case data are linked to the population insurance registry system (henceforth referred to as "registry"), based on a deterministic link of personal health numbers contained in both these systems. This linkage of the registry to the claims combines demographic information with medical transaction data. In order to perform an accurate longitudinal analysis of PD in Alberta, the data are structured in a panel or "profile" form. This profile includes all persons who were defined as PD cases at some time over the study period. The profile is organized as a yearly time-series in which health information and demographic information vary from year to year. This structure facilitates longitudinal analysis, and provides a basis for more accurate measures of incidence and prevalence than independent cross-sectional analyzes. For example, the paneled structure enables one to keep track of changes in residence for cases that move to or from different regions over time.

The year in which a person meets the criteria as a case is treated as the "incident" year. For this and all following years, a case is considered "prevalent" until death or migration out of Alberta.

11.2.2
Analysis

Most of the analysis is based on descriptive tabulations of counts and rates of PD by age, gender, year, and geography. Age is grouped into the following categories:

0–29, 30–39, 40–49, 50–59, 60–69, 70–79, and 80+ years. Temporal analysis is based on the calendar year (i.e., 1st January to 31st December). A descriptive geographical analysis is performed at the level of provincial sub-Regional Health Authorities [25]; these 68 regions have roughly similar populations, and are formed in consultation with officials and stakeholders in the health regions. Temporal and geographic analyzes are age–gender standardized, using the direct method, to the 2001 Alberta Population [54]. Probability maps (e.g., Choynowski 1959 [26]) rather than maps of rates are presented in order to observe the variability in PD incidence and prevalence. Since the numbers of PD cases are fairly large for the regions and time periods under study, deviations of the normal distribution are used as the framework for measuring variations in disease [27]. These deviations or "standard scores" are categorized into five color categories: red (standard score of 2 or more); orange (standard score of 1–2); yellow (standard score of −1 to 1); light green (standard score of −1 to −2); and dark green (standard score of less than −2).

Parkinson-related health service utilization is also described among those persons identified as PD cases. Since the follow-up period is not the same for all subjects (e.g., some are incident at the beginning of the study period, and some are incident at the end of the study period), the time is measured as years from the incident diagnosis. The average number of PD-related claims per person is then calculated for each time period (including the year of incident diagnosis). These estimates are plotted along with 95% confidence bounds.

11.3
Results

Figure 11.1 shows the mean (and 95% CI) number of visits with a PD diagnosis following the first diagnosis available within the administrative health data. In the first year, cases averaged nearly three visits with a diagnosis of PD recorded on the record. The average past this point remained relatively stable at approximately two visits per year with a PD diagnostic code recorded.

11.3.1
Incidence

In the year 2005, there were 1001 incidence cases, with a mean age of 72.9 years that did not show any gender-related difference (males 72.2 years; females 73.9 years). The male : female ratio was 1.47 : 1. Figure 11.2 shows the age- and gender-specific incidence rate for PD for the period 1995 to 2005. Newly diagnosed cases of PD under the age of 50 years were uncommon. The incidence of PD was associated with increasing age, with the highest incidence rate among those aged over 80 years. A separation in the gender-specific rates was evident after the age of 60, with the difference increasing with age.

Both age- and gender-standardized incidence rates are shown in Figure 11.3. In general, the incidence remained stable between 1995 and 2005, although a slight

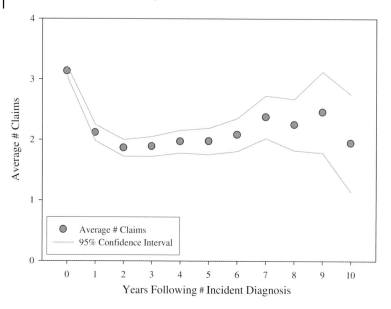

Figure 11.1 Average number of claims per-person between the year of PD onset and loss to follow-up.

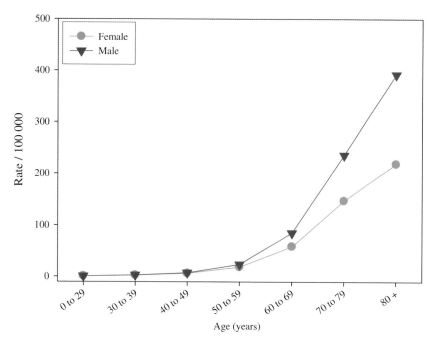

Figure 11.2 Parkinson disease incidence per 100 000 population by age and gender; data from Alberta 1995–2005, combined.

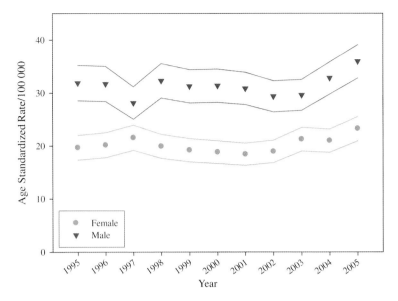

Figure 11.3 Age–gender-standardized incidence of PD by year.

increasing trend appeared between 2003 to 2005 for both genders. Males had a consistently higher incidence rate over the entire study period, however.

The geographic distribution of incidence rates for PD is shown in Figures 11.4 and 11.5 for 1995 and 2005, respectively. Although there appeared to be an increase in the variability observed in the geographic distribution, no geographic areas were identified as being statistically significantly elevated relative to the province rate.

11.3.2
Prevalence

As of 2005, there were 7558 prevalent cases. The mean age of prevalent cases was 75.9 years (74 years for males; 77 years for females; $P < 0.05$). The male:female ratio was 1.56:1 (see Table 11.2).

Figure 11.6 shows the age-standardized prevalence estimates per 100 000 population for the period 1995–2005. The prevalence of PD had remained relatively stable throughout the study period, but increased with age with few prevalent cases being identified before the age of 60 years (see Figure 11.7). Figure 11.8 shows the geographic distribution of PD prevalence in 2005. Variation in the prevalence of PD by geographic area was noted; in particular, the northwestern area of the province appeared to have an elevated prevalence of PD. The two largest cities, Edmonton and Calgary, generally had PD prevalence estimates equal to the provincial rate, or below. Also of note was the somewhat elevated prevalence in the south central areas of the province, both of which have major agricultural activities.

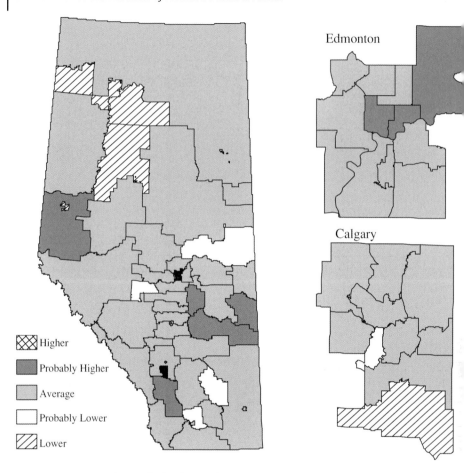

Figure 11.4 Age–gender-standardized map of PD incidence based on Alberta sub-regional health authority boundaries, 1995.

11.4
Discussion

There are a number of limitations that must be acknowledged when using administrative health data for epidemiological purposes. The first is that it was not possible to examine the evidence used by physicians to establish the diagnosis, but to compensate for this multiple service events were used for the diagnosis. This approach should improve the specificity of the surveillance case definition at the expense of sensitivity. In other words, the approach was designed to lead to an underestimate of both the incidence and prevalence of PD. It is also important to note that, among those cases identified using this approach, the mean number of visits in the year of diagnosis was three, but that this fell and stabilized at two visits per year for the first 10 years after diagnosis. This suggests that those cases

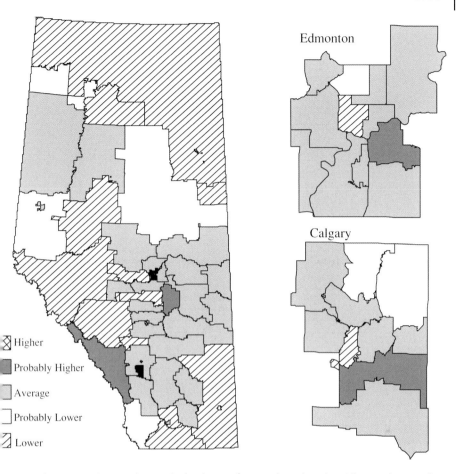

Figure 11.5 Age–gender-standardized map of PD incidence based on Alberta sub-regional health authority boundaries, 2005.

Table 11.2 Age-standardized incidence and prevalence of PD per 100 000 population by gender, Alberta.

Gender	Incidence (%)	95% CI	Prevalence (%)	95% CI
Female	20.2	19.6, 20.9	148.4	142.7, 154.1
Male	31.5	30.5, 32.4	223.6	215.7, 231.4

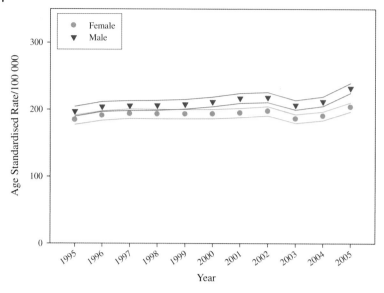

Figure 11.6   Age-standardized prevalence of PD per 100 000 population for Alberta, 1995 to 2005.

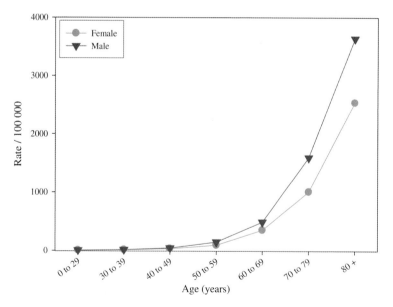

Figure 11.7   Age–gender-specific rates of PD prevalence, Alberta 2005.

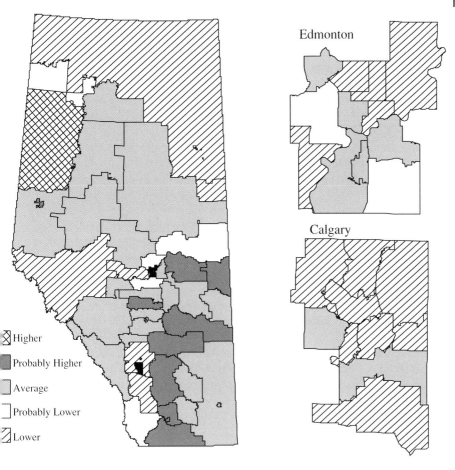

Figure 11.8 Age–gender-standardized map of PD prevalence based on Alberta sub-regional health authority boundaries, 2005.

meeting the surveillance definition were true cases, as the probability of maintaining an incorrect diagnosis for a decade is likely low.

The strengths of the approach taken here were that it was population-based, and that it could be easily replicated and maintained. Instead of relying on a number of point in time studies performed using different methods and time periods, this approach was systematic and can be ongoing. This moves the assessment of incidence and prevalence of PD away from periodic research studies into a surveillance system. Another advantage to this approach was that there was no recall bias involved, and no need to contact individuals directly.

Whilst PD is a relatively common neurological disorder among the elderly, its prevalence can still be considered as low from a survey perspective. The recent Canadian Community Health Survey (CCHS), in which over 130000 Canadians were surveyed, was unable to identify a sufficient number of cases to allow for a comparison to be made across all Canadian provinces and territories. The CCHS also excluded the residents of long-term care facilities which would impact on case ascertainment, particularly for PD. Administrative health data offer the opportunity to develop a public health surveillance system for PD that can support decision making and the development of research hypotheses to be investigated in more detail. Moreover, administrative data have strength over survey data for relatively rare conditions that would normally require a survey sample size that would be cost-prohibitive for the information to be gained.

Similar to other studies, PD prevalence was found to be higher among males [7–12]. In 1993, Svenson *et al.* reported a male:female ratio of 1.2:1 for Alberta, and in the present analysis this ratio has increased to 1.5:1. This increase in the difference between males and females was not surprising. As the incidence of PD is higher among males, this means that the number of newly diagnosed cases each year, when added to the prevalence estimates, will be greater for men than for women. In other words, the higher incidence in males will lead to a faster increase in prevalence. However, care must be taken not to overestimate the importance of changes in the gender distribution of a disease. At any time when the incidence is higher and there is little or no difference in survival, then the gender with the higher incidence will have a higher prevalence, and the difference between the prevalence estimates will continue to widen.

The incidence of PD has generally been constant up until the last three years, when there has appeared to be a slight increasing trend. Even nonstatistically significant increases in incidence can lead to increases in prevalence. Prevalence is a function of the duration of illness, and even small increases will accumulate over time.

Geographically, there was little difference in the distribution of incident cases of PD. The lack of clustering of incident cases of PD was unexpected given that agricultural activity has been identified as a risk factor [24]. In 2005, several geographic areas appeared to have elevated prevalent estimates, and these were in areas with higher agricultural activity. In general, the rural preponderance of prevalent cases was consistent with other studies, but not the lack of clustering for incident rates [9, 12, 24, 28]. Other studies have, generally, examined prevalence geographically and not incidence, and this is important from the perspective of generating etiologic hypotheses. Whilst PD is believed to be a condition with a long latency period, examining its incidence brings one closer to the potential exposures than does using prevalence estimates.

Yiannakoulias *et al.*[29] examined the geographic movements of patients with PD after they had received their first diagnosis. Whilst patients with PD were no more likely to migrate to urban settings than age- and gender-matched controls, there was still some movement. The movement of patients makes it difficult to assess any potential impact of rural living, and it also means that prevalence studies will have only a limited value in generating potential hypotheses related to environmental factors. The role of prevalence studies is well suited for monitoring the burden of PD, its natural history and the planning of health services, but migration makes it difficult to thoroughly assess potential exposures. While case control studies often ask questions related to residential history, this information is limited by recall bias and the lack of data on dose and duration of any particular exposure.

The information that can be derived from administrative health data sources can be used for a number of purposes that include: public health surveillance; planning; policy development; and the evaluation of interventions at a population level. These data function to improve the understanding of geographic patterns and secular trends; administrative health data allow this assessment to occur at a population-based level, and are relatively inexpensive to implement. There is a need to expand the current analysis in Alberta to other provinces and territories in Canada so as to allow for a national perspective on the distribution and burden of PD. Such a system would represent a unique resource internationally, would build on consistent case definitions, and would also provide information needed for the planning of health services and the development of policy options. These will become increasingly important as the population continues to age.

References

1 Parkinson, J. (1817) *An Essay on the Shaking Palsy*, Sherwood, Neely & Jones, London.

2 Charcot, J.M. (1880) *Leçons Sur Les Maladies Du Systeme Nerveux Faites A La Salpetriere*, 4th edn, Bourneville, Paris, p. 6.

3 Charcot, J.M. and Vulpian, A. (1861) De la paralysie agitante. *Gazzetta Hebdom di Medicina e Chirurgia*, **8**, 765–768.

4 Charcot, J.M. and Vulpian, A. (1861) De la paralysie agitante. *Gazzetta Hebdom di Medicina e Chirurgia*, **8**, 816–823.

5 Charcot, J.M. and Vulpian, A. (1862) De la paralysie agitante. *Gazzetta Hebdom di Medicina e Chirurgia*, **9**, 54–64.

6 Barbosa, M.T., Caramelli, P., Palma, D., Cunningham, M.C.Q., Guerra, H.L., Lima-Costa, M.F., and Cardoso, F. (2006) Parkinsonism and Parkinson's disease in the elderly: a community-based survey in Brazil (the Bambuí Study). *Movement Disorders*, **21**, 800–808.

7 Benito-Leon, J., Bermejo-Pareja, F., Rodriguez, J., Molina, J.A., Gabriel, R., and Morales, J.M. (2003) Prevalence of PD and other types of parkinsonism in three elderly populations of central Spain. *Movement Disorders*, **8**, 267–274.

8 Claveria, L.E., Duarte, J., Sevillano, M.D., *et al.* (2002) Prevalence of Parkinson's disease in Cantalejo, Spain:

a door-to-door survey. *Movement Disorders*, **17**, 242–249.

9 Svenson, L.W., Platt, G.H., and Woodhead, S.E. (1993) Geographic variations in the prevalence rates of Parkinson's disease in Alberta. *Canadian Journal of Neurological Sciences*, **20**, 307–311.

10 Mayeux, R., Marder, K., Cote, L.J., *et al.* (1995) The frequency of idiopathic Parkinson's disease by age, ethnic group, and sex in northern Manhattan, 1988–1993. *American Journal of Epidemiology*, **142**, 20–27.

11 Li, S.C., Schoenberg, B.S., Wang, C.C., *et al.* (1985) A prevalence survey of Parkinson's disease and other movement disorders in the People's Republic of China. *Archives of Neurology*, **42**, 655–657.

12 Svenson, L.W. (1991) Regional disparities in the annual prevalence rates of Parkinson's disease in Canada. *Neuroepidemiology*, **10**, 205–210.

13 de Rijk, M.C., Breteler, M.M., Graveland, G.A., *et al.* (1995) Prevalence of Parkinson's disease in the elderly: the Rotterdam Study. *Neurology*, **45**, 2143–2146.

14 Tison, F., Dartigues, J.F., Dubes, I., Zuber, M., Alperovitch, A., and Henry,

P. (1994) Prevalence of Parkinson's disease in the elderly: a population study in Gironde, France. *Acta Neurologica Scandinavica*, **90**, 111–115.

15 Morgante, L., Rocca, W.A., Di Rosa, A.E., *et al.* (1992) Prevalence of Parkinson's disease and other types of parkinsonism: a door-to-door survey in three Sicilian municipalities. *Neurology*, **42**, 1901–1907.

16 de Rijk, M.C., Tzourio, C., Breteler, M.M., *et al.* (1997) Prevalence of parkinsonism and Parkinson's disease in Europe: the Europarkinson Collaborative Study. *Journal of Neurology, Neurosurgery, and Psychiatry*, **62**, 10–15.

17 Langston, J.W., Ballard, P., Tetrud, J.W., and Irwin, I. (1983) Chronic Parkinsonism in humans due to a product of meperidine-analog synthesis. *Science*, **219**, 979–980.

18 Nussbaum, R.L. and Ellis, C.E. (2003) Alzheimer's disease and Parkinson's disease. *New England Journal of Medicine*, **348**, 1356–1364.

19 von Campenhausen, S., Bornschein, B., Wick, R., Bötzel, K., Sampaio, C., Poewe, W., *et al.* (2005) Prevalence and incidence of Parkinson's disease in Europe. *European Neuropsychopharmacology*, **15**, 473–490.

20 Evers, S. and Obladen, M. (1994) Epidemiology and therapy of Parkinson disease in inpatient nursing homes. *Zeitschrift für Gerontologie*, **27**, 270–275.

21 de Lau, L.M.L. and Breteler, M.M.B. (2006) Epidemiology of Parkinson's disease. *Lancet Neurology*, **5**, 525–535.

22 Seidman-Ripley, J. (1993) Monograph series on aging-related diseases: II. Parkinson's disease. *Chronic Diseases of Canada*. **14**, 34–47.

23 Watensson, G., Hagberg, S., Andersson, E., Johnels, B., and Barregård, L. (2006) Parkinson's disease in diphenyl-exposed workers – a causal association? *Parkinsonism and Related Disorders*, **12**, 29–34.

24 Kumar, A., Calne, S.M., Schulzer, M., Mak, E., Wszolek, Z., van Netten, C., *et al.* (2004) Clustering of Parkinson's disease: shared cause or coincidence? *Archives of Neurology*, **61**, 1057–1060.

25 Ellehoj, E. and Schopflocher, D.P. (2003) *A Rate Mapping Template for Alberta Regional Health Authorities*, Alberta Health and Wellness, Edmonton, Canada. Available at: http://www.health.gov.ab.ca/resources/publications/GeoTemplate.pdf (accessed 1 July 2008).

26 Choynowski, M. (1959) Maps based on probabilities. *Journal of the American Statistical Association*, **54**, 385–388.

27 Ellehoj, E. and Schopflocher, D.P. (2003) *Calculating Small Area Analysis: Definition of Sub-regional Geographic Units in Alberta*, Alberta Health and Wellness, Edmonton, Canada. Available at: http://www.health.gov.ab.ca/resources/ publications/pdf/Geo-subRHA.pdf (accessed 1 July 2008).

28 Svenson, L.W. (1990) Geographic distribution of deaths due to Parkinson's disease in Canada: 1979–1986. *Movement Disorders*, **5**, 322–324.

29 Yiannakoulias, N., Schopflocher, D.P., Warren, S.A., and Svenson, L.W. (2007) Parkinson's disease multiple sclerosis and changes of residence in Alberta. *Canadian Journal of Neurological Sciences*, **34**, 343–348.

30 Lai, B.C.L., Schulzer, M., Marion, S., Teschke, K., and Tsui, J.K.C. (2003) The prevalence of Parkinson's disease in British Columbia, Canada, estimated by using drug tracer methodology. *Parkinsonism and Related Disorders*, **9**, 233–238.

31 Strickland, D. and Bertoni, J.M. (2004) Parkinson's prevalence estimated by a state registry. *Movement Disorders*, **19**, 318–323.

32 Taba, P. and Asser, T. (2002) Prevalence of Parkinson's disease in Estonia. *Acta Neurologica Scandinavica*, **106**, 276–282.

33 Wermuth, L., Bech, S., Skaalum Petersen, M., Joensen, P., Wiehe, P., and Grandjean, P. (2008) Prevalence and incidence of Parkinson's disease in the Faroe Islands. *Acta Neurologica Scandinavica*, **118**, 126–131.

34 Wermuth, L., Pakkenberg, H., and Jeune, B. (2002) High age-adjusted prevalence of Parkinson's disease among Inuits in Greenland. *Neurology*, **58**, 1422–1425.

35 Taylor, K.S.M., Counsell, C.E., Harris, C.E., and Gordon, J.C. (2006) Screening for undiagnosed parkinsonism in people

aged 65 years and older in the community. *Parkinsonism and Related Disorders*, **12**, 79–85.

36 Porter, B., Macfarlane, R., Unwin, N., and Walker, R. (2006) The prevalence of Parkinson's disease in an area of North Tyneside in the north-east of England. *Neuroepidemiology*, **26**, 156–161.

37 Bergareche, A., De la Puente, E., de Munain, A.L., Sarasqueta, C., de Arce, A., Poza, J.J., and Martí-Massó, A. (2004) Prevalence of Parkinson's disease and other types of Parkinsonism: a door-to-door survey in Bidasoa, Spain. *Journal of Neurology*, **251**, 340–345.

38 Totaro, R., Marini, C., Pistoia, F., Sacco, T., and Carolei, A. (2005) Prevalence of Parkinson's disease in the L'Aquila district, central Italy. *Acta Neurologica Scandinavica*, **112**, 24–28.

39 Nicoletti, A., Sofia, V., Bartoloni, A., Bartalesi, F., Gamboa Barahon, H., Giuffrida, S., and Reggio, A. (1993) Prevalence of Parkinson's disease: a door-to-door survey in rural Bolivia. *Parkinsonism and Related Disorders*, **10**, 19–21.

40 Saacutenchez, J.L., Buriticaacute, O., Pineda, D., Uribe, C.S., and Palacio, L.G. (2004) Prevalence of Parkinson's disease and parkinsonism in a Colombian population using the capture-recapture method. *International Journal of Neuroscience*, **114**, 175–182.

41 Zhang, Z.-X., Roman, G.C., Hong, Z., Wu, C.-B., Qu, Q.-M., Huang, J.-B., *et al.* (2005) Parkinson's disease in China: prevalence in Beijing, Xian, and Shanghai. *Lancet*, **365**, 595–597.

42 Wang, S.J., Fuh, J.L., Liu, C.Y., Lin, K.P., Chang, R., Yih, J.S., *et al.* (1994) Parkinson's disease in Kin-Hu, Kinmen: a community Survey by neurologists. *Neuroepidemiology*, **13**, 69.

43 Seo, W.K., Koh, S.B., Kim, B.J., Yu, S.W., Park, M.H., Park, K.W., and Lee, D.H. (2007) Prevalence of Parkinson's disease in Korea. *Journal of Clinical Neuroscience*, **14**, 1155–1157.

44 Mehta, P., Kifley, A., Wang, J.J., Rochtchina, E., Mitchell, P., and Sue, C.M. (2007) Population prevalence and incidence of Parkinson's disease in an Australian community. *Internal Medical Journal*, **37**, 812–814.

45 Chan, D.K.Y., Cordato, D., Karr, M., Ong, B., Lei, H., Liu, J., and Hung, W.T. (2005) Prevalence of Parkinson's disease in Sydney. *Acta Neurologica Scandinavica*, **111**, 7–11.

46 Peters, C.M., Gartner, C.E., Silburn, P.A., and Mellick, G.D. (2006) Prevalence of Parkinson's disease in metropolitan and rural Queensland: a general practice survey. *Journal of Clinical Neuroscience*, **13**, 343–348.

47 Caradoc-Davies, T.H., Weatherall, M., Dixon, G.S., Caradoc-Davies, G., and Hantz, P. (1992) Is the prevalence of Parkinson's disease in New Zealand really changing? *Acta Neurologica Scandinavica*, **86**, 40–44.

48 Okubadejo, N.U., Bower, J.H., Rocca, W.A., and Maraganore, D.M. (2006) Parkinson's disease in Africa: a systematic review of epidemiologic and genetic studies. *Movement Disorders*, **21**, 2150–2156.

49 Centers for Disease Control (1990) Guidelines for investigating clusters of health events. *Morbidity and Mortality Weekly Report*, **39** (No. RR-11), 1–23.

50 Duvoisin, R.C. (1992) A brief history of parkinsonism. *Neurology Clinics*, **10**, 301–316.

51 Diamond, S.G., Markham, C.H., Hoehn, M.M., McDowell, F.H., and Muenter, M.D. (1990) An examination of male-female differences in progression and mortality of Parkinson's disease. *Neurology*, **40**, 763–766.

52 Guttman, M., Slaughter, P.M., Theriault, M.E., DeBoer, D.P., and Naylor, C.D. (2001) Parkinsonism in Ontario: increased mortality compared with controls in a large cohort study. *Neurology*, **57**, 2278–2282.

53 D'Amelio, M., Ragonese, P., Morgante, L., Reggio, A., Callari, G., Salemi, G., and Savetteri, G. (2006) Long-term survival of Parkinson's disease: a population-based study. *Journal of Neurology*, **253**, 33–37.

54 Fleiss, J.L. (1981) *Statistical methods for rates and proportions*, 2nd edn. John Wiley & Sons, New York.

A Patient's Story

Who Am I?

Joyce Pinckney

Last week I was a person.
  Someone's friend, a wife, a mother–I had a name.
  I had ideas, aspirations, work to do–I had a life.
  But I had pain.
  "We'll fix it," said the doctor and promptly booked a bed.
  Now, here I am "all fixed"–almost, restricted to the pre-booked bed.
  I'm told I'm not to worry, but no dancing for the minute, for the next two days the bed stays flat and I'm to stay flat in it.
  I know I'm here, for when I came delivered like the head of John the Baptist on a "silver stretcher"–the team assembled.
  Slid me like an omelet from the pan onto the plate.
  Checked my tubes and levels, marked some numbers on the chart, then disappeared.
  I must be hard to see or hear for no one says my name or strokes my hair or holds my hand or seems to care.
  And though they "check my pupils," and shine a bright light in my eyes, no one makes contact, eye to eye.
  Or sees me, soul to soul.

12

Knowledge, Service Access, and the Needs of Individuals Living with Parkinson Disease: The Alberta Case

Katharina Kovacs Burns

12.1
Introduction

This chapter describes the perceptions of individuals living with Parkinson disease (PD) and their caregivers with regards to what information, services and supports are accessed, needed and valued by people diagnosed with PD in Alberta. The hope is that they are not only able to live with and manage their condition, but also to maintain a reasonable quality of life (QoL). Adequate and appropriate information, services and supports must be available and accessible, including access to the "best" medical treatment – if not in their own communities, then within a reasonable distance. These perceptions and realities are captured in an Alberta case study, the results of which indicate some similar or common trends for many people living with PD elsewhere.

12.2
The Alberta Case

At the time of the study, an estimated 5500 people were diagnosed with PD in Alberta [1]. Although the general distribution of people with PD across the province was known, there was no specific information as to which services were actually available or accessed in each health region. Neither was any information available regarding the caregivers' feelings about what the PD patients needed, or what they valued in terms of their treatment, therapy, support, or information. It was these unknowns which became the focus of a research study.

Thus, the aim of the study was to survey individuals living with and affected by PD. As a similar study had been completed previously in Southern Alberta two years earlier [2], the present case study was intended to expand on those findings, and to explore the perceptions and experiences of persons with PD and their caregivers residing throughout Alberta. The objectives were to: (i) determine the demographics and characteristics of individuals living with PD; (ii) assess which support, health, and other services individuals with PD have accessed, or are

Parkinson Disease – A Health Policy Perspective. Edited by Wayne Martin, Oksana Suchowersky,
Katharina Kovacs Burns, and Egon Jonsson
Copyright © 2010 WILEY-VCH Verlag GmbH & Co. KGaA, Weinheim
ISBN: 978-3-527-32779-9

accessing; (iii) determine what information they found most useful; (iv) determine what information and services they felt they needed and where there were gaps and barriers; and (v) determine which services and information the caregivers felt that individuals with PD should have, or need to have access to.

12.3
Background and Context for Study

Although the surveillance and prevalence data are important to know for the context of the current and future status of information and service provision for persons with PD, this study did not focus on this area, other than to obtain the number of individuals diagnosed with PD across Alberta.

There was also relevant information in the literature concerning the information and service needs and challenges of persons with PD and their caregivers. This closely relates to the economic burden of the disease, as well as to the capacity of persons with PD and their caregivers to manage the disease and cope with the challenges it presents.

12.4
Parkinson Disease: Its Impact and Costs

There are two types of economic burden of PD: one which reflects the general costs, and one which is specific to the individual. The economic burden of PD has been mapped out by Health Canada in the report, *Economic Burden of Illness in Canada, 1998* [3]. The total cost of PD in Canada for 1998 is given as $558.1 million, of which the direct costs amounted to $87.8 million (hospital care at $39.7 million, drugs at $24.1 million, physician care at $23.0 million, and research at $1.0 million), while indirect costs for premature mortality and long-term disability totaled $470.3 million. Men accounted for over 56% of the total PD costs, and seniors (both men and women) for over 90%. The average cost per capita was about $23 per year. In Alberta, this amount was about $21, for a total cost of $46.6 million, or about 12% of the total cost for PD in Canada. Since 1998, these figures have increased, in parallel with the increased costs of healthcare service delivery and treatment, including drugs. Additional support services are not covered under the public government coverage plan and must, therefore, be paid for by the patient unless he or she has employment-related or personally paid private insurance plan which pays for such services.

Other population-based studies confirm that parkinsonism leads to a burden of illness and cost to society, some of which is difficult to quantify. In Ontario, Guttman *et al.* [4] identified specific burdens and costs; compared to individuals without PD, those with PD had higher costs: "Physician costs were 1.4 times more, there were 1.44 times more hospital admissions, admissions were on average 1.19 times longer, and drug costs were 3.0 times more for parkinsonian cases (p. 313)".

Guttman and colleagues concluded that the substantially higher physician and drug costs and also the hospitalization rates, when compared to controls, clearly suggest that parkinsonism is associated with large direct costs to society. Their key message was that additional information must be aggressively pursued by research groups, government agencies, industry, and the voluntary sector on an international basis, in the hope of reducing the burden of PD.

In a more recent study on the QoL of Canadian patients with PD, Keranen *et al.* [5] identified a significant association between the QoL or cost-of-illness, and the severity of the disease. Specific to the direct and indirect costs of illness, the authors pointed out the following statistics: "... direct costs accounted for 41%, early retirement due to PD 43%, and informal home care 16%. Of the direct costs, hospitalization is the main cost driver accounting for 41%. PD medication accounted for 20%, formal home care 14%, rehabilitation outside hospitalization periods 9%, inpatient care other than hospitalization 7%, and hospital outpatient visits and visits to GPs and specialists 9%, of the direct costs" (p. 165).

They concluded by saying that policies regarding effective treatments which reduce or delay physical disabilities would in turn increase the QoL and, at the same time, decrease some of the economic burden of PD to the individual, as well as to society. In the year 2000, Scheife *et al.* [6] published similar results based on studies conducted in the United States.

The very "real" impact of PD is with the person who lives with the disease. When Marr [7] completed a phenomenological study examining the experience of persons with PD, he found that this experience included the impact of the disease and having to deal with it in order to maintain as much independence and normalcy as possible. This takes a lot of effort on the part of the individual with PD. A loss of independence and normality as a result of a loss of mobility and social activity results in a "changed self-concept".

This latter study was cited in other reports which suggested that a patient's mental health plays a major role in the QoL, including their general health and well-being associated with living with PD. Chrischilles *et al.* [8] concluded that for persons with PD, "... the well-being, general health perceptions, health satisfaction, and overall HRQL (health-related quality of life) are strongly influenced by mental health symptoms and more weakly influenced by physical symptoms." The PD patient's mental state has a huge bearing on their welfare, especially during the late stages of the disease when there are changes in physical and mental health, a loss of autonomy and self-esteem, altered relationships, and social isolation. Both depression and dementia in patients interfered with their care and outcomes. From another perspective, Marras *et al.* [9] suggested that the impact of physical changes and disabilities such as dyskinesias (inappropriate muscle movement) and motor fluctuations on QoL at the various stages of PD is not well understood.

Many of these health-related QoL aspects for persons with PD can be measured using various PD-validated instruments. An example is the 15D, which measures levels of change dimensions such as mobility, vision, hearing, breathing, sleeping, eating, speech, elimination, usual activities, mental function, discomfort and symptoms, depression, distress, vitality, and sexual activity [10]. An alternative instrument is the PDQ-39, which measures eight subscales: mobility; activities of daily living; emotional wellness; stigma; social support; cognition; communication; and bodily discomfort [11]. The latter instrument was used in the present study.

12.4.1
Specific Support and Services Needed by PD Patients and Their Caregivers

The issues for people with PD, as identified by researchers, caregivers, health professionals and others, are also issues with implications for the healthcare system and community services. Some challenges faced not only by persons with PD but also by others with progressive degenerative disabilities are captured in a report called, *In Synchrony: Looking at Disability Supports from a Progressive Disability Perspective* [12]. Generally, the report states that:

> People with progressive disabilities encounter many obstacles to meeting the expectations of our modern world. Access to disability supports is recognized to be a critical factor in ensuring the social participation of people with disabilities. Existing policies and programs designed to support people with disabilities do not address the needs of the sub-population of persons with progressive disabilities. Based on the preliminary interviews, it appears that there are not specific tools or procedures to assess the needs of people living with progressive disabilities. The lack of understanding and inflexibility of the existing service structure demonstrate there is an urgent need for a restructuring of governmental policies to attain the basic principles of independent living promoted by the disability movement. The current situation is probably due to the lack of a clear definition of the concept of progressiveness, or at least its inclusion in the definition of disability. This lack of definition and the literature's silence regarding the issue of people living with progressive disabilities' needs, indicates a general misunderstanding of what people living with progressive disability experience, even by the major contributors involved in disability supports (p. 6).

The report goes on to mention that people with progressive disabilities feel marginalized, and that without appropriate supports these individuals end up with dissatisfied lives, are misunderstood or ignored, and socially deprived. The research for the report also confirmed that the disability supports are full of gaps and are poorly coordinated across the country. Specifically, the disability supports are found to be difficult to find (lack of information available on supports) or to access (multiple providers, rigid procedures and long waiting lists), and effectively unavailable to people in rural settings. Neither was the range of services needed seen to be available, nor sufficiently flexible to meet the individuals' needs.

Parashos *et al.* [13] showed that people with PD are more likely than other patients to access physicians and emergency departments on a frequent basis.

They are also more likely to have a need for home care or nursing homes sooner than other patients. Depending on the demographics, the age of disease onset, their clinical characteristics and response to medication, the survival times of persons with PD is also shorter. Predictors of the use of healthcare and other services are defined by De Boer *et al.* [14] as being the number of visits to a general practitioner, disease severity and a poor QoL, followed by other predictors such as physiotherapy, lack of social supports, and depression. These factors have consequences for care and costs of care primarily related to the multidisciplinary nature of care needed to address these different factors. Kale and Menken [15], Wade and colleagues [16], and Iansek [17] all suggested that people with PD, like most individuals with chronic neurological disorders, need a multidisciplinary team of physicians, pharmacists, nurses, and physiotherapists to help in their overall management of the disease. Moreover, patients would prefer to access these services within their own communities, or as close as possible.

The starting point for designing a strategy for care and follow-up with patient and caregiver, according to Frazier [18], is to assess the best coping strategies for both individuals, and to look at changes anticipated, the stability, and the supports needed. Coping strategies for both the patient and caregiver can be either self-help or supportive resources [19]; the question is whether individuals prefer self-help groups to discuss PD as part of their every day life, or coping on their own by focusing on normal life without giving the disease a central focus. Charlton and Barrow [19] identified several coping methods which individuals with PD and their caregivers have found works, which include: social interaction and developing friendships; social comparison, where individuals share their good fortunes and experiences; living one day at a time; a fighting spirit to maintain as normal a life as possible, not thinking about the illness; a positive outlook; hope; and acceptance. Specifically for those spouses who are caregivers, Habermann [20] has identified their coping strategies to be "... maintaining their own life, encouraging their partners to stay active and involved, and seeing the challenges they experienced as secondary" (p. 1409).

Several studies have recommended that the priority in care for patients and their caregivers be appropriate education, along with supports [2, 21, 22]. Others have suggested that rehabilitation nurses should provide effective education counseling and support for interventions with both patients and caregivers [23–25]. Edwards and Scheetz [26] further recommended that a combination of supports be provided to patients and their caregivers by the healthcare team, including PD management, activities for daily living, appropriate resources to decrease burdens, and support groups to ensure that both the patients and the caregivers are coping. One additional study also examined the advantages and importance for patients and their caregivers to have a suitable environment, as well as influences to support their other educational and treatment routines [27]. Social relationships and challenges within the environment need to be assessed in order that the most appropriate types of influences be supported so as to assist in maintaining positive outlooks by both the patient and caregiver.

Recently, several PD Societies have engaged in surveys with their members to inquire which services they access, and what they need to manage as patients and caregivers. The United Kingdom Parkinson's Disease Society [28] examined the composition of its membership and their members' needs, including their views about the Society. In turn, the Society raised important questions about access to services, both its own and those of other organizations. They found that "... most members with Parkinson Disease are men, between 65 and 84, and married or living with a partner. One in five lived alone. A very small number of men were put into institutional care" (p. ii). Their findings suggested that "... members may not all have an equal opportunity to benefit from the full range of sources of help for persons with PD. However, there did not appear to be many differences in the use of health services by sub-groups of members" (p. iii). They went on to say that:

> Further consideration should be given to why only relatively small propor-
> tions of respondents use formal services. There are a number of possible
> reasons. Members may be unaware that such services exist, or have prob-
> lems accessing them. For example, if they have to fill in difficult forms or
> use the telephone. There may be inadequate local provision, or services may
> not be appropriate to individual needs. Some people may not be able to
> afford to pay charges for services, although PDS members are generally
> relatively comfortably off. For this very reason, they may not be seen as a
> priority by local authorities or may prefer to buy services privately (p. iv).

In Canada, two studies have been performed to review the situation for people with PD and their caregivers. In the first study, which was conducted in 1999 by Thurston *et al.* [2] for The Parkinson's Society of Southern Alberta in Calgary, the aim was to assess the personal and healthcare needs of people with PD (particu-larly by members of the Society) and their caregivers. The response rate of Society members was 65% (157 of 243), and of nonmembers was 24% (7 of 29), whilst among caregivers the response rate was 49% (of 134 approached). The members were aged between 35 and 90 years (average 61), and 61% were men. The study findings were that, in general, all those who responded were doing well, and nobody was going without support. Between 58% and 75% of the members saw a need for information on the causes, treatment and symptoms of PD, while 39–44% saw a need for information on the services and supports available. Since learning about PD was a key reason for most members joining The Parkinson's Society of Southern Alberta, this was suggested as a reason why the drop out rate was as high as 50% in the last year prior to the study. Either way, members were not receiving the information and supports or services expected, or they had received what they wanted but did not wish to continue as members of the Society.

The second study was conducted by the Parkinson's Society of Canada and other organizations in Ontario [12]. This survey, which was distributed to 3000 people with PD and their caregivers, consisted of similar patterns of questions for both the patients and caregivers alike, and focused on evaluating the impact of PD on their daily living, as well as determining the types of services they used, needed, wanted, and valued. Although the results of the study were only accessible on the Society's website, they presented some useful information. Of the 3000 surveys distributed, 911 people with PD (30%) and 678 caregivers responded. The profile of the respondents suggested that 65% of those with PD were aged 70–89 years, 11% were aged 50–59 years, and 2% were aged less than 50. The majority of respondents (63%) were aged 60 or more when they were first diagnosed with PD. The distribution of the respondents was province-wide, with almost 25% living in Southwestern Ontario. Almost three-quarters of respondents with PD said that they had an unpaid caregiver. Overall, the respondents were most likely among the least vulnerable in Ontario, as they had access to the Ontario division of the Parkinson's Society of Canada. Generally, the respondents were accessing doctors, care, drug and medical coverage, and information as needed, and were satisfied with the care they had received. The study provided a number of key conclusions and related recommendations, including dealing with the widespread lack of awareness among persons with PD and caregivers of available services in their area, sustaining support and exercise groups which are the most used and valued services of both persons with PD and caregivers, and looking at ways of enhancing awareness (e.g., website for younger people) and networks (e.g., for free community transportation) to combat feelings and experiences of isolation.

Studies such as these provide a good source of essential information for Parkinson's Societies, healthcare providers and decision makers to use in their planning of services and needed resources so as to meet the needs of persons with PD and their caregivers. If the prediction is correct about the increasing prevalence of PD correlating with an increase in the aging population, then the need for health and social supports by people living with, and affected by PD, will also increase.

12.4.2
Significance of the Study

The 2003 report on *In Synchrony: Looking at Disability Supports from a Progressive Disability Perspective*, was prepared by the Parkinson's Society of Canada, in partnership with other health charities providing services to people with degenerative or progressive disabilities (ALS Society of Canada, Alzheimer Society of Canada, Huntington Society of Canada, Multiple Sclerosis Society of Canada, and Muscular Dystrophy Canada) [12]. The report confirmed that individuals with a progressive disability: (i) experience many gaps in disability supports; (ii) find that the services between provinces and territories are not coordinated; (iii) perceive disability supports to be poorly advertised and therefore difficult to find, difficult to access and unavailable to many individuals living in rural or remote areas, rigidly structured, unresponsive to individual needs, and lacking flexibility of range of supports available; and (iv) overlook the economic impact of living with a progressive disease or disability. The study also showed that, although the number and variety of disability and other supports have increased and broadened over the years, there is still a need to have these supports synchronized with the progression of the disease and disabilities experienced. Every individual progresses through the disease differently, and will need some different supports. However, there are some supports which are universally needed by persons with PD as well as their families and/or caregivers.

Some of the Parkinson's Societies in Canada (in Southern Alberta and Ontario, for example), and in other parts of the world such as the United Kingdom, have conducted similar studies and reported similar findings around the need to improve information on PD and services available, and to improve service access and availability geared to capacities rather than disabilities. In the UK, it was discovered that individuals use formal services less because of other issues, such as transportation [2, 12, 29].

The significance of this study was that there has been an identification of the need to survey persons with PD and their families and caregivers concerning their issues, information and services needs, and gaps and barriers to access services. At the time, it was felt that the recommendations based on the study results would be of benefit to decision makers, to inform them about where the gaps are in the health system, including what services and resources are needed, and how the regional health authorities and other aspects of the healthcare system can better accommodate the needs of those affected by PD in rural and urban areas of Northern Alberta. It was also felt that the results would be useful to healthcare and service providers to improve practices, and also to administrators who make program policies and funding decisions with the intent of making positive changes to meet the needs of individuals affected by PD. As a progressively disabling degenerative disease, social and economic impact increases over time for the patient, family, and the healthcare system.

The results of this study will also contribute to the growing evidence in the literature which demonstrates the impact that debilitating conditions such as PD can have on individuals living with the disorder, their caregivers, and on the healthcare system and community-based services. The planning of acute, community-based, and continuing or long-term supportive care must consider the impact of an aging population, and the high prevalence of PD among those aged 60 and over. The need for access to adequate and appropriate health care and treatment, social supports, as well as financial assistance for individuals with PD and their caregivers, will also need to be examined [30]. Health and social science professionals and community service providers must be included in the awareness of the potential implications, and the need to plan accordingly.

12.5
Study Design and Methodology

The research design chosen was a quantitative case study focusing on basic frequencies and numbers of persons with PD responding to PD-related questions.

Surveys were used to explore the perceptions of two targeted groups affected by PD: those living with it; and the caregivers of those with PD. The research questions developed for this project reflect back to the purpose and objectives stated in the introduction, and are as follows: (i) What are the demographics and characteristics of individuals living with PD across Alberta?; (ii) What are the services (i.e., support, health, and others) which individuals with PD access, and which of these services do they find most useful or beneficial?; (iii) What additional information and services do they need? What are the identified gaps in services, and barriers to access?; and (iv) What issues, concerns, and needs do caregivers say that individuals with PD have (i.e., caregivers are family members and/or non-professionals)?

Two questionnaires were developed – one for individuals living with PD, and the other for caregivers of individuals with PD. The proposed project borrowed from and modified several instruments (Parkinson's Disease Questionnaire 39 and PDQ 8), as well as surveys/questionnaires completed in other Canadian jurisdictions. The questions were added as needed. The surveys referenced from other studies included: (i) An Assessment of the Personal and Health Care Needs of Persons with Parkinson's and Their Caregivers, completed for the Parkinson's Society of Southern Alberta [2]; (ii) A Survey of People with PD and Survey of Caregivers for People with PD prepared for The Parkinson's Society Canada, Ontario Division [12]; and (iii) A Survey of Members of the Parkinson's Disease Society, Parkinson's Society of the United Kingdom [28].

Each of the two questionnaires is targeted to a different group, but focuses on some similar questions. For persons with PD, the questionnaire focuses on:

- Personal information about the individual including where they live, age, gender, age at diagnosis, living arrangement, earnings, and other information.
- Employment information and sources of income, as well challenges at work.
- Treatment, medical and healthcare services accessed.
- Community care including home care or long-term/continuing care.
- Medical and other expenses and costs related to living with PD.
- Living with PD, generally and specifically.
- Services needed by people with PD.
- Affiliation with the Parkinson's Society of Alberta.

The general focus of the questions for caregivers related to the service use and needs of those with PD includes:

- Some personal information about the caregiver.
- Community and other services accessed and valued by persons with PD.
- Information and services needed.
- Affiliation with the Parkinson Societies in Alberta.

Participant numbers were based on the estimated 5500 persons with PD living in Alberta during the timeframe of the study [1]. Based on the literature, it was estimated that between 66% and 70% of people with PD would have informal caregivers, which would translate into approximately 3740 caregivers.

Participants were recruited through a variety of sources, including the Parkinson's Societies in Edmonton and Calgary, clinics specific for management of PD or other movement disorders, home care services and long-term/continuing care in cities and rural communities. Service providers within six of the nine regional health authorities (i.e., those located in Central and Northern Alberta) agreed to participate and support the distribution of the surveys to their clients with PD and caregivers, targeting about 3320 persons with PD and their caregivers directly. The other three regions were targeted through bulletins distributed through clinics. In addition, advertisements were placed in a number of free newspapers that circulated across Alberta.

Individuals who participated by completing their questionnaires and sending them back in the provided stamped and addressed envelopes voluntarily consented to do so. There was no means of following up with individuals after the initial distribution of the surveys.

Databases were set up for the two groups, namely persons with PD and their caregivers. Quantitative analyses were conducted on the data using SPSS.

12.5.1
Limitations and Challenges

One of the biggest challenges faced by the research teams was to reach the number of participants to achieve the needed return rate. The 1999 study in Southern Alberta had about a 46% response rate, but the individuals were members of the Parkinson's Society of Southern Alberta [2]. Factors which must be considered in analyzing the response rate included that some persons with PD may not be well enough or have physical limitations which would prevent them from completing the survey. There was also the perceived limitation as to what the subjects might be able to say without feeling they could jeopardize their standing with either the Parkinson's Societies or Movement Disorder Clinics [31].

The surveys were basically a one-time ask for information. Therefore, the questionnaires were more comprehensive than originally intended, which may also have had a negative impact on persons with PD and their caregivers to fill out the entire questionnaires. Other limitations and challenges also existed, and were managed accordingly.

12.5.2
Study Results

12.5.2.1 Responses to the Survey
Considering the various challenges of locating and accessing people with PD and their caregivers, 1000 surveys for each group (i.e., persons with PD and caregivers) were distributed broadly and via request from individuals and groups. Responses from across Alberta totaled 524 persons with PD and 413 caregivers.

12.5.2.2 **Demographic Information**

The majority of persons with PD who responded to the survey were males (66%); the average age was about 70 years, with a range of 41 to 94 years. The findings were similar to those of other Alberta studies and those conducted in Ontario and elsewhere. The majority (70%) of the caregivers were female; about 32% of them were aged 66–75 years, and 25% were aged 56–66 years. The large majority of the caregivers (90%) were aged 46–85 years. These values were are similar to those of the studies conducted in Calgary [2] and the UK [28].

The respondents were distributed across Alberta; their distribution was determined by the first three letters of their postal code, and using Regional Health Authority boundaries [2] to categorize both the persons with PD and the caregivers. The results from the study (see Table 12.1) were compared with the 2005 prevalence data on people diagnosed with PD, as provided through data from Alberta Health and Wellness [1]. The number of persons with PD diagnosed in each of the nine regional health authorities (based on 2005 data), and the numbers who responded to the survey are provided in Table 12.1. The response rate varied across the regions, ranging from 3% to 15%, with the total number of respondents comprising about 10% of the total number of persons with PD in Alberta. The numbers of caregiver respondents in each regional health authority are also shown, although the actual numbers in each region were unknown.

The average age of diagnosis of persons with PD was 61.6 years; one person claimed to have been diagnosed at the age of 8 years, but the majority were in their late 50s to late 70s. Three-quarters of persons with PD were married, and another 15% were widowed. When asked about their living arrangements, 63%

Table 12.1 The number of persons with PD diagnosed in each of the nine regional health authorities.

Regional health authority	No. of persons with PD (response rate, %) Total = 524 (10%)	No. of caregivers who participated (*n* = 413)	Statistics on number persons diagnosed with PD in health regions [1]
David Thompson Health Authority	34 (5%)	31	621
East Central Health Authority	35 (10%)	28	360
Capital Health Region	260 (15%)	187	1783
Aspen Health region	22 (8%)	15	281
Peace Country Health Authority	7 (3%)	5	247
Northern Lights Health Region	1 (4%)	1	28
Calgary Health Authority	54 (3%)	42	1605
Chinook Health Region	33 (8%)	26	396
Palliser Health region	23 (10%)	16	240
Totals	469	351	5500
Missing postal code information	55	62	–

said they lived with their spouse or partner, while the remainder had a variety of living accommodations which included 12% living in continuing care or long-term care facilities, and 9% in retirement homes. Of those living with family or on their own, 67% had an unpaid caregiver. These demographic findings were similar to those reported elsewhere in the literature.

Whether or not there was any correlation, about one-quarter of persons with PD identified other family members with PD (as shown in Figure 12.1). Uncles, aunts, and mothers were identified most often as having had PD.

About 60% of the caregivers indicated that they have been assuming their role for between one and just less than 10 years, while 14% had been caregivers for 10–15 years. The majority of these caregivers were spouses of the persons with PD (83%). About 68% lived with the people with PD, while 16% lived with other family members. Others had various other living arrangements, including 3% in continuing or long-term care and another 3% in retirement homes.

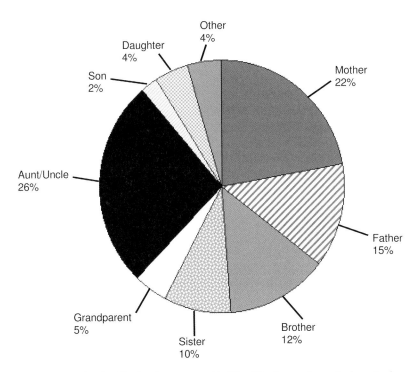

Figure 12.1 The identification by persons with PD, of family members who have (or have had) PD.

12.5.3
Education, Employment, and Income

Among the 524 persons with PD who responded to the present study, 41% had attended high school or less, and about 23% had graduated from high school. A number also had a university or college education, with about 18% having graduated with a degree or diploma, while 6% had obtained post-graduate degrees. The majority of persons with PD were fluent at speaking, reading, and writing English. Details of their current income are shown in Figure 12.2.

About 37% (*n* = 194) of the persons with PD claimed to have an annual income of less than $30 000, which in Alberta at that time was just above the low-income or poverty line. What should be explored further with these latter individuals are their actual expenses or costs that they are unable to pay for out-of-pocket, and which become a concern if these items are essential for treatment or care. Further analysis is also needed to examine the average burden of personal costs for persons with PD, regardless of their income level.

The employment picture provides some reasons for the lower incomes of persons with PD. The majority of persons with PD were retired (75%), 5% were employed full time, 5% were self-employed, and 12% were on long-term disability. Less than one-quarter of the persons with PD had told their employers about their diagnosis, but of those that had only 15% found their employers to be somewhat or very supportive.

Some PD respondents did not answer the questions related to their employment or employer situation. Of the 63% that responded (*n* = 346), 23% said that the job requirements were getting difficult to fulfill, and 11% had to have their jobs modified. For those who retired or stopped work voluntarily, about 32% (*n* = 106) said that PD was somewhat of or a major contributing factor. Only 6% said

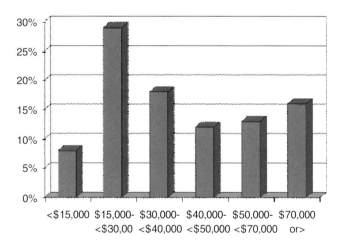

Figure 12.2 Household (pre-tax) income of persons with PD, in 2004. Note: 3% of individuals did not respond to this question.

that their spouses had to start or continue to work because of the situation. For the persons with PD, the average age when they stopped working was 60 years, which correlates closely with the average age at which they were diagnosed (average 62 years). Therefore it is important to note that, on average, most people with PD were diagnosed very shortly after their retirement or within two to three years.

There were different sources of income identified by people with PD, including employment for 52 respondents (10%), disability income from the Alberta Income for the Severely Handicapped program or AISH for six individuals (1%), employment insurance (four individuals), investments including Registered Retirement Savings Plans (RRSPs) ($n = 246$; 47%), work pension ($n = 246$; 47%), Canada Pension Plan (CPP) ($n = 346$; 63%), CPP disability ($n = 54$; 11%), private insurance ($n = 31$; 6%), seniors' supplement ($n = 121$; 23%), and family members ($n = 52$; 10%). The majority of individuals had not applied for any type of long-term disability benefits through work or the CPP (about 78%), although of the 18% who had done so very few had any difficulties or had minor difficulties with the process before receiving any benefits.

12.5.4
The Impact of Parkinson Disease on the Person with Parkinson Disease and Caregivers

Both, the persons with PD and their caregivers indicated that they had been impacted by PD in a number of ways. Many of the persons with PD felt that at the time of the survey they were mild to moderately impaired with physical and other changes (58%), while about 28% felt their impairment was significant, and some (8%) were confined to their bed or wheelchair. As PD progresses in individuals, there are likely more tasks that the caregivers assume because the person with PD can no longer do them. For example, there are a number of personal and other tasks which the person with PD may find challenging to do personally and will require assistance from their caregiver, including dressing/undressing (26%), bathing/showering (20%), eating and drinking (17%), turning in bed (13%), using the toilet (13%), and washing (10%).

The responses to the types of challenges and difficulties often identified with people who have PD are summarized in Table 12.2. The extent of the challenges or difficulties is directly linked with the stage of disease. In summary, there were more people with PD who often had challenges or problems than those that never had them. There were a few items that one-third or more of persons with PD felt they had never experienced at the time of the survey, including difficulty with eating or swallowing, feeling angry, feeling lonely or isolated, feeling embarrassed in public, feeling that they had no support from family or friends, hiding their PD, or having concerns with sexuality. In contrast, close to 50% of persons with PD had experienced frequent difficulties with such PDQ-39 items as getting around, worried about falling, difficulty dressing and writing clearly, loss of independence, and feeling frustrated.

Table 12.2 Challenges and concerns of persons with PD ($n = 524$). All values are given as percentages.

	Often	Sometimes	Never
1. Had difficulty getting around	34	17	21
2. Been worried about falling	33	19	19
3. Had difficulty dressing	29	18	18
4. Had difficulty with eating or swallowing	16	16	32
5. Had difficulty writing clearly	49	20	8
6. Felt a loss of independence	37	17	18
7. Felt frustrated	35	21	10
8. Felt depressed	25	16	23
9. Felt angry	18	14	32
10. Felt lonely and isolated	16	18	32
11. Felt anxious	23	17	16
12. Withdrawn from social activities	24	23	21
13. Felt unmotivated	24	18	20
14. Felt embarrassed in public	15	21	27
15. Tried to hide your PD	15	15	38
16. Had difficulty having your speech understood	27	19	22
17. Had difficulty with concentration	22	22	18
18. Had difficulty with memory	25	20	17
19. Felt a lack of support from family and friends	5	8	54
20. Had physical discomfort	29	20	16
21. Had concerns with sexuality	16	11	36

12.5.5
Medical and Health Care Services Accessed

Caregivers and persons with PD were asked about their satisfaction with the overall level of medical care. Those with PD indicated that they were generally "very satisfied" (46%) or "somewhat satisfied" (44%); less than 10% were dissatisfied or very dissatisfied with the level of medical care. The caregivers responded in similar fashion to the persons with PD; they were generally very satisfied (44%) or somewhat satisfied (41%) with the services which persons with PD received; less than 9% of caregivers were dissatisfied in any way.

The majority of persons with PD had family doctors (96%) who they believed were very knowledgeable (21%) or somewhat knowledgeable (56%), but about 17% questioned the knowledge level of their family doctors. A variety of reasons was given by those persons with PD who did not have a family doctor, including: no doctors in the area were accepting new patients; being placed on a waiting list; physically unable to travel to the doctor; and having no means of transportation. These people generally went to a walk-in clinic (5%) or emergency department at a hospital (3%). Although family physicians diagnosed PD for 33% of persons with PD, 60% of the diagnoses were made by neurologists. Family physicians also referred the person with PD to a specialist, such as a general neurologist (43%) or a specialized neurologist at a movement disorder clinic (68%). It is likely that the person with PD would go to the specialist more often than to the family physician, because the specialist (e.g., the movement disorder neurologist) prescribed and managed the person's medication on 55% of occasions. The family physicians appeared to prescribe medications to persons with PD less than one-fifth of the time. At the time of the survey, over 92% of persons with PD were receiving drug treatment for their PD, primarily Sinemet (55%) or Sinemet CR (40%). Nearly 67% of the persons with PD felt that their medications had been adequately explained to them.

The number of visits which a person with PD will make to the family doctor, neurologist or nurse clinician for medications or other issues is summarized in Table 12.3. The majority of persons with PD visit their neurologist (64%) and family physicians (59%) at least two to three times within the same year. Face-to-face visits are preferred more by persons with PD as compared to telephone or e-mail use, or accessing nurse clinicians at the clinics. On average, people with PD had had to travel between 1 to 30 km to see their family doctor, and between 1 and 150 km to see their neurologist. The literature also supported these findings, namely that persons with PD continue to visit their doctors and are generally satisfied with the care they received [12].

In some cases, the person with PD must be hospitalized, although this does not happen often. Only 13% of those with PD said they had been hospitalized during the previous 12 months of the survey (2004–2005).

There are also other healthcare providers which the person with PD will be referred to by family doctors, specialists, community home care provider, or others. Details of the services referred to, and the responses of persons with PD as to how helpful these healthcare providers have been, are listed in Table 12.4. In the past, physical therapists have been the most referred service for persons with PD (38%), and found to be very or somewhat helpful to 31% of responding persons with PD. Speech and language therapists were referred to 23% of respondents, and found very or somewhat helpful by about 16%. There were several other therapies to which at least 10% of persons with PD were referred, and were found to be relatively helpful. However, many other therapies, such as psychologist,

Table 12.3 Number of times persons with PD visited health professionals ($n = 524$). All values are given as percentages.

Professional visited	No. of visits			
	0	1	2	≥3
Neurologist, face-to-face	10	18	44	18
Neurologist, by telephone	27	3	2	2
Nurse clinician at PD clinic	17	7	10	9
Neurologist, by e-mail	23	0.7	0.2	0
Family doctor	6	9	15	48

Table 12.4 Referrals to (i) and helpfulness of (ii) healthcare providers (*n* = 524; some no responses). All values are given as percentages.

	Have been referred	Helpfulness			
		Very helpful	Somewhat helpful	Not very helpful	Not helpful at all
Physical therapist	38	20	12	7	4
Occupational therapist	16	8	7	1	1
Dietician/Nutritionist	12	5	5	2	0.7
Speech and language therapist	23	8	8	3	1
Homemaker service	9	4	2	0.5	0.5
Psychiatrist	9	3	3	1	1
Social worker	7	1	3	1	1
Swallowing specialist	15	6	4	1	1
Sleep specialist	4	0.7	0.5	0.7	0.7
Psychologist	5	0.7	1	1	0.7
Day program	8	4	2	2	1
Massage therapist	10	4	3	1	1
Public health nurse	7	3	2	0.7	0.7
Sexual therapist	2	0	0	0.2	0.5
Neuropsychologist	3	0.2	0.7	0.2	0.5

psychiatrist, social worker, day program, sleep specialist or public health nurse, to which persons with PD were referred less frequently. Not having more referrals to these latter services is in contradiction to the high value rating and need for these services expressed by persons with PD to enhance or sustain their ability to function and have some quality of life.

Generally, in order to access these healthcare providers, it is necessary that the person with PD or the caregiver has access to transportation. In about 49% of cases, the persons with PD drive themselves, while 40% prefer to be driven; only 3% utilize the community disabled services. When PD makes it difficult for individuals to drive (20% of respondents) they will ask others to drive them. For example, in addition to family members who might be available, service groups (which were available to 33% of persons with PD) were utilized by about 13% of individuals to attend their appointments. A summary of the ability to go to different places, depending on the stage of the PD is shown in Table 12.5. Whenever respondents were not having specific difficulties with driving, they answered "doesn't apply" (see Table 12.5).

12.5.5.1 Community Care: Home Care or Long-Term/Continuing Care?

When traveling or driving becomes an issue for persons with PD and caregivers, or if additional support is needed in the home, individuals can access home care or long-term/continuing care. Almost two-thirds of persons with PD had

Table 12.5 The inability of persons with PD to travel as a result of their disease. The data were not related to urban versus rural locations (n = 524; some no responses). All values are given as percentages.

Problem encountered	PD is ...				
	A major factor	Somewhat of a factor	Not really a factor	Not a factor at all	Does not apply
I have difficulty driving a car	20	14	13	14	30
My driver's license was removed	13	0.5	1	8	64
My driver's license is under suspension	3	0.7	0.2	8	71
I have difficulty carrying out day- to-day tasks (e.g., grocery shopping)	22	17	8	12	31
I visit with friends less frequently	22	24	9	14	21
I leave home less frequently	24	23	9	13	23
I never leave home	5	9	4	15	51
I have given up regular social activities outside of the home	17	22	8	14	29
I feel more isolated	17	23	9	15	27

not used home care services, but of those who had one-quarter were "somewhat" or "very satisfied" with the services they had received. Between 4 and 8 hours of home care services were being utilized by persons with PD, and this was acceptable by about 19% of the individuals who received such services. The main advantage here for about 8% of people with PD was that they could continue to live in their own homes, but for others this was not a factor in using home care services.

For those persons with PD who currently live in a nursing home or long-term care facility, their needs are different. When asked how satisfied they were with the care they were receiving in the nursing home or long-term care facility, they indicated their general satisfaction with various aspects, including the level of knowledge about PD of the nursing staff at the facility, the incidence of receiving their PD medications at the correct times, the availability of daily exercise routines, availability of rehabilitation (physiotherapy, occupational therapy, speech therapy), and the overall level of care and support that they received.

12.5.6
Medical and Other Expenses

Looking after a person with PD, as with any other similar chronic condition, requires financial support in order to cover costs beyond those paid for by insurance plans. Medical expenses were covered for about 84% of the persons with PD, with the majority covered by Alberta Health Care, Blue Cross, or Employer group plans, and about 11% having e a combination plan. Depending on the needs of the person with PD, the range of insurance paid per month by companies ranged from $50 to over $1000 per month. Additional out-of-pocket costs were paid personally by the persons with PD, with the amount being based on the medications used. Most persons with PD will, pay out-of-pocket, between $1 and $25 per month, with very few individuals paying more than $200. In addition to prescription drugs, 11% of individuals also paid out $20–30 per month for nonprescription supplements such as vitamins or herbals, many of which were relevant to their PD treatment plan. These findings were on par with those of other studies, including the *Economic Burden of Illness in Canada 1998* report.

When persons with PD were asked if they would not buy their PD medications due to cost, the very large majority (92%) said "no." So, essentially 8% of respondents would not buy their PD medications if they had to pay more out of pocket than what they pay currently. The same applies to the purchase of assistive devices needed by the person with PD; about 85% of respondents said they would still purchase any assistive devices needed, regardless of the personal cost. Presently, one-third were paying for their assistive devices. Additional expenses were also incurred by persons with PD; the proportions of persons with PD purchasing various services and paying out of pocket for them, are shown in Figure 12.3.

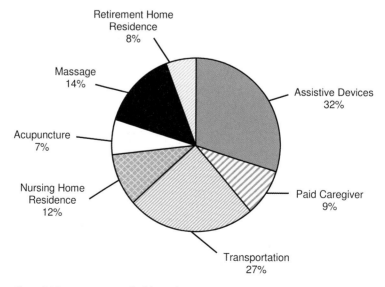

Figure 12.3   Proportions of additional expenses incurred by persons with PD (*n* = 524).

As mentioned above, assistive devices which persons with PD use and/or need, but may not have, are also those which are not always reimbursed by the insurance companies or plans, such that individuals end up paying out-of-pocket. Examples include bathing aids (75%), toilet aids (47%), walkers (67%), and manual wheel-chairs (28%). The list of assistive devices (see Table 12.6) includes such items as bathing bars and chairs, bath lifts, raised toilet seats, walkers, scooters, wheel-chairs, communication aids for talking and/or hearing, eating, and dressing aids. The most common assistive devices used, needed, and sometimes reim-bursed – though not always – include those for the bathroom or for mobility (e.g., wheelchairs or walkers). In addition to these devices, persons with PD need their homes to be adapted so as to improve accessibility, often with the use of inside and outside ramps. About 82% of respondents had their homes accessible-ready. As shown in Table 12.6, a large number of persons with PD indicated that, at the time of the survey, they did not require any of these types of assistive devices or adaptations for their homes; conversely, there were very few that needed the assis-tive devices but did not have them.

12.5.7
Services Needed and Valued by People with Parkinson Disease

People with PD require specific services, and find some more valuable than others. These different services and the responses of persons with PD are detailed in Table 12.7, although only a small proportion of persons with PD actually currently use these various services. The two services that currently are utilized by 19% of persons with PD are the Parkinson Clinic and the local or area office of the Par-kinson's Societies (located in Edmonton and Calgary); two other support services, namely support groups and massage therapists, were each used by 14%. There were, however, more individuals who said that if the services were available in their community they would "very likely" or "somewhat likely" use them. These included exercise groups, toll-free numbers to call for information about PD, a PD clinic, free transportation to appointments, homemaker service, speech therapy, and massage therapy. On the other hand, a large proportion of persons with PD also said that it was "very unlikely" or "somewhat unlikely" that they would utilize the various services if they were available within their community. These services included access to exercise groups, toll-free number, adult day care center, free transportation, homemaker service, written information about PD in a language other then English or French, meals on wheels, respite care, social worker, or volunteer visitors, and others. From these responses, it can be deduced that it is not necessary to have all the listed services available in communities where persons with PD live, because there is only a select few (about one-third) of the services that they would use or very likely use. If people said they would "somewhat use" or "somewhat unlikely" use the services, this could be interpreted as either unsure or uncertain, and may be a 50/50 chance of going either way.

When persons with PD were asked to take this same list of services and to state how valuable (if at all) they believed these to be for them, there were some differ-ent responses; these are detailed in Table 12.8. Most items on the list were rated

Table 12.6 Assistive devices used and needed by persons with PD (*n* = 524). All values are given as percentages.

Assistive aid(s)	Requirement					
	Current use	Purchased personally	Supplied by home care	Supplied by aids to daily living	Need, but do not have	Do not need
Bathing aids (e.g., bars, chairs)	31	18	9	12	3	27
Bath lift	4	1	1	1	1	35
Toileting aids (e.g., bars, raised seats)	23	11	7	11	4	28
Walker	23	17	3	10	2	30
Scooter	6	5	1	1	2	34
Wheelchair (manual)	17	10	3	8	1	34
Wheelchair (electric)	3	3	0	1	2	36
Communication aids (e.g., voice amplifier)	2	1	1	1	3	35
Communication aids (type/ computer assistive device)	3	2	0	1	2	37
Communication aids (adapted telephone)	3	4	0	1	3	35
Communication aids (hearing aid)	5	3	0	2	4	34
Communication aids (call or alarm button)	10	6	2	2	4	32
Eating aids	5	4	1	1	2	35
Dressing aids	6	4	2	2	4	32
Ramp(s) or lifts in house	3	2	1	0	3	34
Ramp(s) or lifts outside house	3	2	1	1	4	33
Modified vehicle	2	2	0	1	2	35
Other (please name)	6	4	1	3	0	24

Table 12.7 Availability of services and their current and likely use by persons with PD. All values are given as percentages.

Service	Level of use				
	Very likely	Somewhat likely	Somewhat unlikely	Very unlikely	Already use
Exercise group	20	24	8	23	14
Toll-free number to call for information about PD	20	23	11	23	8
Support group	19	25	14	16	14
PD clinics (doctors, nurses, etc.)	37	21	6	6	19
Local or area office of Parkinson Society of Alberta	18	24	12	11	19
Adult day care center	13	15	13	36	7
Free transportation to appointments	29	17	9	28	2
Homemaker service	20	16	12	30	4
Written information about PD in a language other than English or French	7	3	3	66	3
Meals on wheels	8	12	14	47	2
Speech therapy	20	23	11	23	7
Occupational therapy	18	21	11	27	6
Dietitian/nutritionist	17	18	17	26	4
Massage therapy	28	23	12	18	6
Respite care	13	16	14	33	6
Counseling	12	27	15	28	5
Caregiver training	10	18	15	34	2
Long-term planning	13	24	15	28	2
Psychologist	8	14	19	37	2
Social worker	7	14	18	38	4
Volunteer visitors	7	16	17	28	1
Other (please specify)					

Table 12.8 Value rating of the services, as indicated by persons with PD (*n* = 524). All values are given as percentages.

Service	Rating			
	Very valuable	Somewhat valuable	Not very valuable	Not valuable at all
Exercise group	60	22	3	2
Toll-free number to call for information about PD	46	29	7	4
Support group	47	33	4	2
PD clinics (doctors, nurses, etc.)	67	16	1	2
Local or area office of Parkinson Society	44	31	4	2
Adult day care center	34	33	9	7
Free transportation to appointments	53	22	6	4
Homemaker service	45	26	7	4
Written information about PD in a language other than English or French	18	25	12	25
Meals on wheels	35	30	11	6
Speech therapy	45	29	6	4
Occupational therapy	39	30	9	3
Dietitian/nutritionist	35	33	7	4
Massage therapy	43	32	5	3
Respite care	36	30	9	4
Counseling	35	34	8	4
Caregiver training	36	31	6	5
Long-term planning	37	32	8	4
Psychologist	37	34	13	5
Social worker	26	35	15	5
Volunteer visitors	25	33	12	7
Other (please specify)[a]				

a) For the "Other" category, persons with PD identified chiropractor, physiotherapy/physical therapy, information for family on how to deal with PD, reflexology, and more research.

as "very valuable," especially the PD clinic and exercise groups (66% and 61%, respectively). About 53% of people with PD said they would find free transportation to appointments very valuable, while a few other services were considered very valuable by 43–47% of the respondents.

12.5.8
What Caregivers said About the Services Needed by Persons with PD, and Their Value

Caregivers were given the same lists for services as the persons with PD respondents had received, and asked similar questions about whether or not the person with PD currently uses any or all of the services, and how likely that individual would use these and other services if they were available in his/her area. The caregivers' responses to both questions for the list are included in Tables 12.9 and 12.10. The items rated "very likely" and similar to persons with PD responses, included exercise groups, toll-free numbers to call for information about PD, PD clinic, free transportation, homemaker service, speech therapy, and massage therapy. However, there were other services which caregivers rated as "very likely" to be used by individuals if available, that were not acknowledged by persons with PD as being something they would very likely use. These services included a local or area office of the Parkinson Society, occupation therapy, dietitian/nutritionist, respite care, counseling, caregiver training, and long-term planning. The two most items "very unlikely" to be used by persons with PD, according to caregivers, were written information about PD in a language other than English or French, and meals on wheels. Some persons with PD were already using the various services to varying degrees, with the PD clinic being used by 20%, and the Parkinson Societies by 18%.

Caregivers were also asked to rate the value of the services for persons with PD, as shown in Table 12.9; their responses are summarized in Table 12.10. Caregivers felt that all the services listed would be "very valuable" for persons with PD. Every service identified in the list was rated this way by the majority of the caregivers, which was both significant and noteworthy.

Often, there are reasons why persons with PD and their caregivers are unable to or do not access the services they identify as being needed or something they would use and value, if the services were available in their community. Some of the more common reasons for not accessing services, as identified by the caregivers, are that they do not have transportation to get to the services (14%), they cannot afford the cost of the service, especially if paid for by the person with PD (14%), and the service is not available in their communities (28%). Almost half of the caregivers said they do not access services if they do not need them (46%).

12.5.9
Information Needed and Accessed

People with PD and their caregivers were asked about what type of information they needed about PD or other issues, and where they have accessed or need to access this information. People with PD indicated that they needed information on such things as symptoms of PD over time (56%) and changes they could expect with the disease (46%). They also wanted information on how to live well with PD (46%), as well as treatment (49%), and other specific and personal items.

Caregivers viewed the need for different types of information in a very similar way to persons with PD. However, the one difference which stood out for 47% of

Table 12.9 Caregivers' perceptions concerning the services persons with PD currently access, and would likely access if available (*n* = 413). All values are given as percentages.

Service	Level of use				
	Very likely	Somewhat likely	Somewhat unlikely	Very unlikely	Already use
Exercise group	21	22	9	16	12
Toll-free number to call for information about PD	25	21	9	14	12
Support group	21	24	11	9	14
PD clinics (doctors, nurses, etc.)	41	14	3	5	21
Local or area office of Parkinson Society of Alberta	23	25	7	7	19
Adult day care center (supervised day care by hospital, nursing home, etc.)	17	21	16	20	8
Free transportation to appointments	27	17	10	24	3
Homemaker service	23	20	13	22	4
Written information about PD in a language other than English or French	7	3	2	62	3
Meals on wheels	9	17	23	42	2
Speech therapy	22	20	7	22	9
Occupational therapy	22	22	8	21	6
Dietitian/nutritionist	20	22	14	18	6
Massage therapy	31	24	8	13	6
Respite care (short-term, supervised, overnight care)	20	21	10	23	5
Counseling	21	28	15	13	2
Caregiver training	24	26	10	19	6
Long-term planning	22	26	15	17	2
Psychologist	15	21	18	22	2
Social worker	11	20	20	24	2
Volunteer visitors	12	17	20	24	1
Other (please specify)	2	0.9	0.6	3	2

Table 12.10 Caregivers rating of the value of services for people with PD ($n = 413$). All values are given as percentages.

Service	Rating			
	Very valuable	Somewhat valuable	Not very valuable	Not valuable at all
Exercise group	65	17	2	2
Toll-free number to call for information about PD	48	24	7	3
Support group	57	22	5	2
PD clinics (doctors, nurses, etc.)	75	11	0.6	0.9
Local or area office of Parkinson Society of Alberta	48	30	7	0.6
Adult day care center (supervised day care by hospital, nursing home, etc.)	51	27	5	2
Free transportation to appointments	54	21	6	3
Homemaker service	48	23	5	3
Written information about PD in a language other than English or French	23	16	12	25
Meals on wheels	39	29	9	5
Speech therapy	53	22	5	3
Occupational therapy	51	22	7	3
Dietitian/nutritionist	47	25	6	2
Massage therapy	57	20	5	2
Respite care (short-term, supervised, overnight care)	55	20	5	3
Counseling	45	27	7	3
Caregiver training	44	28	7	4
Long-term planning	43	29	7	3
Psychologist	38	27	12	3
Social worker	32	32	13	5
Volunteer visitors	34	26	11	7
Other (please specify	2	0.6	0.3	0.9

caregivers as opposed to 45% of persons with PD was the changes expected with PD. The different types of information which both groups said persons with PD would need are shown in Figure 12.4.

When persons with PD were asked about where and to whom they go to for this information, over half said that they went to their neurologist (63%) or family doctor (51%). Other sources of information are shown in Figure 12.5. The Parkinson's Societies were viewed as good sources of information by about 43% of respondents. This is supported by the earlier "very valuable" rating given to the Parkinson Societies by 45% of persons with PD. The library seemed to be the least likely place for persons with PD to go for their information. Support groups were also not rated very highly.

Caregivers also need information for caregiving for persons with PD, and for their own needs as caregivers. The different types of information which caregivers say they need, in comparison to persons with PD, are illustrated graphically in Figure 12.4. In addition (as noted in Figure 12.5), the majority of caregivers suggest that they obtain most of their information from the neurologist and family doctor. However, in contrast to persons with PD, more caregivers use the Internet (30%) or contact support groups (24%) to obtain their information.

12.5.10
Parkinson's Societies in Alberta: Persons with PD and Caregivers' Connections

The majority of respondents (414 with PD, 329 caregivers) were from Central and Northern Alberta and commented on the Parkinson Society of Alberta in

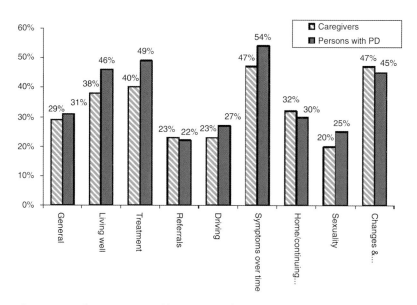

Figure 12.4 Information required by persons with PD, and their caregivers.

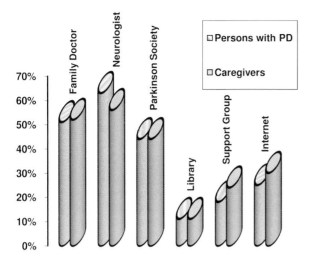

Figure 12.5 Sources of information used by persons with PD and their caregivers.

Edmonton. Of the 194 respondents from Southern Alberta (110 with PD, 84 caregivers), less than half responded to questions about the Parkinson Society of Southern Alberta in Calgary, although most knew of its existence.

When all of the persons with PD and caregivers were asked whether or not they had heard about the Parkinson's Society either in Edmonton or Calgary before completing this survey, about 74% from both groups said "yes." In addition, both groups also said they had made contact with the Society. They had first learned about the Parkinson's Societies in Alberta primarily through their doctor or health professional (30% persons with PD indicated this, and 34% of caregivers). Other respondents had learned about the society in other ways, including newspapers/ magazines and newsletters (17% with PD, 19% caregivers), and through a relative or friend (10% with PD, 15% caregivers). Television, radio, and another member of the Society were ranked low in terms of making persons with PD and caregivers aware of the Parkinson's Society nearest to them. Of the respondents with PD, about 54% indicated that they were members of the Society, while 45% of caregivers were members.

Respondents had various reasons for contacting the Parkinson's Societies. Persons with PD said that one reason for contacting the Society closest to them was because they had been recently diagnosed (27%); likewise, caregivers said they made contact with the Society when someone they cared for was recently diagnosed with PD (30%). The diagnosis was what made them want to seek out and connect with others, particularly other people with PD and their caregivers. About 22% of persons with PD wanted to connect with others, and about 23% of caregivers wanted to meet not only other persons with PD but also other caregivers. The majority of respondents in both groups wanted general information about PD, and one-quarter of respondents in both groups specifically wanted information about support groups. About one-quarter of persons with PD who responded also wanted information about medications and exercise groups. Both groups wanted to donate money to the Society (23% of both groups). Other reasons for connecting with the Parkinson's Societies are summarized in Table 12.11.

Both groups identified what they found most useful. Themes which were evident from the comments of persons with PD included resources of information on PD and who to see for referrals, education sessions, support groups and self-help, staff support, events, and programs (speech and exercise). For caregivers, the themes around what they found most useful in connecting with the Societies included library, newsletter, website for information, literature available, interaction with others (especially through support groups), education sessions, accessibility to Societies when needed, volunteer work as in special events, and medical and healthcare services accessed through the Societies. About 23% of persons with PD and caregivers who responded said that they attended the Societies' support groups, while 43% of those with PD and 35% of caregivers said that they would like to see a support group in their immediate area. The majority of caregivers also said that support groups should really be for both the person with PD and

Table 12.11 Reasons for persons with PD and caregivers contacting the Parkinson's Societies in Alberta. All values are given as percentages.

Reason for contact	Persons with PD (*n* = 524)	Caregivers (*n* = 413)
Information about support groups	23	24
Information about treatment	22	19
Information about speech	21	19
Information about special events	16	19
Information about medications	25	17
Information about exercise groups	24	16
Information about PD in general	43	33
Information about driving (advice, assessment)	8	5
Information about interventions (e.g., physiotherapy, other therapies)	16	15
To use the telephone help line	2	3
To volunteer	9	10
To donate money	22	22
To obtain recommendations for doctors or neurologists in the area	9	8
Was referred by a doctor	14	11
To talk with support staff	15	14

the caregiver, together with some separate discussion time (92%). The value of the support groups was indicated by caregivers and persons with PD in previous discussions (see Tables 12.8 and 12.10).

For those persons with PD and caregivers who indicated that they were members of the either the Parkinson Society of Alberta (located in Edmonton) or the Parkinson Society of Southern Alberta (located in Calgary), they were asked to rate how valuable they found the current programs, activities and services offered by the Society. These findings are summarized in Table 12.12. Free information packages and brochures and the *"Parkinson's Perspectives"* newsletter were value-rated the highest.

Caregivers were asked additional questions about what programs, services, or activities they would like to see offered by the Parkinson Societies in Alberta. The themes identified in their comments included more information sessions (awareness of disease, research) offered by different means (newsletters, e-mail help line, library lending services, more resources), more programs (day care, exercise, special clinics for speech and physiotherapy), more support for newly diagnosed and for issues concerning sexuality and decision making, professional access (psychologist, social worker, community services, knowledgeable staff), and others (events, greater focus on the young population with PD, financial assistance, respite, drivers, outreach).

12.6
Concluding Comments and Recommendations

The present case study, by using surveys with persons with PD and their caregivers, provided: (i) demographics and characteristics of individuals living with PD; (ii) support, health, and other services individuals living with PD accessed including those provided by the Parkinson's Society of Alberta; (iii) information that individuals with PD found most useful, and where they accessed the information they needed; and (iv) gaps and barriers in service and information access.

Of the surveys distributed to persons with PD and to caregivers the response rates, at 524 for persons with PD and 413 for caregivers, were within the estimated number needed for the study, considering that there was no follow-up mechanism in place for survey recipients. The demographics of the respondents in this case study survey reflected those of other studies and their participants in general. There were more males with PD in most studies, and the majority are aged 65–70 years. The caregivers were primarily female, and ranged in age from 41 to 95 years, with some being spouses and others daughters or other relations to the person with PD. These demographics are important, and will remain important for decision makers to consider in their planning the types of programs and services needed, as well as allocating budgets for them. As PD is primarily, but not totally, a disease that impacts upon people at retirement age, these individuals will not be working, nor will they have a fixed income. While some of their spouses had to

Table 12.12 Programs, activities and services of the Parkinson's Societies in Alberta; value-rated by persons with PD (PWP; $n = 524$) and caregivers (C; $n = 413$). All values are given as percentages.

Activity/Service	Very valuable		Somewhat valuable		Not very valuable		Not at all valuable		Do not know	
	PWP	C	PWP	C	PWP	C	PWP	C	PWP	C
Free information packages and brochures	41	33	13	12	1	2	0.7	0.6	3	4
Toll-free number to call for information about PD	19	16	14	10	5	4	2	2	10	12
Support groups	21	21	15	8	5	2	2	2	10	11
Walk-in, appointment, or phone staff support	15	15	14	9	5	3	2	3	13	14
Newsletter *Parkinson's Perspectives*	42	33	10	14	1	0.6	0.7	1	2	3
Referral to community resources	12	15	15	10	4	3	2	2	14	13
Speech education program	18	16	13	7	4	2	1	2	14	14
Education sessions for health professionals	13	11	11	10	4	2	1	2	17	20
Educational lectures	17	15	13	11	4	2	1	2	49	15
Social events (e.g., Christmas party)	13	11	15	15	6	2	2	3	13	15
Resource/lending library	16	13	15	10	6	3	2	2	13	14
Awareness/ fundraising events (e.g., SuperWalk, Tulip Sales)	26	23	12	11	3	2	1	2	9	9
Donations to research (to national or local)	31	27	10	8	1	1	1	3	7	9

go to work to help maintain their income, in most cases the spouse had to stop working to become a full-time caregiver, with the result being a much lower income. Those with an annual income less than $30 000 are nearing low-income status, and may encounter more burden in paying for all the necessities, treatment, assistive aids, and therapies needed to manage or control PD. The majority of respondents had some type of insurance or assistance with covering medications, but some did pay differences in costs of medications and for nonprescriptive supplements. Paying out-of-pocket for various of the needed care items was common for persons with PD; these included walkers, massage, physiotherapy, bathroom aids, and some adaptation to the home.

The burden of the cost of PD is borne out in the many changes and accommodations that persons with PD and their caregiver, whether spouse or family, have had to make. Persons with PD expressed concerns over the many challenges of living with PD, which included just getting around without falling or needing help to dress or eat. Difficulties with writing, speaking, and a loss of independence generally lead to withdrawal and isolation as well as to depression, frustration, and anger. At this stage, the access to services, therapies for speech and muscle tone, and support groups is critical in order to manage the disease and live with some dignity and quality of life. Those patients in rural settings will encounter more challenges in accessing services and programs, and must drive greater distances to access these. In fact, transportation was highlighted as one of the major barriers to accessing needed services, with those persons with PD who had transportation (i.e., they could still drive or had drivers) being more inclined to take an active part in the services. This is an important consideration for not only those persons with PD but also for others with challenges of transportation and of accessing the needed services, particularly when these are not close to hand in the community.

Some of the key highlights of the responses from persons with PD and their caregivers concerned actual services accessed, valued, and needed. Persons with PD valued their visits with their neurologists (44% saw their neurologists at least twice a year, while almost 18% saw them three or more times per year) and family physicians (48% saw their family physicians three or more times a year) for not only the treatment but also the information provided.

Persons with PD vary in their access and value for certain health and support services. There are some things they value but will not likely use because of out-of-pocket costs attached or lack of access. Most persons with PD would pay out of pocket for assistive devices, medications, and services. However, on analyzing the various responses for services valued, used or likely to use if available, there was some discrepancy. Many persons with PD rated the various services as valuable, but far fewer indicated that they already used the services or would use/access them if available.

For caregivers specifically, the main issue was to ensure that the person with PD had access to a variety of programs and services which were seen as needed and valued for controlling and managing the disease. PD impacts on both the person with PD and the caregiver and, therefore, the desire of the caregiver is that both parties have access to the same information and services. Again, for program and policy decision makers, consideration for making services available and accessible to persons with PD and their caregivers is important. Although the focus in this chapter is not on caregivers, it is important to not forget them.

There may be areas identified in the survey findings which might be perceived to be of value for further research. For example, longer-term effectiveness of many treatment or support strategies and the usefulness of QoL instruments are critical for future research [32]. There are also economic or cost analysis studies of what having PD actually costs the healthcare system or society, or even the individual with PD or the caregiver. With the transformation of the healthcare system in Alberta from nine regional health authorities to one Alberta Health Services (AHS), there will be some implications for persons with PD and their caregivers. The Continuum of Care which is proposed in the new AHS, with rural as well as urban focus, has the potential of ensuring that the service needs of people with PD can be provided for. It will be important for persons with PD, their caregivers, the Parkinson's Societies in Alberta, healthcare providers and others, to monitor this new approach.

Recommendations based on the findings and results of this study include:

- The need for a plan for the enhancement and expansion of programs and services as the population ages and the incidence of PD increases.
- A need more awareness of the services available, and where these are located for the persons with PD and caregivers to access.
- A need for a province-wide PD Registry to capture surveillance data relating to the incidence and prevalence of PD.
- A need for more resources in rural communities or an alternate mobile service plan.
- A need for the support of regional and provincial decision/policy makers to examine programs and services along with persons with PD, caregivers, health professionals, and other service providers.
- A need to explore whether the Alberta Telehealth or Primary Care Networks that recently were implemented, will provide assistance with identified information and service access gaps.
- To explore the translation of this information for all service providers and decision makers at regional and provincial levels.
- To determine the need for policies regarding service provision and chronic disease management programs for PD and other chronic diseases.
- For caregivers to receive special attention to address their personal needs, and for researching other relevant questions.

References

1 Svenson, L. (2006) Prevalence from surveillance data. Oral Report.
2 Thurston, W.E., Andersen, D., and Emmett, J. (1999) *An Assessment of the* *Personal and Health Care Needs of Persons With Parkinson's and Their Caregivers,* The Parkinson's Society of Southern Alberta.

3 Health Canada (2002) *Economic Burden of Illness in Canada, 1998*, Health Canada, Ottawa.

4 Guttman, M., Slaughter, P.M., Theriault, M., DeBoer, D.P., Math, M., and Naylor, C.D. (2003) Parkinsonism in Ontario: comorbidity associated with hospitalization in a large cohort. *Movement Disorders*, **19** (1), 49–53.

5 Keranen, T., Kaakkola, S., Sotaniemi, K., Laulumaa, V., Haapaniemi, T., Jol, T., *et al.* (2003) Economic burden and quality of life impairment increase with severity of PD. *Parkinsonism and Related Disorders*, **9** (3), 163–168.

6 Scheife, R.T., Schumock, G.T., Burstein, A., Gottwald, M.D., and Luer, M.S. (2000) Impact of Parkinson's disease and its pharmacologic treatment, quality of life and economic outcomes. *American Journal of Health-System Pharmacy*, **57** (10), 953–962.

7 Marr, J.A. (1991) The experience of living with Parkinson's disease. *Journal of Neuroscience Nursing*, **23** (5), 325–329.

8 Chrischilles, E.A., Rubenstein, L.M., Voelker, M.D., Wallace, R.B., and Rodnitzky, R.L. (2002) Linking clinical variables to health-related quality of life in Parkinson's disease. *Parkinsonism and Related Disorders*, **8**, 199–209.

9 Marras, C., Lang, A., Krahn, M., Tomlinson, G., Naglie, G., and The Parkinson Study Group (2004) Quality of life in early Parkinson's disease: impact of dyskinesias and motor fluctuations. *Movement Disorders*, **19** (1), 22–28.

10 Haapaniemi, T.H., Sotaniemi, K.A., Sintonen, H., Taimela, E. for the EcoPD Study Group (2004) The generic 15D instrument is valid and feasible for measuring health related quality of life in Parkinson's disease. *Journal of Neurology, Neurosurgery, and Psychiatry*, **75**, 976–983.

11 Peto, V., Jenkinson, C., Fitzpatrick, R., and Greenhall, R. (1995) The development and validation of a short measure of functioning and well being for individuals with Parkinson's disease. *Quality of Life Research*, **4**, 241–248.

12 Parkinson Society Canada, ALS Society of Canada, Alzheimer Society of Canada, Huntington Society of Canada, Multiple Sclerosis of Canada, and Muscular Dystrophy Canada (2003) Synchrony: Looking at Disability Supports from a Progressive Disability Perspective. Executive Summary, October, 2003.

13 Paraashos, S.A., Maraganore, D.M., O'Brien, P.C., and Rocca, W.A. (2002) Medical services utilization and prognosis in Parkinson disease: population-based study. *Mayo Clinic Proceedings*, **77** (9), 918–995.

14 De Boer, A.G., Sprangers, M.A., Speelman, H.D., and de Haes, H.C. (1999) Predictors of health care use in patients with Parkinson's disease: a longitudinal study. *Movement Disorders*, **14** (5), 772–779.

15 Kale, R. (ed.) (2004) Who should look after people with Parkinson's disease? *British Medical Journal*, **328**, 62–63.

16 Wade, D.T., Gage, H., Owen, C., Trend, P., Grossmith, C., and Kaye, J. (2003) Multidisciplinary rehabilitation for people with Parkinson's disease: a randomized controlled study. *Journal of Neurology, Neurosurgery, and Psychiatry*, **74** (2), 158–162.

17 Iansek, R. (1999) Key points in the management of Parkinson's disease. *Australian Family Physician*, **28** (9), 897–901.

18 Frazier, L.D. (2002) Stability and change in patterns of coping with Parkinson's disease. *International Journal of Aging and Human Development*, **55** (3), 207–231.

19 Charlton, G.S. and Barrow, C.L. (2002) Coping and self-help group membership in Parkinson's disease: an exploratory qualitative study. *Health and Social Care in the Community*, **10** (6), 472–478.

20 Haberman, B. (2000) Spousal perspective of Parkinson's disease in middle life. *Journal of Advanced Nursing*, **31** (6), 1409–1415.

21 Reid, J. (2003) Diagnosis of Parkinson's disease: why patient education matter. *Professional Nurse*, **19** (1), 33–35.

22 Lee, K.S., Merriman, A., Owen, A., Chew, B., and Tan, T.C. (1994) The medical, social, and functional profile of Parkinson's disease in patients. *Singapore Medical Journal*, **35** (3), 265–268.

23 Haberman, B. (1996) Day-to-day demands of Parkinson's disease. *Western Journal of Nursing Research*, **18** (4), 397–413.

24 Edwards, N.E. and Ruettiger, K.M. (2002) The influence of caregiver burden on patients' management of Parkinson's disease: implications for rehabilitation nursing. *Rehabilitation Nursing*, **27** (5), 182–186.

25 Calne, S.M. and Kumar, A. (2003) Nursing care of patients with late-stage Parkinson's disease. *Journal of Neuroscience Nursing*, **35** (5), 242–251.

26 Edwards, N.E. and Scheetz, P.S. (2002) Predictors of burden for caregivers of patients with Parkinson's disease. *Journal of Neuroscience Nursing*, **34** (4), 184–190.

27 Sunvisson, H. and Ekman, S.L. (2001) Environmental influences on the experiences of people with Parkinson's disease. *Nursing Inquiry*, **8** (1), 41–50.

28 Yarrow, S. (1999) *Survey of Members of the Parkinson's Disease Society*, Parkinson's Disease Society of the United Kingdom and Policy Studies Institute, London.

29 Allen, I., Hogg, D., and Pease, S. (1999) *Elderly People: Choice, Participation and Satisfaction*, Policy Studies Institute, London.

30 Gordon, M. (2001) Challenges of an aging population. *Annals of the Royal College of Physicians and Surgeons of Canada*, **34** (5), 306–308.

31 Guttman, M., Slaugher, P.M., Theriault, M.E., De Boer, D.P., and Naylor, C.D. (2003) Burden of parkinsonism: a population-based study. *Movement Disorders*, **18** (3), 313–319.

32 Rubenstein, L.M., Chrischilles, E.A., and Voelker, M.D. (1997) The impact of Parkinson's disease on health status, health expenditures, and productivity. Estimates from the National Medical Expenditure Survey. *Pharmacoeconomics*, **12** (4), 486–498.

A Patient's Story

We Don't Choose Parkinson's – It Chooses Us

Jackie Bodie

I was diagnosed with Parkinson's disease (PD) at the age of 33, when my first son was just 2 months old. Although I knew nothing about PD, other than it involved "shaking," I had suspected for at least a year that PD was the reason my pinkie finger trembled uncontrollably. I was told about *the* Parkinson Society of Southern Alberta (PSSA) by my neurologist, but did not call until a year later when I was eight months pregnant with my second son. No one other than my husband knew about my condition. I was not ready to tell family or friends, but was reaching a point of despair that prompted me to call the PSSA. I was advised to seek individual counseling before attending a support group meeting. I had so many questions that neither the counselor, my neurologist, nor the numerous books on PD that I had read, could answer. So, a few months after that phone call I reluctantly dragged my husband and my new 11-week-old baby to my first support group meeting. Although I was fearful of what I might find, I needed to see for myself what someone living with PD looked like. I am a person that needs to know as much as possible about everything. In hindsight, this personality trait has been a blessing and a curse.

As it turned out, walking into a room full of strangers sitting around a table was almost more than I could handle. My feelings of shame and embarrassment, coupled with the looks of sympathy and surprise on the faces of everyone in the room, nearly caused me to turn and run. I am a very proud person and do not want anyone to feel sorry for me. I can only assume the others were surprised at how young I looked, or perhaps it was the sight of my baby. I don't really know, but at this point, it doesn't much matter. As the meeting progressed, and the attendees took turns to tell their stories, I scanned their faces, assessing their symptoms and trying to guess their ages. One woman, in particular, didn't look much older than me, and when she started to tell her story I burst uncontrollably into tears. I realized that I was looking at my future, and this was more than I could bear. I cried for the remainder of the meeting, as the others continued talking. I don't really know what enabled me to stay in that room. Part of me thinks it was my morbid sense of curiosity. I had to listen to other people's experiences just for the sake of knowing what I should expect. As I mentioned, my thirst for information has been a negative and a positive. Walking into that room was the hardest thing I've ever had to do.

At the end of the meeting however, as various people sat down and talked to me, hugged me, and fed me positive words of support and encouragement, I realized that these were people who understood what I was going through. Contrary to my belief, I wasn't the only one suffering. That was two years ago, and although I couldn't see it at the time, when I look back to that day, I realize that attending that support group meeting took courage that I didn't even know

I had. But it was the best thing I could have done for my mental health, and it marked the start of a new journey for me.

Since that day, I've made a whole new group of friends with PD, traveled to Parkinson's conferences, and been introduced to a whole new Parkinson's community that I didn't even know existed. Talking about my PD has motivated me to try to help others rather than feel sorry for myself, and that's been extremely therapeutic. I don't know that I've fully accepted my illness yet, but I'm definitely at a better place than I was two years ago.

Accepting a diagnosis of a chronic, degenerative disease is a huge challenge that no one should try to deal with alone. During times of adversity, everyone needs some type of support network. I think that to deny yourself such, will only prolong the painful process that leads to the final acceptance of this illness. One thing I've learned is that, although a person living with PD needs the support of family and friends, it is crucial to build a support network of other people with Parkinson's. No one can better understand the slowness or tremor you feel inside, or the frustration at not being able to read your handwriting, than someone who has also experienced it. You're not alone ..."

We don't choose Parkinson's – it chooses us. But how well we live with it is our choice.

13
Caregivers of Persons with Parkinson Disease: Experiences and Perspectives

Katharina Kovacs Burns

Besides the persons with Parkinson disease (PD) being impacted physically, mentally and socially, others that are substantially impacted by the disease include the family members and close friends, many of whom are also the informal or unpaid caregivers of the persons with PD. The term *caregiver* "... refers to anyone who provides assistance to someone else who needs it to maintain an optimal level of independence" [1]. For anyone who takes on caregiving, there needs to be an understanding that the person who is the caregiver also has physical, mental, social, and other needs. During the past decade, there has been a general increase in amount of research conducted with caregivers, and more specifically with caregivers of individuals living with certain chronic illnesses or conditions such as Alzheimer's disease and, more recently, PD. Today, with 20–25% of all households providing care to someone aged 50 years or more, there is a need to explore the experiences and perspectives of caregivers, and to ensure that they receive the support that they need to sustain their own health and well-being [1].

In this chapter, a review is presented of the literature on caregivers in general, along with some of the more specific references and studies on caregivers of persons with PD. A section has also been dedicated to spousal caregivers for persons with PD, as a good proportion (≥33%) of caregivers fit into this category [1]. A specific case study with caregivers of persons with PD is also described, together with an analysis of a survey that parallels the one described in Chapter 12, which relates to persons with PD and their knowledge and service needs, uses and values, as well as the "gaps." The aim of surveying these caregivers was to not only establish a profile of this specific group of caregivers, including their general characteristics and demographics, but to also determine their perceptions and experiences with regards to their caregiving role, the challenges they face daily and generally, and their use and need for specific services and information. An analysis and comparison is provided for the responses from the caregivers with other studies and findings in the literature and various reports for caregiver support and care. Consideration will also be given to policy and program interventions, which currently vary in their translation and implementation for caregivers across provinces and countries.

Parkinson Disease – A Health Policy Perspective. Edited by Wayne Martin, Oksana Suchowersky,
Katharina Kovacs Burns, and Egon Jonsson
Copyright © 2010 WILEY-VCH Verlag GmbH & Co. KGaA, Weinheim
ISBN: 978-3-527-32779-9

13.1
Appreciating the Relevance of the Caregivers' Experiences

As the population ages, the importance of caregivers will become more acknowledged and valued. Family members and close relatives provide the vast majority of care, estimated at 85% [1]. There are several different ways of looking at the statistics related to family caregivers. Almost one out of every four households provides care to a relative or friend aged 50 years or more; about 23% of Canadians aged 45 to 64 years provide care to Seniors [2]; and an estimated 2.85 million adult Canadians find themselves in a caregiver role [3]. Of these caregivers, about 70% are still employed while caregiving, and almost three-fourths are female [1, 4–6]. The hours of caregiving varies, with about 48% of caregivers providing eight or less hours per week, while 17% provide more than 40 hours per week [6].

Taking on a caregiver role means that the individual will be going through a transition and reorganization of personal goals, time, commitments, behaviors, and responsibilities [7]. Whilst the circumstances which bring individuals to this caregiver's role vary, one thing which has been mentioned repeatedly is that nobody feels or comes prepared for the different tasks demanded of them.

As mentioned previously, there has been a growing interest in exploring the perceptions and experiences of informal or unpaid caregivers generally, and more specifically as related to caring for someone with a chronic illness or condition. The ability to understand these experiences and the varied expectations, could shed light on what types of program might be of value to new caregivers, to help them face each challenge as it comes. Not only has research expanded in this area and provided some valuable insights for those concerned, but it also provides the much-needed incentive to establish support groups, resource networks, and societies or associations that are specifically focused on the needs of caregivers. Examples of this include the Caregiver Resource Network [8], the Canadian Caregivers Coalition, the Canadian Hospice Palliative Care Association, Care Services Improvement Partnership, Victorian Order of Nurses, National Alliance for Caregiving, and others that can be explored on the Internet.

Although the costs of caregiving in terms of time, economics, physical and mental stresses, and other considerations are recognized today as part of the burden of cost identified with chronic diseases, illnesses or conditions, it was for many centuries and generations a hidden cost. Today, it has been estimated that the 2.85 million Canadian caregivers save the healthcare system more than $5 billion annually by providing vital, supportive care to loved ones who may otherwise be institutionalized [9]. What are the facts and general experiences which should be captured and presented on caregivers for persons with PD? To whom should the information regarding the costs and burdens borne by caregivers be directed, to ensure that supports and solutions are not only considered for the persons with PD but also for their caregivers? These and other questions warrant a review of the current literature and the initiation of related research.

13.2
Caregiver Burden: A Review of the Literature

Whetten-Goldstein *et al.* [10] have indicated that, on average, the family caregivers of persons with PD provide 22 hours per week of informal care, while the General Social Survey [2] has indicated that, on average, Canadians spend about 23 hours of unpaid caregiving per month (29 hours by women, 16 hours by men). In some cases, this translates into an earnings loss and may affect not only the family income but also relationships. The National Alliance for Caregiving [6] and the article "Caring for Elderly Can Hurt Careers" in *The Grande Rapids Press* newspaper [11], found caregivers rating their financial burdens high, at four or five on a five-point scale. In fact, for those caregivers who spent more than 8 hours per week providing unpaid care, the average loss in income over a lifetime was calculated at $659 139 in wages, pension, and Security Benefits.

The majority of initial costs to caregivers, however, are either indirect or hidden, and are represented by a number of issues including formal changes in roles [10], increased stress and anxiety, psychosocial burdens such as disorganization of household routines, difficulties going away for holidays, restrictions on social life, and disturbances of sleep [12]. For caregivers, the costs associated with PD may not be direct initially in terms of economic implications, treatment, hospitalization or physician services, but they could be if no interventions are made available or prescribed.

There are known health issues and other impacts associated with providing long-term care. Carter and colleagues [20] demonstrated that specific types of caregiver indirect and direct costs increased significantly or accumulated as the patient's disease stage progressed. In 1990, Pearlin and colleagues [13] developed a stress process model which has been used to guide major longitudinal investigations of caregivers of dementia patients. This model has been applied with various caregivers to reflect long-term caregiving as a "career," and the associated transitional changes which caregivers undergo as the person with the chronic illness/ condition progresses through advanced stages.

13.2.1
Spousal Caregivers and Their Experiences

Although the general theories and models apply across all caregivers, more attention has been paid lately to spousal caregivers. Burton *et al.* [14] explored the details of career spousal caregivers over five years as they transitioned into and within their caregiving roles. Burton and coworkers expanded on the many studies which documented the mental and health effects of spousal caregiving by assessing the longitudinal transitioning of caregivers, not only at one point in time but also across years of caregiving and aligned with the progression of the disease of the person they were caring for. Edwards and Scheetz [15] showed specifically that for spousal caregivers there are four major factors which significantly predict their perceived burden: activities of daily living; perceived social support; psychological well-being; and marital satisfaction. Another common component of spousal caregiver burden is the couple's or family's financial situation. A loss of earnings – primarily due to premature retirement – is associated with financial difficulties [10, 16] that often lead to relationship conflicts and marital difficulties.

As mentioned above, in many studies correlations have been identified between spousal caregiving and health effects. In a study conducted by O'Reilly *et al.* [17], it was found that spouses who were caregivers experienced more social (fewer outings, contacts, holidays), psychological (fivefold increase in psychiatric morbidity), and physical (more medical problems and chronic illness) issues or problems. Happe and Berger [18] identified direct ill-health signs and symptoms in caregivers, especially sleep disturbances, nocturnal pain, and cramps. Added to this list are emotional strain and depression [19, 20–24], which have been shown to intensify as the spouse's PD advances and the care needed increases. Other physical issues or problems of the caregivers also intensify with advanced-stage PD of spouses [20, 25]. The caregiver's functional ability, social ability and hours of caregiving are closely associated with the stages of PD [19].

When asked about the most significant challenges and how they coped, spousal caregivers indicated that it was watching their partners struggle, be frustrated, and renegotiating their lives. The most frequently used coping strategies were trying to maintain their own life, encouraging their partner to stay active and involved, and seeing the challenges as secondary [26]. When the circumstances of spousal caregivers for people with PD were compared with those of caregivers of people with dementia and stroke, Thommessen *et al.* [12] found a heavier burden of care associated with PD.

13.2.2
Specific Caregiver Burden and Costs

All of the above-mentioned burdens and challenges of spousal caregivers are similar to the indirect and direct costs experienced by caregivers in general, and are additional to their need to demonstrate that they have the strength to cope. One additional consideration which was highlighted in a study conducted by Zhang and colleagues [27] was the influence of gender and chronic stress on the coping ability, and on the overall health outcomes of caregivers generally. Here, it was contended that male and female caregivers fared differently in their roles and in their personal outcomes. Most studies, however, do not differentiate between genders when discussing the indirect and direct costs of caregiving.

In one survey study with caregivers conducted by the Alberta Caregiver's Association [28], eight issue-themes were identified. These were: handling negative thoughts and emotions; disturbed sleep; physical impacts on caregivers; adjusting perceptions of one's relationship with the care recipient; coping with difficult family dynamics; physical environment barriers to social interaction; navigating the service systems; and financial hardships. Other studies instigated by Schrag and colleagues [29], Happe and Berger [18], and by Carter and colleagues [20] confirmed the above findings as well as those which reported a significant increase of caregiver-burden with increasing PD severity. Notably, the costs for caregivers increased as the PD progressed.

These hidden costs, the researchers maintained, form a large component of the family and caregiver burdens of PD, which will have implications for targeting interventions or programs for caregivers as well as for people with PD. If some of these costs are to be minimized, it is essential for early preventive interventions to be employed, including home care, counseling, and PD support groups.

When focusing on both the person with PD and their caregivers, there are additional challenges to overcome and additional supports needed. A well-established link has already been identified between the caregiver needs and burden, and the functional status of the person with PD [25], which must also be considered with the planning of supports needed for both groups. In order to optimize the care plans for persons with PD and decrease the stress and anxiety for the caregivers, it has been suggested that nursing and other health practitioners include the senior caregiver in the development of the care plans [19].

13.2.3
Services and Supports for Caregivers

The assessment and determination of burden and other problems associated with caregiving is critical in order for appropriate and effective interventions to be developed and implemented. The types of service, location and affiliation with other agencies or programs will need to be determined with caregivers and service providers [30, 31]. There are, in fact, many supports identified as being of value and importance to caregivers in different sectors, including recognition for caregiving, information about services and supports (counseling, educational and others), training for caregivers to increase skills and sensitivity, respite care (in-home, day care, extended or out-of-home), help with daily caregiving activities, and financial support as needed [30, 31]. Support groups for caregivers are also very popular and effective in meeting the needs of caregivers, not only their well-being but also their social needs [30]. During the past decade, a greater emphasis has been placed on respite for caregivers, which could be in the form of replacement caregiving or direct service to the caregiver [32]. The intention of respite is to reduce anxiety and, at the same time, to give the caregiver a break or relief from routine or allow them to catch up on personal tasks and responsibilities. Chappell *et al.* [33] claimed that the interpretation of respite should really be the caregiver's and not the provider's. Caregivers have their own individual needs, and respite should accommodate that rather than be generic. However, this may be difficult to achieve if the caregivers have different definitions and interpretations of respite, based on their context and communities. This was found to be the case in a study conducted by Chappell *et al.* [33]. For many caregivers, respite means stolen moments (48%), while for others it means external relief (18%), or mental/physical boost (11%), or having connections (9%), or even having an angst-free care recipient (1%). Knowing *what* the caregiver means by respite is therefore important for providing what that person needs. The Victorian Order of Nurses (VON) of Canada has suggested the use of "optimal care for families" as opposed to respite, because of the confusion with the concept of respite (2001, p. ix).

There are also other interventions that have proven to be helpful to caregivers and given them the skills, knowledge, and tools to carry out self-care and behavior modifications [34]. There are stress management programs [35], telephone support systems [36], and other supports and therapies, all of which need to be assessed for their effectiveness. One meta-analysis of many common interventions has shown an on average success in alleviating burden and depression, increasing personally rated well-being, and increasing the caregivers' abilities and knowledge over a long period of time [37]. Chappell and Reid [38] took an opposite approach to caregiver intervention, and examined the caeregivers' well-being and its relationship to burden. In this case, social supports were found to be strongly related to well-being but not to burden, which suggested that quality of life (QoL) interventions could help caregivers remain well, even in the presence of burdens.

Myers [39] assessed a similar approach to dealing with caregivers' stress by presenting wellness as a caregiver-empowering tool, by developing a wellness-oriented, strengths-based model in which wellness interventions were applied with caregivers and they were engaged in their wellness planning.

Specifically for caregivers, the United Kingdom Parkinson's Disease Society study [40] has stated that caregivers or carers "... did not tend to complain about lack of support from formal services or friends or family. Carers also did not often comment that such support was helpful. Instead, support from others seemed to play a relatively minor role in caring. Further research or analysis could explore carers' needs for help and whether services are accessible to them" (p.v).

One Canadian study conducted in 1999 by Thurston *et al.* [41] for The Parkinson's Society of Southern Alberta in Calgary, assessed the personal and healthcare needs of persons with PD, particularly by members of the Society, and their caregivers. In the part of the study involving member and nonmember caregivers, the majority were women (over 70%), ranging in age from 26 to 86 years. The majority of caregivers said they needed information and resources on PD, and on how to care for people with PD. Over two-thirds of the caregivers had received information from the Parkinson's Society, as well as from family doctors, neurologists, family, and friends. A small proportion of caregivers, whether members or not, were likely to get help for stress, anxiety, or depression. A significant number of caregivers expressed a need for practical and personal help, including financial help. Members were more likely to express these needs than nonmembers; some caregivers (14% members and 19% nonmembers) also made use of support and discussion groups. A number of barriers to accessing services were also identified, including a lack of awareness, distance, transportation, fatigue, and wheelchair accessibility. Many individuals accessed complementary therapies and supports elsewhere.

A second Canadian-based study was conducted by the Parkinson's Society of Canada, Ontario division [42]. This survey was distributed to 3000 people with PD and their caregivers, who were primarily members on existing databases of the Ontario Division and other regions. A total of 678 caregivers responded. The surveys consisted of similar patterns of questions for both persons with PD and their caregivers, and focused on evaluating the impact of PD on their daily living, as well as determining the types of services they used, needed, wanted, and valued. Although the results of the study have not been published, they presented some useful information. The caregivers indicated that PD has been a major factor in their experiencing more stress and worry, inability to take vacation, visit with others, or take up regular social activities. The study provided a number of key conclusions and related recommendations, including: (i) dealing with the widespread lack of awareness among persons with PD and caregivers of available services in their area; (ii) sustaining support and exercise groups which are the most used and valued services of both persons with PD and caregivers; and (iii) looking at ways of enhancing awareness (e.g., website for younger people) and networks (e.g., for free community transportation) to combat feelings and experiences of isolation.

13.3
Results of an Alberta Study Involving Caregivers

As a brief background to the Alberta Study, a survey was conducted across Alberta's nine regional health authorities that existed at the time of the study, focusing on the caregivers and their relationship with persons with PD. Based on a 2005 estimate of 5500 people with PD [43], about 68% of whom would have caregivers, there should be about 3740 caregivers in Alberta. In total, 1000 specifically designed caregiver surveys (using various validated PD questionnaires) were distributed broadly across the nine regional health authorities in different ways; the response rate was 41%, with 413 surveys returned.

The majority of caregiver respondents were female (70%), of which 32% were aged 66–75 years and 27% were aged 56–66 years. These numbers were similar to those in other studies, including that conducted in Calgary, Alberta [41], and the United Kingdom [40].

In terms of education, 27% of caregivers had some experience of high school (or less), while 26% had graduated from high school. About 19% of the caregivers had a university degree or college diploma, and 7% a post-graduate degree.

About 65% ($n = 368$) of the caregivers indicated that they were retired, so that questions related to work were not applicable. However, about 14% were working full-time at the time of the survey, and 10% worked part-time. About 14% indicated that they had had to retire or stop working when they became caregivers, and this was a fairly major factor for them. At the other extreme, 5% had started a job because their spouse/partner was unable to work due to their PD. This percentage correlated closely with the 5% of people with PD who indicated the same response with regards to their spouses having to go to work. Very few caregivers had to change jobs (3%), or take on a new job with less pay (2%). The stated income of the caregivers was, on average, better than that of the persons with PD. Caregivers were about 5% better off at the $40 000 and higher income levels, but were about the same as persons with PD with regards to income below $40 000. About 35%

of caregivers had incomes of $30000 or less which, at the time in Alberta, was considered to be at the low-income level.

At the time of the survey, over 90% of caregivers had been in this role for one year or more, while only 3% had been caregivers for less than one year. More specifically, about 62% of caregivers indicated that they had been caregivers for persons with PD for 1 to 10 years, and 13% had been so for 10–15 years.

Over 20% of caregivers said that the person with PD they looked after could not be left unattended at any time, but at the other end of the scale about 39% said they could leave the PD patient unattended for more than 24 hours. There were numerous variations in responses over 24 hours. When caregivers themselves needed a break (which was the case for about 26% of them), there were others who would come in to replace them. Figure 13.1 shows who, and to what extent, others assisted with this break for the caregivers. However, it should be noted that 74% of caregivers said that they actually did not have anyone else to care for the person with PD when the caregiver was unable to do so. Some of these ended up utilizing adult day care for the person with PD (about 33%).

For approximately 42% (*n* = 174) of the caregivers, respite care was available in their area. There were also a variety of other support services available for about 14% of caregivers, but only 12% of them actually used the respite care and only 9% accessed the adult day care center in their area. This discrepancy in use may be due to the fact that there is an out-of-pocket cost to both services which, if linked back to income, may suggest that persons with PD and their caregivers have not accessed these and other services because of the cost involved, even though the services may be needed and valued. About 39% (*n* = 161) of caregivers also said they were not sure what respite care was available, although this could mean either that they did not know what respite care was, or that respite care was actually not available near to them.

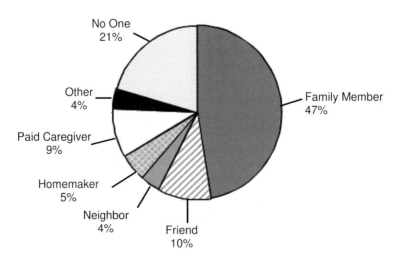

Figure 13.1 Categories of people available to stay with persons with PD when the caregiver is unable to attend (*n* = 413).

As PD progresses, there are likely more tasks that the caregivers assume because the affected individual can no longer do them. There was also a number of personal and other tasks which caregivers assumed when their partners or spouses had PD for any length of time with progression to advanced stages (see Figure 13.2).

In addition to assisting with these activities, caregivers also have other household management tasks which they assume around the house with and for the person with PD, as well as outside of the home, such as paying bills, gardening, shopping, and taking the affected individual to the doctor or hospital, or elsewhere. Together, the number of different activities taken on by the individual is quite substantial; the various activities of the caregiver, in addition to assisting the person with PD directly, are depicted in Figure 13.3.

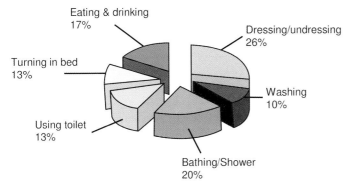

Figure 13.2 Caregiver-assisted activities in persons with PD as the disease progresses ($n = 413$).

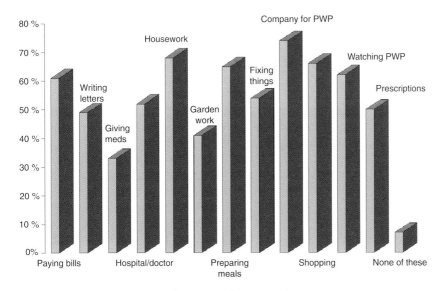

Figure 13.3 Additional activities of caregivers of persons with PD ($n = 413$).

Caregivers were also asked to discuss the impact which PD has had on them, and on the person with PD whom they cared for. About 56% (*n* = 231) of the caregivers said that having to look after someone with PD had made no difference to their own health, but 34% (*n* = 140) said the opposite, that the situation had made their health worse. These findings were consistent with other reports [15, 17, 18, 20]. The research group has termed these challenges as direct and indirect personal costs experienced by the caregivers.

When asked if their family doctors understood the impact which living with and/or looking after someone with PD has had on them, 40% of the caregivers had not discussed this with their doctors, while 49% said that their family doctors understood their predicament fairly well to very well. The extent to which living with and caring for someone with PD had impacted them with things other than their health was also identified (see Table 13.1). Between 11% and 30% of care-

Table 13.1 Impact of caring for persons with PD on the caregiver (*n* = 413).

Problem encountered	PD was or is ...				
	A major factor	Somewhat of a factor	Not really a factor	Not a factor at all	Does not apply
Difficulty in carrying out day-to-day tasks, such as grocery shopping	5%	14%	13%	26%	30%
Visit with friends less frequently	14%	27%	10%	16%	25%
Leave home less frequently	15%	27%	9%	12%	26%
Have given up regular social activities	11%	26%	12%	16%	27%
Feel more isolated	13%	19%	15%	18%	25%
Less time to pursue personal hobbies	14%	25%	14%	15%	21%
Experience more stress and worry	32%	37%	8%	4%	11%
More difficult to make financial ends meet	9%	9%	20%	25%	26%
Unable to take vacations	21%	20%	12%	17%	21%
Anger and resentment	8%	22%	17%	23%	20%
Tired/exhausted	17%	26%	14%	15%	18%
Loss of freedom	17%	28%	13%	16%	18%

givers (depending on the impact item) claimed that certain things were not impacted as a result of their caring for a person with PD.

When caregivers identified any of the changes as being "somewhat of a factor" or "a major factor," they implied that they are experiencing some major issues which needed to be addressed if they were not to end up with poor health or other problems. About 69% of caregivers said they experienced more stress and worry, and over 40% were unable to take vacations, visit with friends as frequently, or leave home as much, while 43–45% said they were more tired and exhausted, and felt a loss of freedom. These points were all very significant to caregivers, and could lead to serious physical and emotional health, and social consequences.

Caregivers also need information or tips for the caregiving of persons with PD, and for their own needs as caregivers. Almost half of all the caregiver respondents indicated that they needed and wanted information on the PD symptoms and changes that could be expected over a period of time, or as the PD advanced in stages. About 42% of them said they also wanted information on PD treatment and on how to live well with PD or have some quality of life. Another one-third wanted information on home care, continuing care and general PD information, and about one-fourth also wanted information on driving, referrals, and sexuality for persons with PD. The majority of caregivers suggested that they got most of their information from the neurologist (64%) and family doctor (51%) attending to the person with PD, but they also relied on the Internet (32%) and support groups (23%) for additional information.

Specifically related to the needs of caregivers, they were asked about what types of support they felt they personally needed. More than one-third of caregivers indicated a need for emotional support (42%), but 32% said they did not need any support. About one-fourth of caregivers said that they needed practical support or help with daily activities, and another 11% said they needed financial support.

Caregivers were asked additional questions about programs, services, or activities they would like to see offered by the Parkinson's Societies in Alberta. The themes identified in their comments included more information sessions (awareness of disease, research) offered by different means (newsletters, e-mail help line, library lending services, more resources), more programs (day care, exercise, special clinics for speech and physiotherapy), more support for the newly diagnosed and for issues concerning sexuality and decision making, professional access (psychologist, social worker, community services, knowledgeable staff, and others (events, more focus on young population with PD, financial assistance, respite, drivers, outreach). And, finally, when asked how well the Parkinson's Societies were known in their community, the caregivers' responses showed the following breakdown (Figure 13.4), with 40% of the respondents generally knowing about them. Among the caregiver respondents from Southern Alberta specifically (84 of the 413), only 19 who lived in close proximity to Calgary (via postal code) indicated they were aware of and utilized the Parkinson's Society of Southern Alberta located in Calgary.

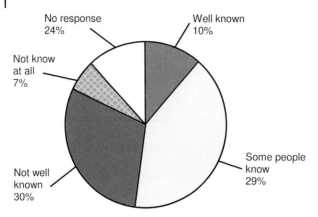

Figure 13.4 Caregivers' perceptions of how well known the Parkinson's Societies are in their communities (*n* = 413).

13.4
Analysis, Conclusions and Recommendations

As society ages and individuals live longer as a result of advanced technologies and treatments to help manage chronic conditions and illnesses, individuals and families must be prepared to become caregivers and/or recipients of caregiving. Caregiving is a complex role with multidimensional considerations, not only for providing caregiving assistance to a family member, friend or spouse, but also for personal transitional changes, all of which require different types of care and attention depending upon the issues (i.e., personal mental and physical health, finances, access to respite or support, and others). The challenge is to appropriately assess each caregiver's issues and needs, and to align services so as to address or accommodate these needs. The additional considerations for planning and delivering programs and services for caregivers includes geographic location (i.e., urban versus rural), gender differences in managing caregiving stresses, access to services approved and available, and the cost-efficient delivery of services, programs and supports.

Based on the burdens and costs identified in the literature, and with the Alberta case study concerning the caregiving role and outcomes for not only caregivers, but also their families, healthcare and social support providers, decision makers, and society in general, it is imperative that more attention be given to caregivers. Policies and program plans must reflect a commitment to ensuring that caregivers are given the support they need. With the number of hours they provide in caregiving, and the costs they save society and the healthcare system, it makes sense to be proactive and to support the caregivers as much as possible across the caregiving cycle. However, ways and means are also needed to measure the effectiveness of programs and services received by caregivers.

Based on the literature review on caregiving and the Alberta case study, there are several areas where recommendations can be made for consideration by program planners and decision makers, including:

- Assessing the caregiver–caregiving recipient relationship, family dynamics if available, and supports needed to manage burdens and costs.
- Assessing the caregiver's overall health, both mental and physical well-being, as well as other considerations including finances, social networks, and information accessibility.
- Determining best practices and gaps (as determined by research or community/ practice studies) in all areas of care and services needed by caregiver personally and for caregiving responsibilities.
- Evaluating different programs and services for their effectiveness in meeting the needs of caregivers, and generally addressing the burdens and costs associated with caregiving.
- Translating findings from various levels of care, service delivery and caregivers' perspectives/experiences for healthcare providers and decision makers.
- Finding ways to be inclusive of all interested stakeholders in the planning and provision of various programs and supports for caregivers, especially spousal and family caregivers.
- Recommending further research around identified gaps in the available information and practices.
- Recommending to healthcare and government decision makers that policies be considered specifically around caregivers and their caregiving roles or careers, to ensure that their burdens and costs can be eased.

An elaboration of these recommendations follows under major themes.

13.4.1
Caregiver Burden, Needs, and Quality of Life

It appears from the case study findings and the results of other studies that the trends, demographics, identified burdens and issues, and needs for services and information are similar across the majority of different caregivers of people with chronic diseases or conditions. Although a generalization from one group of caregivers to another is not a valid approach, it is reasonable to make some assumptions based on similar research statistics and findings.

Whilst different practitioners and researchers have used a variety of tools and instruments to assess or determine caregivers' burdens, costs and needs, there is no one tool that has been developed and validated, and which is comprehensive in inquiring about the key aspects of caregiving, yet be used with ease at the same time [44]. Decken *et al.* [44] have described eight common instruments used to assess caregiver and family needs. Others have also described specific instruments for determining caregiver burden either generally [29] or with subjective and objective burdens of care [45], and the QoL of caregivers, along with patients in some cases [46–50].

However, without a more comprehensive instrument it is difficult to determine any correlation or general relationship among and between diverse measures of health and other aspects that would provide the multidimensional focus needed for a more holistic care [27]. These tools would be especially valuable to the health-care providers who work closely with the patients and caregivers. Not only are providers encouraged to ask questions and listen carefully to what caregivers and care recipients tell them about all aspects of their relationships, challenges, issues or concern, and needs, but they are also encouraged to determine levels of urgency and provide individualized care plans with information about services available and referrals [30, 44]. In summary, comprehensive validated instruments – when used in the practice settings – can assist the providers to work closely with care-givers and patients so as to identify the stresses and burdens that can be addressed through various services and referrals.

13.4.2
Best Practices: Programs, Services, and Care for Caregivers

The identification of best practices in assessing and providing appropriate services, programs and care for caregivers is critical for best outcomes in health and social well-being. The identification of gaps in best practices is equally important, as determined by the lack of continuity in services or having the specific needs of caregivers and patients go unmet or unattended. Besides the usual types of serv-ices and programs identified as needed and valued by caregivers, and mentioned in the literature (examples include support or counseling groups, mutual help groups, educational programs of various types, psychotherapeutic interventions for emotional stress, societies to call or locate on the Internet, and respite in the form of home care services or day centers), there are other less well-known or new programs and services which could be explored.

Respite is an important service for caregivers. Yet, caregivers appear to interpret respite in different ways, with implications for the type and value of the respite provided. Chappell and colleagues [33] suggested that service providers and policy makers redefined respite as an outcome rather than a service, taking into account the caregivers' experiences and needs. Something similar was suggested by VON Canada [32], with the addition of speaking of optimal care for families as opposed to respite. This would avoid the misinterpretation and disappointment when receiving something different than was expected.

Other newer services mentioned in the literature have included an automated telephone support system to assist caregivers with their burdens and anxieties [36]. This intervention was found to be effective in providing caregivers access to information when they needed it the most, and when there were no time con-straints or other barriers for people to contend with. The suggestion has been made to link this system with a network of service providers or expert panels. An optimal mix of technology, content information, and human interface is recom-mended, which would reduce the fears or frustrations often associated with tech-nology of this type.

When considering a broader plan to manage the multiple issues, burdens and costs experienced by caregivers, Myers [39] suggested the use of a wellness-oriented, strengths-based approach for family counselors. This model is based on a premise of holistic wellness and interventions planning to meet the needs of the individual as caregiver, but requires further testing.

13.4.3
Engaging Caregivers and Stakeholders

One of the key ways to ensure that caregivers and people with PD become more involved in their management of care and well-being is to encourage them to be part of the discussions, planning and design of the care plan to manage issues, burdens, costs, healthcare, and social needs. Today, there is a growing movement and desire for patients and caregivers to become more actively and meaningfully engaged in the decisions taken that concern their treatment and care plans and ongoing assessments, particularly self-reporting assessments [51]. Some of these individuals may also become involved in discussions and consultations with healthcare and government decision makers, such as on citizen panels or advisory groups [52].

13.4.4
Program and Service Evaluation for Effectiveness and Outcomes

It is not enough simply to put programs and services into place for caregivers; rather, these programs and services must be evaluated for their effectiveness in meeting the needs of caregivers and alleviating ongoing stresses, burdens, and costs. If the latter continue to be bothersome, despite the services or programs, then they have not met the needs of the caregivers. Today, evaluation research is becoming more popular as a means of assessing programs and services and their outcomes and benefits to caregivers, patients, and generally families. Assessing programs and services provides the information needed to make changes as needed to improve them.

Sorensen and colleagues [37] conducted a meta-analysis on qualifying studies to determine the effectiveness of a number of different interventions used with caregivers to address caregiver burden, caregiver depression, well-being, ability/ knowledge, and health-related symptoms. Subsequently, it was found that interventions generally were shown to be effective in alleviating stress, burden and depression, and increasing caregiver subjectivity of well-being and ability/knowledge. Spousal caregivers benefited less from existing interventions than others for a number of reasons, some of which included their knowledge and experience as caregivers generally, risk factors for distress such as shrinking social networks, lower income, and health problems. Individual interventions were more effective at enhancing well-being, while group interventions improved care-recipient symptoms. Such findings are relevant to service providers such as home care nurses [53] and multidisciplinary rehabilitation specialists [54], who work with patients and families in customizing the interventions through planning and helping the caregiver to manage problems and stressors, as well as introducing new resources and interventions as needed [55].

Another type of specific program assessment was conducted by Lopez and colleagues [35] on a stress management intervention designed specifically for caregivers of dependent older adults. The program was assessed as not effective in meeting the needs of caregivers, since it was too intensive and complex in teaching caregivers to self-manage their problems. Caregivers preferred to have sessions or programs which were simple in nature and did not add stress on top of their other stressors. This type of assessment is critical to the program developers, as they will need to make significant adjustments to the program if it is to serve as a successful intervention for caregivers.

Another more recent intervention implemented and tested by Won Won *et al.* [34] is the community-based "powerful tools," which was designed to empower caregivers and families to maintain their own health. The program was found to facilitate self-care by caregivers, regardless of age, keeping caregivers healthier and able to provide a higher quality of care, and therefore reduce costs for both the caregiver and care-recipient.

13.4.5
Research Gaps and Recommendations

There are many areas concerning caregivers and people with PD that have not been investigated or evidenced for process, outcomes or other aspects. There are also challenges to conducting well-designed studies with caregivers, particularly if there is interest in capturing the life experiences of caregivers. The vulnerability of caregivers makes the planning of interviews uncertain, and rescheduling more likely [56]. Gaining access to caregivers to hear their stories represents a large gap in the research, although a number of studies have been conducted on the perspectives and general experiences of caregivers of persons with PD. Nonetheless, further studies are required in this area, particularly with regards to the implementation of interventions and the assessment of their effectiveness.

Additional studies are also required to assess the impact of PD on the emotions and health of caregivers. Along with this is a need to examine influential factors such as gender and chronic stress on measures of mental and physical health and well-being. Today, there is a large gap in caregiver studies [27], and the variety of limitations in such studies must be identified, taking into consideration the subjectivity associated with many of the measures of personal health and well-being.

More specific research needed with caregivers includes pilot studies on interventions for caregivers of people with PD or other neurological disorders, to determine their experiences in implementing certain interventions to manage various identified health and social challenges or problems, the effectiveness of the different interventions in improving health and other outcomes of caregivers, and changes needed to make the selected effective interventions more available or accessible for caregivers, regardless of where they live [26]. Further research into the application of wellness or caregiver burden models is also required, there having been a surge in the number of these models or frameworks, such as the "Caregiver

Burden Model" presented by Chou [45], the burden and well-being conceptual model by Yates and colleagues [57], and the "Wheel of Wellness" by Myers [39]. Determining which of these is/are feasible to use or apply, and which is/are unrealistic, is important for the future planning of programs, services, interventions, and policies.

13.4.6
Knowledge Translation for Decision Makers

Knowledge translation or transfer or exchange is becoming a central point of the discussion, not only in practice settings but also in the education of healthcare professionals, patients and caregivers, and in research. The latter three are linked in terms of where and what knowledge is created or developed, and how it is best disseminated and implemented in practice. More knowledge translation and utilization approaches are being explored with patients and caregivers, and need to be applied with caregivers to help them manage their burdens and stresses and with practitioners who are working with caregivers and providing the services and programs required. Knowledge translation should be capable of providing a bridge between what works, what does not work, and where there are gaps. This should be an area of ongoing discussion and exploration with caregivers and others involved with PD.

13.4.7
Caregiving Program and Policy Considerations and Implications

There exist certain key policy considerations and implications for decision/policy makers who have a mandate for chronic disease management. Currently, there is no policy which provides the support needed by caregivers and the recipients of care with PD. One reason for this is that PD is not really on the "radar" of government decision makers in terms of priority funding allocations or program and service delivery. In the past very little was known about the prevalence of PD and, until very recently, also its incidence. Hence, a provincial and national surveillance or monitoring system is needed to gather these data and to allow for updates as needed. Clearly, PD is not a condition which will be disappearing; rather, its prevalence is expected to increase as the population continues to age and to live longer. However, caregivers of persons with PD represent only one subset of a much larger group of caregivers that should be targeted with regards to policies and programs.

As caregivers contribute many volunteer hours and save the healthcare system millions of dollars, it is important that policies are put in place to provide them with the support and services they need to continue their efforts [34]. These policies should also have funding allocated for specific caregiver interventions, including respite. Whilst respite still needs to be defined and understood, it also requires a framework and infrastructure such that caregivers are able to link into the respite service that they need, when they need it [33, 32]. Resource portals represent yet another service deserving of supportive policies, along with investments in education, research, and community supports [32]. Tax credits and breaks would also be helpful to alleviate the financial burden of many caregivers, particularly as many of them have either to leave their employment to become full-time caregivers or return to work in order to supplement their income. Clearly, work and caregiving are important ongoing issues for caregivers [58].

In order to develop any policies and service plans, caregivers should be actively engaged in the appropriate discussions and decisions [32, 52]. Information should not only be made available to the patients and their caregivers or families [59], but the decision makers should be informed by these people. As an example, the challenges and experiences of caregivers would provide the decision makers with the necessary insights not otherwise captured in the statistical information that is often provided. The patients and caregivers alike should be involved and be invited to participate in healthcare decisions that, in time, will impact upon them [51].

A *best practices framework* is something which decision makers might appreciate, as this helps to guide best practices, sustainable funding, client-centered care, and evidence-based decision making [59]. The principles could be defined to guide the policy framework, along with goals and directions for best practices concerning caregivers. A round table on caregiving policy in Canada was conducted in 2005 [31], in the summary report of which a number of recommendations for policy development were made, including the proposal to keep the scope broad so as to address the wide range of needs of caregivers at the community level.

In conclusion, this chapter has provided an overview of the caregivers' needs, burdens, costs, and potential interventions. The complexity of caregiving requires that a broad perspective be provided to cover the full range of discussion, from the caregiver to the decision makers. A continuum of a full range of care and supports is needed not only for the person with PD but also for the caregiver. With the reform of the Alberta healthcare system, it will be important for the Ministry of Health and Alberta Health Services to include policies supporting caregivers associated with all areas of chronic and other diseases or conditions. This needs to become a priority for Public Health as the shift is made from a local to provincial integration of services.

References

1 American Society on Aging (2003) Facts about caregivers. The Care Guide. Available at: www.asaging.org (accessed 10 May 2008).

2 Statistics Canada (2002) *General Social Survey – Cycle 16*, Statistics Canada, Ottawa.

3 VON Canada (2006) Touching Lives Since 1897. VON's submission to the House of Commons Standing Committee on Finance in preparation for Budget 2007, Ottawa.

4 Kropf, N.P., and the Home Health and Community Services (2006) *Gerontological Social Work: Settings and Special Populations*, Brooks/Cole, Belmont, California, pp. 167–190.

5 Jans, L., and Stoddard, S. (1999) Chartbook on Women and Disability in the United States. An InforUse Report.

U.S. National Institute on Disability and Rehabilitation Research, Washington, DC.

6 National Alliance for Caregiving and AARP (2004) Caregiving in the U.S. National Alliance for Caregiving and AARP, Bethesda, MD.

7 Lund, M. (2005) Caregiver, take care. *Geriatric Nursing*, **26** (3), 152–153.

8 Caregiver Resource Network (2004) Sample Research Data on Caregiving. Available at: www.caregiverresource.net (accessed 6 April 2008).

9 Eales, J., Keating, N., and Fast, J. (2001) *Analysis of the Impact of Federal, Provincial and Regional Policies on the Economic Well-Being of Informal Caregivers of Frail Seniors*, Federal/Provincial/Territorial Committee of Officials (Seniors), pp. 1–99.

10 Whetten-Goldstein, K., Sloan, F., Kulas, E., Cutson, T., and Schenkman, M. (1997) The burden of Parkinson's disease on society, family and the individual. *Journal of the American Geriatric Society*, **45** (7), 844–849.

11 Anonymous (1999) *Caring for Elderly Can Hurt Careers*, The Grand Rapids Press, p. A6.

12 Thommassen, B., Aarsland, D., Braekhus, A., Oksengaard, A.R., Engedal, K., and Laake, K. (2002) The psychosocial burden on spouses of the elderly with stroke, dementia and Parkinson's disease. *International Journal of Geriatric Psychiatry*, **17** (1), 78–84.

13 Pearlin, L.I., Mullan, J.T., Semple, S.J., and Skaff, M.M. (1990) Caregiving and the stress process: an overview of concepts and their measures. *Gerontologist*, **30**, 583–594.

14 Burton, L.C., Zdaniiuk, B., Schulz, R., Jackson, S., and Hirsch, C. (2003) Transitions in spousal caregiving. *Gerontologist*, **43** (2), 230–241.

15 Edwards, N.E. and Scheetz, P.S. (2002) Predictors of burden for caregivers of patients with Parkinson's disease. *Journal of Neuroscience Nursing*, **34** (4), 184–190.

16 Clarke, M.C. (1997) A causal functional explanation of maintaining a dependent elder in the community. *Research in Nursing and Health*, **20**, 515–526.

17 O'Reilly, F., Finnan, F., Allwright, S., Smith, G.D., and Ben-Shlomo, Y. (1996) The effects of caring for a spouse with Parkinson's disease on social, psychological and physical well-being. *British Journal of General Practice*, **46** (410), 507–512.

18 Happe, S. and Berger, K. (2002) The association between caregiver burden and sleep disturbances in partners of patients with Parkinson's disease. *Age and Ageing*, **31**, 349–354.

19 Berry, R.A., and Murphy, J.F. (1995) Well-being of caregivers of spouses with Parkinson's disease. *Clinical Nursing Research*, **4** (4), 373–386.

20 Carter, J.H., Stewart, B.J., Archbold, P.G., Inoue, I., Jaglin, J., Lannon, M., *et al.* (1998) *Living with a Person Who has Parkinson's Disease: The Spouse's Perspective by Stage of Disease*, Parkinson's Study Group.

21 Ellgring, H., Seiler, S., and Perletth, B. (1993) Psychosocial aspects of Parkinson's disease. *Neurology*, **43**, 641–644.

22 Gallagher, D., Rose, J., Rivera, P., Lovett, S., and Thompson, L. (1989) Prevalence of depression in family caregivers. *Gerontologist*, **29**, 449–456.

23 Human Resources and Social Development Canada (2006) *Caregivers – Backgrounder*, Government of Canada.

24 Aarsland, D., Larsen, J.P., Karlsen, K., Lim, N.G., and Tandberg, E. (1999) Mental symptoms in Parkinson's disease are important contributors to caregiver distress. *International Journal of Geriatric Psychiatry*, **14** (10), 866–874.

25 Caap-Ahlgren, M., and Dehlin, O. (2002) Factors of importance to the caregiver burden experienced by family caregivers of Parkinson's disease patients. *Aging Clinical and Experimental Research*, **14** (5), 371–377.

26 Habermann, B., and Lindsey Davis, L. (2006) Lessons learned from a Parkinson's disease caregiver intervention pilot study. *Applied Nursing Research*, **19**, 212–215.

27 Zhang, J., Vitaliano, P.P., and Lin, H.H. (2006) Relations of caregiving stress and health depend on the health indicators used and gender. *International Journal of Behavioral Medicine*, **13** (2), 173–181.

28 Alberta Caregivers' Association (2003) *Freedom and Friendship*, AB, Edmonton.

29 Schrag, A., Hovris, A., Morley, D., Quinn, N., and Jahanshahi, M. (2005) Caregiver-burden in Parkinson's disease is closely associated with psychiatric symptoms, falls, and disability. *Parkinsonism and Related Disorders*, **12**, 35–41.

30 Emlet, C.A. (1996) Assessing the informal caregiver: team member or hidden patient? *Home Care Provider*, **1** (5), 255–262.

31 Varga-Toth, J. (2005) *A Healthy Balance: A Summary Report on a National Roundtable on Caregiving Policy in Canada*, Canadian Policy Research Networks Inc, Ottawa.

32 VON Canada (2004) *Caring for Family Caregivers: The Unmet Need for Respite as a Break, Time Out or Relief from Caregiving. Case Study*, VOICE in health policy, Ottawa.

33 Chappell, N.L., Reid, C., and Dow, E. (2001) Respite reconsidered: a typology of meanings based on the caregiver's point of view. *Journal of Aging Studies*, **15**, 201–216.

34 Won Won, C., Sizer Fitts, S., Favaro, S., Olsen, P., and Phelan, E. (2008) Community-based "powerful tools" intervention enhances health of caregivers. *Archives of Gerontology and Geriatrics*, **46**, 89–100.

35 Lopez, J., Crespo, M., and Zarit, S.H. (2007) Assessment of the efficacy of a stress management program for informal caregivers of dependent older adults. *Gerontologist*, **47** (2), 205–214.

36 Mahoney, D.F., Tarlow, B.J., and Jones, R.N. (2003) Effects of an automated telephone support system on caregiver burden and anxiety: findings from the REACH for TLC Intervention Study. *Gerontologist*, **43** (4), 556–567.

37 Sorensen, S., Drhabil, M.P., and Duberstein, P. (2002) How effective are interventions with caregivers? An updated meta-analysis. *Gerontologist*, **42** (3), 356–372.

38 Chappell, N.L., and Reid, C. (2002) Burden and well-being among caregivers: examining the distinction. *Gerontologist*, **42** (6), 772–780.

39 Myers, J.E. (2003) Coping with caregiving stress: a wellness-oriented, strengths-based approach for family counselors. *The Family Journal*, **11**, 153–161.

40 Yarrow, S. (1999) *Survey of Members of the Parkinson's Disease Society*, Policy Studies Institute for the Parkinson's Society of the United Kingdom, p. 101 and appendices.

41 Thurston, W.E., Andersen, D., and Emmett, J. (1999) *An Assessment of the Personal and Health Care Needs of Persons with Parkinson's and their Caregivers*, The Parkinson's Society of Southern Alberta.

42 Parkinson Society of Canada–Ontario (2002) A Study with People Living with Parkinson's Disease and their Caregivers. Parkinson Society of Canada, Toronto.

43 Svenson, L. (2005) Prevalence from surveillance data.

44 Decken, J.F., Taylor, K.L., Mangan, P., Yabroff, K.R., and Ingham, J.M. (2003) Care for the caregivers: a review of self-report instruments developed to measure the burden, needs, and quality of life in informal caregivers. *Journal of Pain and Symptomatic Management*, **26** (4), 922–953.

45 Chou, K.R. (2000) Caregiver burden: a concept analysis. *International Pediatric Nursing*, **15** (6), 398–407.

46 Daminano, A.M., Snyder, C., Strausser, B., and Willian, M.K. (1999) A review of health-related quality-of-life concepts and measures for Parkinson's Disease. *Quality of Life Research*, **8**, 235–243.

47 Martinez-Martin, P., Benito-Leon, J., Alonso, F., Catalan, M.J., Pondal, M., Zamarbide, I., *et al.* (2005) Quality of life of caregivers in Parkinson's Disease. *Quality Life Research*, **14**, 463–472.

48 Glozman, J.M., Bicheva, K.G., and Fedorova, N.V. (1998) Scale of quality of life of care-givers (SQLC). *Journal of Neurology*, **245** (Suppl. 1), S39–S41.

49 Fleming, A., Dook, K.F., Nelson, N.D., and Lai, E.C. (2005) Proxy reports in Parkinson's disease: caregiver and

patient self-reports of quality of life and physical activity. *Movement Disorders*, **20** (11), 1462–1468.

50 McRae, C., Diem, G., Vo, A., O'Brien, C., and Seeberger, L. (2002) Reliability of measurements of patient health status: a comparison of physician, patient, and caregiver ratings. *Parkinsonism and Related Disorders*, **8**, 187–192.

51 Kovacs Burns, K., and Best Medicines Coalition (2006) The Voluntary Health Sector as Participants in the Public Health System: Defining the Role and Impact. Report submitted to the Public Health Agency of Canada, National Voluntary Health Organizations.

52 Integrated Care Network (2006) *Strengthening Service User and Carer Involvement: A Guide for Partnerships*, Department of Health, London. Available at: www.icn.csip.org.uk (accessed 8 April 2008).

53 Sisk, R.J. (2000) Caregiver burden and health promotion. *International Journal of Nursing Studies*, **37**, 37–43.

54 Trend, P., Kaye, J., Gage, H., Owen, C., and Wade, D. (2002) Short-term effectiveness of intensive multidisciplinary rehabilitation for people with Parkinson's disease and their caregivers. *Clinical Rehabilitation*, **16** (7), 717–725.

55 Zarit, S.H., Davey, A., Edwards, A.B., Femia, E.E., and Jarrott, S.E. (1998) Family caregiving: research findings and clinical implications, in *Comprehensive Clinical Psychology: Volume 7. Clinical Geropsychology* (ed. B.A. Edelstein), Elsevier Science Ltd., Oxford, UK, pp. 499–523.

56 Sheriff, J.N. and Chenoweth, L. (2003) Challenges in conducting research to improve the health of people with Parkinson's disease and the well-being of their family carers. *International Journal of Rehabilitation Medicine*, **26** (3), 201–205.

57 Yates, M.E., Tennstedt, S., and Chang, R.H. (1999) Contributors to and mediators of psychological well-being for informal caregivers. *Journal of Gerontology Psychological Science*, **54B**, 12–22.

58 Arksey, H. and Glendinning, C. (2007) Combining work and care: carers' decision-making in the context of competing policy pressures. *Social Policy and Administration*, **42** (1), 1–18.

59 Hollander, M.J. and Prince, M.J. (2008) A best practices framework. *Healthcare Quarterly*, **11** (1), 45–54.

A Caregiver's Story

Parkinson's and Wayne Hale

Carol Hale

My introduction to Parkinson's disease began when my husband Wayne was diagnosed at the age of 47 years and, with no formal training, I took on the role of Wayne's primary caregiver. The learning curve has been steep, but with both of our involvements in the "Parkinson's Community" we have learned a lot. Wayne has participated in a number of programs at the Community Rehabilitation Interdisciplinary Services (CRIS) Clinic, such as physical, occupational, and exercise therapy, and acupuncture. He was also involved in the Movement Disorder Clinic with Doctors Martin, Camicioli, and Germaine. However, it was the Speech Therapy program which has served as the greatest asset in stabilizing his health. Without this support, Wayne and I would be far less knowledgeable about the disease. Being a member of the Parkinson's Society board has helped Wayne remain positive and connected with the Parkinson's Society, and made him realize that we're not alone in the fight. Once I retire, I fully intend to become more involved in the Parkinson's Society.

Prior to attending the caregiver program, there were a number of obstacles we faced as Wayne struggled with his condition and the loss of physical and motor skills. For example, use of the phone, remote controls, brushing teeth, bathing, shaving, and making the bed require a lot more time than they used to. The computer is no longer possible as he struggles to dial numbers, press buttons, and type characters on the keyboard effectively. Using basic kitchen appliances such as can openers and microwaves has become increasingly difficult, and causes a great deal of stress in the home for everyone.

As Wayne's primary caregiver, there are a number of things that I need to do to make each day more convenient. I make a list of to-do's, lay out his medications, prepare his meals, organize a daily calendar to remember events, manage all financial issues, and plan our social life. In order to help Wayne be ready and able to face each day, he must take his medications properly and on time so that he can have a restful night's sleep. This year, Wayne failed his driver's test and is required to be assessed on an annual basis. Last year, we sold our home in St Albert and moved into an apartment close to my daughter and her family. The move has helped to support Wayne in his everyday tasks, such as going to the store, the bank, walking the dog, and visiting his mom. Wayne has always been an active member of the society, and we have always used any available resources to help us cope.

Over the last couple of years, Wayne's Parkinson's has progressed considerably, which has proven difficult to handle our emotions and feelings about the disease. We can no longer put the disease to the back of our minds, as Wayne's mobility, speech and dementia makes it impossible to ignore. We both have had to accept changes in our life and try our best to move forward, although without the support of our family and friends we would not survive.

Without the help of family, friends, doctors and the Parkinson's Society of Alberta, we would not have been able to manage as well as we have. We have also been fortunate in the fact that Wayne's progression has been very slow, and it has only been the last couple of years that our lives have been severely impacted by this disease. Watching Wayne's progression has been painful for me as well as our family and friends. An article about Parkinson's disease is nothing new to this newsletter, so I reached out to our family and a friend to see the changes that they have noticed in Wayne since his diagnosis 14 years ago.

From our daughter, Denise: I first started noticing changes in my stepfather, Wayne in 1994. Since then, the physical symptoms have progressed to include a loss of hearing and fine motor skills, hand tremors, shuffling walk, poor speech, choking, vacant eyes, dementia, and weight loss. Presently, and more importantly, I see a very loving man fighting to keep his pride and independence. It reminds me of a book I read by Margaret Laurence called the *Stone Angel*. In it, she makes a reference to chains that I believe can be used as a metaphor for those who both suffer from, and stand in support of, individuals who have Parkinson's disease.

> "I was alone, never anything else, and never free, for I carried my chains within me, and they spread out from me and shackled all I touched" (p. 292). *Stone Angel*

And from our dear friends and neighbors, Marvin and Marilyn Rice: Wayne Hale has impacted our lives in so many ways. When Wayne bought the cabin next to us our lives changed. Wayne was the nicest, friendliest person we could meet, and it was because of Wayne that 58 St became the block to live on at Alberta Beach. It was Wayne who brought all of us neighbors together. It is with great pain that we have watched Wayne change due to Parkinson's. He is still the kindest, sweetest man you could ever meet, but he has changed —he has trouble carrying on a simple conversation, especially in a large group, he gets frustrated because Carol has to ask the neighbors to help out with things that he easily used to do—not that anyone minds, as we are there for him 100%. He doesn't go golfing with the boys much anymore, which they all miss. As well, we have watched Carol go through so much with Wayne and struggle to hold it all together, but she does it with great determination and love. We truly love Wayne and so wish that we could wave a magic wand and make him all better, but we can't so we just love him for the person he is today and continue to be there for him and Carol.

From Ray Williams, Executive Director of The Parkinson's Society of Alberta (PSA): I came to know Wayne when I started with PSA in the fall of 2006. Over this short period of time I have come to truly appreciate both Wayne's and Carol's enthusiasm and dedication to the society and to the other people living with Parkinson's. Wayne, though his Parkinson's has progressed, is still a very valuable member of the board and a tremendous asset to PSA. Wayne, like a lot of people living with Parkinson's, has a very positive attitude. It is difficult to watch the progression of Parkinson's as it takes a stronger and stronger hold on those you love and respect. The staff and volunteers of The Parkinson's Society of Alberta strive to meet the needs of people like Wayne and Carol by providing education, support services, advocacy and promoting research. The PSA thanks Wayne and Carol for their dedication and service to the Society—thank you for helping make a difference.

To finish this article I can't give any advice except for to use an old cliché—live for today. Don't wait to go on that trip or try that new restaurant, because you just never know how quickly you will not be able to enjoy even the simplest things in life—and NEVER take for granted those who love and support you. Despite the obstacles we've had to face, Wayne and I decided that we would live life to the fullest and make the best of what we have been dealt. And now, when I look back it, was the smartest decision we ever made.

14
Health-Related Quality of Life in Parkinson Disease: An Introduction to Concepts and Measures

Marguerite Wieler and Allyson Jones

A primary goal for treating patients with Parkinson disease (PD) is to ensure the best possible health-related quality of life (HRQoL), despite the myriad of symptoms and treatment-related complications associated with this chronic neurodegenerative disease. Traditionally, outcome indicators in PD have included mortality, health service-utilization measures, laboratory investigations, clinical scales, and economic indicators. If the primary goal is to improve a patient's function or how they feel, then the direct measurement of HRQoL is a means of measuring the effectiveness of a treatment or evaluating the clinical decision-making in PD.

Over the past decade, there has been an ever-increasing acceptance of patient-based measures within the PD clinical and research communities. The evaluation of HRQoL in chronic diseases such as PD requires measures that reflect a broad array of dimensions. In turn, the measurement of HRQoL provides clinically valuable information on how this disease impacts upon health. Health-related QoL information can be used to assist in the management of patients, for clinical policy, research, health policy, and decision making.

The aim of this chapter is to provide an introduction to the literature on HRQoL in PD, and to summarize the most frequently used HRQoL measures in this patient population. The effect of specific therapeutic or pharmacological interventions will not be discussed.

14.1
What Are the Symptomatic Features?

As shown in Table 14.1, persons with PD may experience diverse symptoms which impact upon their overall HRQoL. Symptoms can be classified as either motor or non-motor. *Motor symptoms* include tremor, rigidity, bradykinsesia, postural instability and gait disturbances such as shuffling gait. Other motor symptoms include difficulties with swallowing, speech (reduced volume and articulation), micrographia (small handwriting), difficulty turning in bed, drooling and facial masking. The constellation of non-motor complications affect a number of systems. *Non-motor symptoms* seen in PD include cognitive impairment, visuospatial diffi-

Parkinson Disease – A Health Policy Perspective. Edited by Wayne Martin, Oksana Suchowersky, Katharina Kovacs Burns, and Egon Jonsson
Copyright © 2010 WILEY-VCH Verlag GmbH & Co. KGaA, Weinheim
ISBN: 978-3-527-32779-9

Table 14.1 Health-related quality-of-life areas associated with Parkinson disease and its management.

Physical function	Communication
Self-care activities	Speech
Ambulation	Facial expressions
Mobility	Lack of body language
Bodily discomfort/pain	Handwriting
	Typing
Mental health/emotional well-being	Sleep and rest
Depression	Problems falling asleep
Paranoia	Waking during night
Anxiety	Waking too early
Panic disorders	Daytime drowsiness and dozing
Loneliness	Nightmares, vivid dreams
Embarrassment	Sleep walking
Fear of social stigma	Eating
Isolation	Using utensils
Sense of autonomy/control	Chewing
Sense of loss	Swallowing
Frustration	Reduced appetite
Self-image	Role function
Social function	Employment
Participation in social activities	Home management
Interpersonal relationships	Energy/fatigue
Health-related distress	Sexual function
Cognitive function	Perceived attractiveness
Concentration	Impotence
Memory	Decreased libido
Languages skills	Hypersexuality
Alertness	
Confusion	
Visual hallucination	

Reproduced from Ref. [12].Reproduced from Ref. [12].

culties, emotional lability, alertness, and psychological problems such as anxiety and depression. *Autonomic* problems also include constipation, urinary frequency/urgency, male erectile dysfunction, orthostatic hypotension, and sleep disturbances. Moreover, in many patients, the side effects caused by pharmacological treatments may result in many complications, including motor fluctuations, dose-failures (where medication fails to reduce parkinsonian symptoms), painful early-morning dystonia, excessive sleepiness, and hallucinations. A combination of movement difficulties and the effects of the non-motor issues often lead to problems with activities of daily living (ADL), instrumental activities of daily living (IADL), social functioning, and employment.

Not everyone presenting with parkinsonian symptoms will have idiopathic PD. The constellation of motor impairments, that includes bradykinesia, rigidity and postural instability, is seen in any number of conditions that disrupt the nigrostriatal circuitry in the basal ganglia secondary to a decrease in available dopamine. Each will have a different prognosis and treatment path from PD. While it is important to stress that these non-idiopathic PD syndromes may have different prognoses, the effect on the HRQoL remains similar.

14.2
Health-Related Quality of Life

A primary goal of health care for any chronic disease, including PD, is to maintain or improve the HRQoL [1]. There are many paradigms that attempt to define health and quality of life. A widely accepted definition of health is the one of The World Health Organization (WHO), which describes health as a "... state of complete physical, mental, social and spiritual well-being and not merely the absence of disease or infirmity" [2]. A recent shift in the conceptual model of disease has moved from viewing the "consequences of disease" or the impact of health to components of health.

Health-related QoL is a complex and multidimensional concept that is only one component of the overall paradigm of quality of life. Patrick and Erikson defined HRQoL as "... the value assigned to duration of life as modified by the impairments, functional states, perceptions, and social opportunities that are influenced by disease, injury, treatment, or policy" [3]. It represents those domains that are directly related to the health of a person, including symptoms, mental health, physical functioning, role functioning, and an overall perception of health [4]. The concept of HRQoL embodies not only physical components but also psychological and social factors which are viewed as integral components of health.

One conceptual model of quality of life was developed by Wilson and Cleary (see Figure 14.1) [5]. The model includes components of HRQoL: biological and physiological components; symptom status including emotional; cognitive and physical symptoms; functional status consisting of physical, social, role and psychological functioning; general health perceptions or a subjective evaluation of the preceding components; and lastly, quality of life – that is, overall how satisfied a person is with life. This model emphasizes that HRQoL relates not only to physical health, and all model components require input from a variety of sources. Perhaps more importantly, a person's experience is a central feature of this model. Measures of HRQoL rarely distinguish among these components.

Although an array of motor and non-motor symptoms, along with associated treatment for PD may affect the HRQoL, traditional outcomes of PD have been clinical measures primarily directed at symptoms and disability. A comprehensive evaluation of HRQoL has been more recently advocated to evaluate health from the patient's perspective. The HRQoL measures capture a wide range of quality of life dimensions. By consensus, the primary source of information should be the patient; however, proxy respondents can also provide useful information, especially when patients are unable to respond on their own behalf.

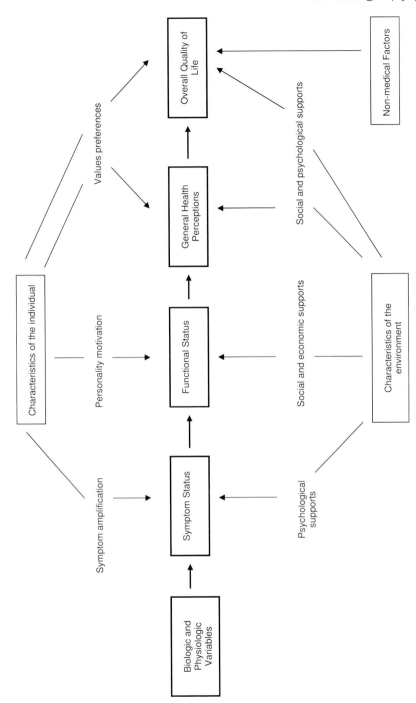

Figure 14.1 Health-related quality of life conceptual model: Relationship among measures of patient outcomes.

Because HRQoL is a subjective concept, its measurement can be challenging. According to one taxonomy, HRQoL measures can be classified as either generic or specific [6]. *Generic measures* apply to virtually any adult population, while *specific measures* apply to a particular population, such as those with a specific disease or disorder. These two types of measure differ in their content and rationale; both contribute distinctive clinical information regarding the burden of disease (Table 14.2). However, the selection of the type of measure is dependent upon its purpose: clinical, research, and health decision-making. For instance, a clinician most likely would require a disease-specific or a patient-specific measure to provide information pertinent to the treatment of a patient. The vast majority of HRQoL measures reported within the literature for PD are disease-specific [12]. A generic measure would be more practical to provide an evaluation at the group rather than the individual level, whereas the economic evaluation of an intervention would benefit from a preference-based measure.

14.3
Generic Measures

The generic health measures can be classified as health-profile or preference-based measures. Both types of measure provide a general view of health across a variety of conditions, and measure several dimensions of health. The wide spectrum of health domains permits the comparison of HRQoL across a variety of patient populations. For example, HRQoL scores can be used as baseline or norm-based estimates against which the efficacy, effectiveness or efficiency of pharmacologic or surgical interventions for PD may be evaluated. Examples of generic health profile measures used in persons with PD include the Medical Outcomes Study 36-Item Short Form (SF-36) [13–15], the Nottingham Health Profile (NHP) [16], and the Sickness Impact Profile (SIP) [17, 18] (see also Table 14.2).

14.3.1
Preference-Based Measures

A preference-based measure places an overall value on a health state. An assumption of HRQoL is that individuals have preferences for alternative health outcomes, with scores being anchored on a scale in which dead = 0.00 to perfect health = 1.00. From an economic perspective, a preference-based measure may be useful to assess the HRQoL. A preference-based measure may have several advantages. First, the single summary score provides the ability to deal with any conflicting changes in various dimensions of health states; for instance, an improvement in function accompanied by a dramatic increase in pain. Second, a single index value can be generated for cost-effectiveness analyses. Mortality and morbidity effects can be integrated by estimating quality-adjusted life years (QALY) [19]. Examples of preference-based measures used in PD patient population are the EQ-5D [20, 21] and the Health Utilities Index Mark 2 (HUI2) [22] (see Table 14.2).

Table 14.2 Summary of frequently used health measures in Parkinson disease.

Type	Measure	Domains		No. of items	Comments
Generic-preference	EQ-5D (Dolan, 1997: 1095–1108 [7]; Shaw, 2005: 203–220 [8])	Mobility Self care Usual activities Anxiety/depression Pain		1 1 1 1 1	Indirect measure of utility. 243 Health states. Scoring function based on TTO. Modified linear additive score. For the United Kingdom scoring system, overall utility score ranges from −0.59 to 1.00. For the US scoring system, scores range from −0.11 to 1.00.
Generic-preference	HUI2/3 (Torrance, 1996: 702–722 [9]; Feeny, 2002: 113–128 [10])	HUI3 Vision Hearing Speech Ambulation Dexterity Emotion Cognition Pain	HUI2 Sensation Self-care Mobility Emotion Cognition Pain	15	Generic preference-based measure that has been used in PD. Indirect measure of utility. Scoring function based on SG. Multiplicative score. Overall HUI3 utility score ranges from −0.36 to 1.00. Overall HUI2 utility score ranges from −0.03 to 1.00.

Generic-health profile	SF-36 (Ware, Jr, 1992: 473–483 [11])	Physical Health
		  Physical function
		  Role function-physical
		  Bodily pain
		  General health
		Mental Health
		  Mental health
		  Role function-emotional
		  Social function
		  Vitality
				10
				4
				2
				5
				5
				3
				2
				4
					Generic profile measure that has been used in PD. Provides eight domains and two summary scores.

Disease-specific	PDQ-39	Mobility Activities of daily living Emotional well-being Stigma Social support Cognition Communication Bodily discomfort		10 6 6 4 3 4 3 3	Omits items on sleep and sexuality; role functioning superficially covered
Disease-specific	PDQL	Parkinsonian symptoms Systemic symptoms Emotional function Social function		14 7 9 7	Omits items on self care; role functioning, close relationships superficially covered

Table 14.2 *Continued*

Type	Measure	Domains	No. of items	Comments
Disease-specific	PDQUALIF	Social role	9	Most recently developed scale. Provides an evaluation of social and related health domains to the effects of PD
		Self-image/sexuality	7	
		Sleep	3	
		Outlook	4	
		Physical function	5	
		Independence	2	
		Urinary function	2	
Disease-specific	PIMS	Feelings of self (positive and negative)	10	Available in Canadian English and Canadian French. Completed three times, one month apart. The scale has 10 items each rated on a 0–4 scale (no change to severe change), and is completed three times, one month apart. The items in the PIMS are broadly formulated and concern domains rather than specific situations. Higher scores reflect a lower HRQL. It does take into account fluctuations in response to medications. Omits items on self care, transfers, walking and other PD-related motor features; cognitive and social stigma superficially covered
		Family Relationships		
		Community Relationships		
		Work		
		Travel		
		Leisure		
		Safety		
		Sexuality (optional)		
		Financial security (optional)		
Disease-specific	PLQ	Depression	5	Validated only in German. Construct validity and responsiveness insufficiently assessed. Omits items on speech and transfers; relationships and role functioning superficially covered
		Physical achievement	5	
		Concentration	4	
		Leisure	5	
		Restlessness	4	
		Activity limitation	6	
		Insecurity	5	
		Social integration	5	
		Anxiety	5	

Because generic measures are multidimensional, they may lack the sensitivity of some areas of interest and have a lower responsiveness than specific measures. A well-validated generic health measure will, however, permit the detection of unanticipated effects. For example, mobility and tremor are primary concerns of patients with PD; however, the use a generic health measure may identify other patient concerns, such as fatigue and anxiety that clinicians or policy makers did not foresee. Generic measures also provide for comparisons across different conditions, which have implications for health resource utilization and policy decisions.

14.4
Disease-Specific Measures

Disease-specific measures focus on patients with the same condition, and are by far the most commonly used HRQoL measures for PD. Five main disease-specific HRQoL measures have been reported for use in PD: the Parkinson Disease Questionnaire-39 (PDQ-39); the Parkinson's Disease Quality of Life Questionnaire (PDQL); the Parkinson Impact Scale (PIMS); the Parkinson Life Quality (PLQ); and the Parkinson's Disease Quality of Life Scale (PDQUALIF). All measures were developed using direct input from patients with the exception of the PIMS, the content of which was developed based on the consensus of a group of ten movement-disorder specialist nurses. These measures were designed to be completed by the patient, typically in 10–45 minutes. The domains covered by each scale differ both in content and in depth.

14.4.1
Parkinson Disease Questionnaire

The Parkinson's Disease Questionnaire-39 (PDQ-39) [23] is perhaps the mostly widely used disease-specific HRQoL measure used in PD. Developed and validated in the United Kingdom in 1995 by Peto *et al.*, it has been translated into more than 40 languages, and has been used in both clinical practice and multicenter international clinical trials [24, 25]. A short-version, the PDQ-8, has also been shown to be valid and reliable [26–28], and can be used in settings where a longer questionnaire would place an excessive burden on the respondent.

The PDQ-39 consists of 39 items covering eight "domains": mobility; activities of daily living; emotional well-being; stigma; social support; cognition; communication; and bodily discomfort. A higher score reflects a larger impact of PD on the HRQoL. The data can be evaluated in a variety of ways; as a total score; as a subscore of each domain; or transformed into a linear scale ranging from 0 to 100 after being summarized into an index.

14.4.2
Parkinson's Disease Quality of Life Questionnaire

Another validated disease specific scale in use is the Parkinson's Disease Quality of Life Questionnaire (PDQL) [29, 30]. This measure contains a total of 37 items which are subdivided into four subscales: parkinsonian symptoms; systemic symptoms; social functioning; and emotional functioning. Here, a low score reflects a poorer HRQoL. The PDQL has been translated into a number of languages, making it amenable for implementation in multinational clinical trials.

14.4.2.1 Parkinson's Impact Scale

The Parkinson's Impact Scale (PIMS) [31] is a validated tool that evaluates ten broad domains. A low score reflects a higher HRQoL. The number of times that questions are completed depends on the presence/absence of motor fluctuations; for example, if a patient is stable then all ten questions are completed only once. However, if they experience "on" and "off" times, then the items are scored twice, once for each state. The PIMS is validated in Canadian English and French, and has not been widely used in clinical trials.

14.4.3
Parkinson Quality of Life

The Parkinson Quality of Life (PQL) is a German measure consisting of 44 questions covering nine domains: depression; physical achievement (five items); concentration (four items); leisure (five items); restlessness; activity limitation; insecurity; social integration; and anxiety. The lack of validated translations makes this scale useful only in German-speaking settings.

14.4.4
Parkinson's Disease Quality of Life Scale (PDQUALIF)

The Parkinson's disease quality of life scale (PDQUALIF) [32] was developed and validated by Welsh, in conjunction with the Parkinson's Study Group, and consists of 33 self-administered questions using a five-point Likert scale. It covers seven domains, including social role, self-image/sexuality, sleep, outlook, physical function, independence, and urinary function. The total range of scores is 0 to 128, where a lower scores reflect a higher HRQoL. Although this measure has not been widely used, and few reports of its use have been made, it has been employed in two studies supported by the Parkinson's Study Group [33, 34].

According to a systematic review [35], which did not include the PDQUALIF, the PDQ-39, PDQL, PIMS, and PQL measures have all been shown to have good internal consistency and test–retest reliability, with the exception of PDQL, which had inadequate data. Only the PDQ-39 showed moderate to good content and construct validity and responsiveness, along with having satisfactory evaluative and discriminative properties.

The recommendation made by Marinus and colleagues was that the PDQ-39 was the best available HRQoL disease-specific measure for both clinical and research purposes. This recommendation was based on the scheme's adequate clinimetric characteristics, the availability of many translations, its widespread testing, and its use in a large number of clinical trials.

14.4.5
Patient-Specific Measures

Patient-specific measures are less-frequently used when evaluating HRQoL, but are conceptually attractive [36]. Although more common HRQoL measures are used within research and clinical settings, patient-generated outcome measure is directed at the individual's perception of HRQoL and the prioritization of which health-related dimensions/attributes. These instruments do not consist of any predefined dimensions; rather, the dimensions are ascertained by the patient. Patients identify the items that are relevant to their condition, and for this reason they are driven by the patient's judgment of importance, and are individualized measures. Each patient identifies the domains for severity and importance, which makes this type of measure particularly suited for clinical practice. The major concerns of patient-specific measures are the respondent burden and the challenge of comparing scores across individuals and groups. In other words, the lack of standardization between individuals makes the comparison of results a challenge. Although no evidence was found of any patient-specific measures being used with PD patients, this does offer another approach to measuring the HRQoL. Perhaps more practically, it may be useful as a supplement to the standardized measures of HRQoL. Examples of patient-specific measures include the Patient-Generated Index [37], Patient-Specific Index [38], and the Patient Specific Functional Scale [39].

14.5
Conclusions

Within the PD community, the importance of HRQoL measures in the clinical and research realms is accepted, with several disease-specific measures having been developed over the past decade. The shift towards HRQoL measures indicates the acceptance of the patient's perception as an outcome. Although a number of HRQoL measures can be used in PD, further research is needed in all aspects of HRQoL in this condition. From a patient perspective, however, HRQoL measures need to gain clinical acceptance.

Today, clinicians and investigators alike are confronted with selecting among several instruments that are directed specifically towards measuring the HRQoL in PD. Whilst comparisons of different PD HRQoL measures have been summarized by others, the most frequently used health measures in PD patient populations are discussed in this chapter.

Acknowledgments

The authors wish to express their gratitude to Dr D. Feeny for his thoughtful comments.

References

1 Osoba, D. and King, M. (2005) Meaningful differences, in *Assessing Quality of Life in Clinical Trials* (eds P. Fayers and R. Hays), Oxford University Press, Oxford, pp. 243–257.

2 Patrick, D.L. and Erickson, P. (1993) *Health Status and Health Policy: Quality of Life in Health Care Evaluation and Resource Allocation*, Oxford University Press, New York, p. 19.

3 Patrick, D.L. and Erickson, P. (1993) *Health Status and Health Policy: Quality of Life in Health Care Evaluation and Resource Allocation*, Oxford University Press, New York, p. 22.

4 Wilson, I.B. and Kaplan, S. (1995) Clinical practice and patients' health status: how are the two related? *Medical Care*, 33, AS209–AS214.

5 Wilson, I.B. and Cleary, P.D. (1995) Linking clinical variables with health-related quality of life. A conceptual model of patient outcomes. *Journal of the American Medical Association*, 273, 59–65.

6 Guyatt, G.H., Feeny, D.H., and Patrick, D.L. (1993) Measuring health-related quality of life. *Annals of Internal Medicine*, 118, 622–629.

7 Dolan, P. (1997) Modeling valuations for EuroQoL health states. *Medical Care*, 35, 1095–1108.

8 Shaw, J.W., Johnson, J.A., and Coons, S.J. (2005) US valuation of the EQ-5D health states: development and testing of the D1 valuation model. *Medical Care*, 43, 203–220.

9 Torrance, G.W., Feeny, D.H., Furlong, W.J., Barr, R.D., Zhang, Y., and Wang, Q. (1996) Multiattribute utility function for a comprehensive health status classification system. Health Utilities Index Mark 2. *Medical Care*, 34, 702–722.

10 Feeny, D., Furlong, W., Torrance, G.W., Goldsmith, C.H., Zhu, Z., DePauw, S., Denton, M., and Boyle, M. (2002) Multiattribute and single-attribute utility functions for the health utilities index mark 3 system. *Medical Care*, 40, 113–128.

11 Ware, J.E., Jr and Sherbourne, C.D. (1992) The MOS 36-item short-form health survey (SF-36). I. Conceptual framework and item selection. *Medical Care*, 30, 473–483.

12 Damiano, A.M., Snyder, C., Strausser, B., Willian, M.K., Damiano, A.M., Snyder, C., et al. (1999) A review of health-related quality-of-life concepts and measures for Parkinson's disease. *Quality of Life Research*, 8, 235–243.

13 Rubenstein, L.M., Chrischilles, E.A., Voelker, M.D., Rubenstein, L.M., Chrischilles, E.A., and Voelker, M.D. (1997) The impact of Parkinson's disease on health status, health expenditures, and productivity. Estimates from the National Medical Expenditure Survey. *Pharmacoeconomics*, 12, 486–498.

14 Schrag, A., Jahanshahi, M., Quinn, N., Schrag, A., Jahanshahi, M., and Quinn, N. (2000) How does Parkinson's disease affect quality of life? A comparison with quality of life in the general population. *Movement Disorders*, 15, 1112–1118.

15 Kuopio, A.M., Marttila, R.J., Helenius, H., Toivonen, M., Rinne, U.K., Kuopio, A.M., et al. (2000) The quality of life in Parkinson's disease. *Movement Disorders*, 15, 216–223.

16 Karlsen, K.H., Tandberg, E., Arsland, D., Larsen, J.P., Karlsen, K.H., Tandberg, E., et al. (2000) Health-related quality of life in Parkinson's disease: a prospective longitudinal study. *Journal of Neurology, Neurosurgery, and Psychiatry*, 69, 584–589.

17 Welsh, M.D., Dorflinger, E., Chernik, D., Waters, C., Welsh, M.D., Dorflinger, E., et al. (2000) Illness impact and adjustment to Parkinson's disease: before and after treatment with tolcapone. *Movement Disorders*, 15, 497–502.

18 Ellis, T., de Goede, C.J., Feldman, R.G., Wolters, E.C., Kwakkel, G., Wagenaar, R.C., et al. (2005) Efficacy of a physical therapy program in patients with Parkinson's disease: a randomized controlled trial. *Archives of Physical Medicine and Rehabilitation*, 86, 626–632.

19 Dowding, C.H., Shenton, C.L., and Salek, S.S. (2006) A review of the

health-related quality of life and economic impact of Parkinson's disease. *Drugs and Aging*, **23**, 693–721.

20 Schrag, A., Selai, C., Jahanshahi, M., Quinn, N.P., Schrag, A., Selai, C., *et al.* (2000) The EQ-5D–a generic quality of life measure–is a useful instrument to measure quality of life in patients with Parkinson's disease. *Journal of Neurology, Neurosurgery, and Psychiatry*, **69**, 67–73.

21 Reuther, M., Spottke, E.A., Klotsche, J., Riedel, O., Peter, H., Berger, K., *et al.* (2007) Assessing health-related quality of life in patients with Parkinson's disease in a prospective longitudinal study. *Parkinsonism and Related Disorders*, **13**, 108–114.

22 Siderowf, A., Ravina, B., Glick, H.A., Siderowf, A., Ravina, B., and Glick, H.A. (2002) Preference-based quality-of-life in patients with Parkinson's disease. *Neurology*, **59**, 103–108.

23 Peto, V., Jenkinson, C., Fitzpatrick, R., and Greenhall, R. (1995) The development and validation of a short measure of functioning and well being for individuals with Parkinson's disease. *Quality of Life Research*, **4**, 241–248.

24 Wade, D.T., Gage, H., Owen, C., Trend, P., Grossmith, C., and Kaye, J. (2003) Multidisciplinary rehabilitation for people with Parkinson's disease: a randomised controlled study. *Journal of Neurology, Neurosurgery, and Psychiatry*, **74**, 158–162.

25 Gershanik, O., Emre, M., Bernhard, G., and Sauer, D. (2003) Efficacy and safety of levodopa with entacapone in Parkinson's disease patients suboptimally controlled with levodopa alone, in daily clinical practice: an international, multicentre, open-label study. *Progress in Neuropsychopharmacology and Biological Psychiatry*, **27**, 963–971.

26 Jenkinson, C., Fitzpatrick, R., and Peto, V. (1998) *The Parkinson's Disease Questionnaire: User Manual for the PDQ-39, PDQ-8 and the PDQ Summary Index*, University of Oxford Health Services Research Unit, Oxford.

27 Jenkinson, C. and Fitzpatrick, R. (2007) Cross-cultural evaluation of the short form 8-item Parkinson's Disease Questionnaire (PDQ-8): results from America, Canada, Japan, Italy and Spain. *Parkinsonism and Related Disorders*, **13**, 22–28.

28 Tan, L.C., Lau, P.N., Au, W.L., and Luo, N. (2007) Validation of PDQ-8 as an independent instrument in English and Chinese. *Journal of Neurological Science*, **255**, 77–80.

29 de Boer, A.G., Wijker, W., Speelman, J.D., and de Haes, J.C. (1996) Quality of life in patients with Parkinson's disease: development of a questionnaire. *Journal of Neurology, Neurosurgery, and Psychiatry*, **61**, 70–74.

30 Hobson, P., Holden, A., Meara, J., Hobson, P., Holden, A., and Meara, J. (1999) Measuring the impact of Parkinson's disease with the Parkinson's Disease Quality of Life questionnaire. *Age and Ageing*, **28**, 341–346.

31 Calne, S., Schulzer, M., Mak, E., Guyette, C., Rohs, G., Hatchard, S., *et al.* (1996) Validating a quality of life rating scale for idiopathic parkinsonism: Parkinson's Impact Scale (PIMS). *Parkinsonism and Related Disorders*, **2**, 55–61.

32 Welsh, M., McDermott, M.P., Holloway, R.G., Plumb, S., Pfeiffer, R., Hubble, J., *et al.* (2003) Development and testing of the Parkinson's disease quality of life scale. *Movement Disorders*, **18**, 637–645.

33 Noyes, K., Dick, A.W., and Holloway, R.G. (2006) Pramipexole versus levodopa in patients with early Parkinson's disease: effect on generic and disease-specific quality of life. *Value Health*, **9**, 28–38.

34 Biglan, K.M., Schwid, S., Eberly, S., Blindauer, K., Fahn, S., Goren, T., *et al.* (2006) Rasagiline improves quality of life in patients with early Parkinson's disease. *Movement Disorders*, **21**, 616–623.

35 Marinus, J., Ramaker, C., van Hilten, J.J., Stiggelbout, A.M., Marinus, J., Ramaker, C., *et al.* (2002) Health related quality of life in Parkinson's disease: a systematic review of disease specific instruments. *Journal of Neurology, Neurosurgery, and Psychiatry*, **72**, 241–248.

36 Patel, K.K., Veenstra, D.L., and Patrick, D.L. (2003) A review of selected patient-generated outcome measures and their application in clinical trials. *Value Health*, **6**, 595–603.

37 Ruta, D.A., Garratt, A.M., Leng, M., Russell, I.T., and MacDonald, L.M. (1994) A new approach to the measurement of quality of life. The Patient-Generated Index. *Medical Care*, **32**, 1109–1126.

38 Wright, J.G. and Young, N.L. (1997) The patient-specific index: asking patients what they want. *American Journal of Bone and Joint Surgery*, **79**, 974–983.

39 Stratford, P.W., Gill, C., Westaway, M.D., and Binkley, J. (1995) Assessing disability and change on individual patients: A report of a patient-specific measure. *Physiotherapy Canada*, **47**, 258–263.

Appendix: Parkinson-Focused Quality of Life Questionnaires

PDQUALIF©
M Welsh and the Parkinson Study Group™, 1996

PLEASE MAKE A CHECK MARK IN THE BOX BELOW THE ANSWER WHICH BEST DESCRIBES YOUR PERSONAL SITUATION.

EXAMPLE: I exercise regularly:

never	rarely	sometimes	occasionally	always
☐	☐	☐	☐	☐

1. Changing position causes me to become lightheaded (lying to standing, or sitting to standing):

never	rarely	sometimes	occasionally	always
☐	☐	☐	☐	☐

2. When walking, I have trouble keeping my balance:

never	rarely	sometimes	occasionally	always
☐	☐	☐	☐	☐

3. When eating, or drinking liquids, I have difficulty swallowing:

never	rarely	sometimes	occasionally	always
☐	☐	☐	☐	☐

4. My Parkingson's symptoms affect my ability to communicate with people:

never	rarely	sometimes	occasionally	always
☐	☐	☐	☐	☐

5. The need to go to the bathroom wakes me in the night:

never	rarely	sometimes	occasionally	always
☐	☐	☐	☐	☐

6. My Parkinson's symptoms affect my ability to show affection in intimate or sexual ways:

never	rarely	sometimes	occasionally	always
☐	☐	☐	☐	☐

7. I have aching/burming/coldness/numbness in my hand/feet:

never	rarely	sometimes	occasionally	always
☐	☐	☐	☐	☐

8. I have difficulty with bladder control (frequency, urgency, inability):

never	rarely	sometimes	occasionally	always
☐	☐	☐	☐	☐

9. Constipation is a problem:

never	rarely	sometimes	occasionally	always
☐	☐	☐	☐	☐

10. My Parkinson's symptoms cause me to have trouble falling asleep, or waking early.

never	rarely	sometimes	occasionally	always
☐	☐	☐	☐	☐

11. I have trouble staying asleep:

never	rarely	sometimes	occasionally	always
☐	☐	☐	☐	☐

12. My Parkinson's symptoms make it hard to maintain a positive outlook:

never	frequently	sometimes	rarely	always
☐	☐	☐	☐	☐

13. My Parkinson's symptoms cause me to feel like a burden to other people:

never	rarely	sometimes	occasionally	always
☐	☐	☐	☐	☐

14. My Parkinson's symptoms have affected my social life:

never	rarely	sometimes	occasionally	always
☐	☐	☐	☐	☐

15. I worry about what the future has in store:

never	frequently	sometimes	rarely	always
☐	☐	☐	☐	☐

16. Asking others for help is difficult for me:

never	frequently	sometimes	rarely	always
☐	☐	☐	☐	☐

17. Maintaining my independence is important to me:

never	rarely	sometimes	frequently	always
☐	☐	☐	☐	☐

18. It has been difficult to adjust to the changes which have taken place in my body:

very	moderately	somewhat	slightly	not at all
☐	☐	☐	☐	☐

19. My Parkinson's symptoms have not affected my social life:

strongly agree	somewhat agree	agree	somewhat disagree	strongly disagree
☐	☐	☐	☐	☐

20. Travel remains an important part of my leisure activities:

strongly agree	somewhat agree	agree	somewhat disagree	strongly disagree
☐	☐	☐	☐	☐

21. My Parkinson's symptoms have affected my family role and relationship:

strongly agree	somewhat agree	agree	somewhat disagree	strongly disagree
☐	☐	☐	☐	☐

22. My Parkinson's symptoms cause me to stay away from social gatherings:

strongly agree	somewhat agree	agree	somewhat disagree	strongly disagree
☐	☐	☐	☐	☐

23. My spouse/children/friends' view of me has changed because of my illness:

strongly agree	somewhat agree	agree	somewhat disagree	strongly disagree
☐	☐	☐	☐	☐

24. I feel I am less sexually desirable because of my illness:

strongly agree	somewhat agree	agree	somewhat disagree	strongly disagree
☐	☐	☐	☐	☐

IN THE PAST 7 DAYS:

25. In my personal hygiene (bathing, hair care, make up, shaving, or toileting) I have been independent:

everyday	5-6 days	3-4 days	1-2 days	never
☐	☐	☐	☐	☐

26. In food preparation or eating I am independent:

everyday	5-6 days	3-4 days	1-2 days	never
☐	☐	☐	☐	☐

27. Written or spoken communication is a problem for me:

never	rarely	sometimes	frequently	always
☐	☐	☐	☐	☐

28. Fatigue makes participation in activities, household chores, shopping or yard work a problem for me:

always	frequently	sometimes	rarely	never
☐	☐	☐	☐	☐

29. My Parkinson's symptoms interfere with my ability to do my usual share in the home:

always	frequently	sometimes	rarely	never
☐	☐	☐	☐	☐

30. My nighttime symptoms keep me from sleeping with my spouse/partner:

everyday	5-6 days	3-4 days	1-2 days	never
☐	☐	☐	☐	☐

31. My Parkinson's symptoms have interfered with my driving ability:

doesn't apply	rarely	sometimes	frequently	constantly
☐	☐	☐	☐	☐

32. My illness has caused a financiall strain for me and my family:

doesn't apply	rarely a concern	sometimes	frequently	constantly
☐	☐	☐	☐	☐

33. Compared to 6 months ago, my Parkinson's symptoms are:

much better	somewhat better	about the same	somewhat worse	much worse
☐	☐	☐	☐	☐

Parkinson's Impact Scale

Name: Date:
Year symptoms began: Date of Birth:

- Please indicate by a number (0–4) what impact Parkinson's has had on your life.

0 = no change   1 = slight   2 = moderate   3 = moderately severe   4 = severe

- Use the definitions below to help you to measure impact

Self: (positive)	Refers to how positive you feel about yourself (self-worth, happiness, optimism)
Self: (positive)	Refers to how positive you feel about yourself (self-worth, happiness, optimism)
Self: (negative)	Refers to how negative you feel about yourself (level of stress, anxiety, or depression)
Family relationships:	Refers to your spouse, partner, children and relatives that you consider part of your immediate family
Community relationships:	Refers to your neighbors, friends, people you work with and those who provide you with services (store clerk, doctor, pastor, etc.)
Work:	Refers to your job and/or the running of your home and your ability to support yourself and your family
Leisure:	Refers to your ability to continue enjoyable activities (hobbies, sports, volunteering)
Travel:	Refers to your ability to reach your destination, that is, work and/or social
Safety:	Refers to your ability to do what you want without injuring yourself or others (driving, being outdoors, in the kitchen, in the bathroom, etc.)
Financial security:	Refers to your ability to support yourself and your family and pay your medical treatment
Sexuality:	Refers to your ability to maintain a satisfactory sexual relationship

- If your symptoms are stable, complete column 1
- If your symptoms fluctuate, complete columns 2a and 2b (best and worst)

	1 (Stable)	2a (Best)	2b (Worst)
Self: (positive)			
Self: (negative)			
Family relationships:			
Community relationships:			
Safety:			
Leisure:			
Travel:			
Work:			
Financial security:			
Sexuality:			

PDQ-39 QUESTIONNAIRE

Please complete the following

Please tick <u>one</u> box for each question

Due to having Parkinson's disease, how often <u>during the last month</u> have you....

		Never	Occasionally	Sometimes	Often	Always or cannot do at all
1	Had difficulty doing the leisure activities which you would like to do?	☐	☐	☐	☐	☐
2	Had difficulty looking after your home, e.g. DIY, housework, cooking?	☐	☐	☐	☐	☐
3	Had difficulty carrying bags of shopping?	☐	☐	☐	☐	☐
4	Had problems walking half a mile?	☐	☐	☐	☐	☐
5	Had problems walking 100 yards?	☐	☐	☐	☐	☐
6	Had problems getting around the house as easily as you would like?	☐	☐	☐	☐	☐
7	Had difficulty getting around in public?	☐	☐	☐	☐	☐
8	Needed someone else to accompany you when you went out?	☐	☐	☐	☐	☐
9	Felt frightened or worried about falling over in public?	☐	☐	☐	☐	☐
10	Been confined to the house more than you would like?	☐	☐	☐	☐	☐
11	Had difficulty washing yourself?	☐	☐	☐	☐	☐
12	Had difficulty dressing yourself?	☐	☐	☐	☐	☐
13	Had problems doing up your shoe laces?	☐	☐	☐	☐	☐

*Please check that you have ticked **one box for each question** before going on to the next page*

Due to having Parkinson's disease, how often during the last month have you....

Please tick one box for each question

		Never	Occasionally	Sometimes	Often	Always or cannot do at all
14	Had problems writing clearly?	☐	☐	☐	☐	☐
15	Had difficulty cutting up your food?	☐	☐	☐	☐	☐
16	Had difficulty holding a drink without spilling it?	☐	☐	☐	☐	☐
17	Felt depressed?	☐	☐	☐	☐	☐
18	Felt isolated and lonely?	☐	☐	☐	☐	☐
19	Felt weepy or tearful?	☐	☐	☐	☐	☐
20	Felt angry or bitter?	☐	☐	☐	☐	☐
21	Felt anxious?	☐	☐	☐	☐	☐
22	Felt worried about your future?	☐	☐	☐	☐	☐
23	Felt you had to conceal your Parkinson's from people?	☐	☐	☐	☐	☐
24	Avoided situations which involve eating or drinking in public?	☐	☐	☐	☐	☐
25	Felt embarrassed in public due to having Parkinson's disease?	☐	☐	☐	☐	☐
26	Felt worried by other people's reaction to you?	☐	☐	☐	☐	☐
27	Had problems with your close personal relationships?	☐	☐	☐	☐	☐
28	Lacked support in the ways you need from your spouse or partner?	☐	☐	☐	☐	☐
	If you do not have a spouse or partner tick here		☐			
29	Lacked support in the ways you need from your family or close friends?	☐	☐	☐	☐	☐

*Please check that you have ticked **one box for each question** before going on to the next page*

Due to having Parkinson's disease, how often during the last month have you....

Please tick one box for each question

		Never	Occasionally	Sometimes	Often	Always
30	Unexpectedly fallen asleep during the day?	☐	☐	☐	☐	☐
31	Had problems with your concentration, e.g. when reading or watching TV?	☐	☐	☐	☐	☐
32	Felt your memory was bad?	☐	☐	☐	☐	☐
33	Had distressing dreams or hallucinations?	☐	☐	☐	☐	☐
34	Had difficulty with your speech?	☐	☐	☐	☐	☐
35	Felt unable to communicate with people properly?	☐	☐	☐	☐	☐
36	Felt ignored by people?	☐	☐	☐	☐	☐
37	Had painful muscle cramps or spasms?	☐	☐	☐	☐	☐
38	Had aches and pains in your joints or body?	☐	☐	☐	☐	☐
39	Felt unpleasantly hot or cold?	☐	☐	☐	☐	☐

*Please check that you have ticked **one box for each question** before going on to the next page*

Thank you for completing the PDQ 39 questionnaire

A Patient's Story

And Then There Was the Pain Control

Joyce Pinckney

Today I am a number, I must choose one—rate my pain on a scale of 1 to 10. I have traded in my name.

It's important: they will wake me from a dreamless sleep thrice nightly just to ask me, then record the answer on my chart precisely.

If I hesitate in choosing, or they think that I don't get it, they will focus on the scale again: one's no pain, ten's horrific.

But so what? It's just a number meaning nothing with no plan, It's a number with a context they no longer understand.

They've forgotten why they need it: What's my tolerance, what's my goal?

They've forgotten there is more than rating pain to pain control.

No one asks me if I'm hurting, if I could use a hand.

No one calls my name or sees me this carefully sterile land.

Today I am a number, I have traded in my name.

Today I am a number, I have become my pain.

15
Measuring Health-Related Quality of Life in PD: How Does It Compare to the Canadian General Population?

Allyson Jones and Sheri L. Pohar

15.1
Introduction

Parkinson disease (PD) is a leading cause of neurological disability in the adult population [1]. The impact of this chronic progressive condition is substantial [2]. The burden of disease associated with PD includes physical, mental and psychological impairments, which are particularly problematic with the advanced stages of the disease. Although health-related quality of life (HRQoL) has been examined in clinical patient samples, relatively few studies have used large populations to evaluate the impact of PD on HRQoL [3–5]. Rather, HRQoL in PD is more often than not measured in clinical samples using PD-specific measures [6–8], which preclude comparisons to the population without PD and thus limit the external validity. Even fewer large-population studies have adjusted for sociodemographic characteristics beyond controlling for age and gender [5, 9].

From the limited population-based data available, it is apparent that patients with PD were two- to tenfold more likely to have difficulties with self-care, social functioning, mobility and anxiety or depression, and had significantly lower overall HRQoL scores [3]. These findings, however, were compared to published United Kingdom population norms, rather than measuring HRQoL in both the PD and the general population, without the disease at a single point in time. The PD population in this specific cohort was not nationally representative of the UK population; rather, it was representative of a limited geographic area. Similarly, a population-based survey of the American general population reported significant burdens of health in persons with PD as compared to controls [5]. The external validity of this study was limited because of the small sample and subsequent inadequate representation of persons with PD.

Another approach to measuring the burden of disease in PD has been captured, in part, by exploring the economic consequences of the disease in terms of health-care utilization, lost productivity, and caregiver costs [5, 10, 11]. The direct and hidden costs of the disease represent significant burden which have been substantiated in a number of countries [5, 10, 12, 13].

Parkinson Disease – A Health Policy Perspective. Edited by Wayne Martin, Oksana Suchowersky, Katharina Kovacs Burns, and Egon Jonsson
Copyright © 2010 WILEY-VCH Verlag GmbH & Co. KGaA, Weinheim
ISBN: 978-3-527-32779-9

Because of the substantial impact of PD on health status, further investigation of the burden of disease is called for within the literature [2, 14]. A comparison of the HRQoL to the general population represents a useful means of capturing the disease burden from both patient and societal perspectives. The purpose of this study was to compare the health status of community-based Canadians who have PD to those persons without PD, using a nationally representative sample of the general population. This comparison to the general population will provide quantitative estimates of the impact of PD on health status.

15.2
Research Design and Methods

15.2.1
Survey Design

Data from the Canadian Community Health Survey (CCHS) Cycle 1.1 were used in this analysis. Ethical approval was obtained through the University of Alberta Health Research Ethics Board. Approval to access the survey data was obtained from Statistics Canada.

The CCHS 1.1 is a cross-sectional survey of the Canadian population over age 12 years. Data pertaining to health status, determinants of health, and utilization of health services were collected between September 2000 and November 2001 [15]. The survey represented approximately 98% of the Canadian population over 12 years of age. Persons who resided in institutions, on Crown or reserve land, and in some remote areas of the country, as well as full-time members of the Canadian Armed Forces, were excluded [15]. A multistage stratified cluster design combined with random sampling methods was used to select the sample [15]. At the end of Cycle 1.1 a total of 131,535 respondents had been surveyed, with an overall response rate of 84.7% [16].

15.2.2
Sample

Within the CCHS 1.1, approximately 294 respondents reported having a diagnosis of PD; this represented a weighted percentage of 0.2% of the Canadian population. This was comparable to previous prevalence rates reported within the Canadian population [17]. Of the 294 respondents with PD, 261 (89% of the PD population) had complete data for purposes of this analysis. The general population was restricted to respondents over the age of 18 years with complete data ($n = 111,707$).

15.2.3
Health Utilities Index Mark 3 (HUI3)

The HRQoL was assessed with the HUI3, a generic preference-based measure [18]. The HUI3 was administered as a 31-item questionnaire that assessed usual health status. Eight attributes are included in the HUI3 system: vision; hearing; speech; ambulation; dexterity; emotion; cognition; and pain and discomfort. The utility scores for single attributes range from 0.0 to 1.0, with a score of 0.0 representing the lowest level of functioning on an attribute, and a score of 1.0 representing full functional capacity. For instance, a score of 0 within the emotion attribute represents a state so unhappy that life is not worthwhile, while a score of 1 indicates a state that is happy and interested in life. A difference of 0.05 on a single attribute is considered to be clinically important [19].

The HUI3 overall scores for health states ranged from −0.36 to 1.0 (−0.36 = worst possible health, 0.0 = dead, and 1.0 = perfect health) [18]. Differences of greater than 0.03 for HUI3 overall scores were considered to be clinically important [19]. Cross-sectional comparisons between groups of individuals known to differ in their level of HRQoL support this value as clinically important [20–23].

These attributes of HUI3 have a significant overlap with those measured by PD-specific measures of HRQoL, such as the Parkinson's Disease Questionnaire (PDQ-39) which assesses mobility, activities of daily living (ADL), emotional well-being, stigma, social support, cognition, communication, and bodily discomfort [24]. Previous research has demonstrated moderate to strong correlations between HUI scores, disease-specific measures of HRQoL, and clinical measures in PD [25]. The HUI was also able to discriminate between clinically different groups of patients with PD, based on the Hoehn and Yahr stage and Unified Parkinson's Disease Rating Scale scores [25]. These results provide evidence of construct validity of the HUI in PD, and lend support for its use in the disease [25].

Demographics from the CCHS 1.1 were also included in the analysis. Age, gender, marital status, and socioeconomic status were compared between the Canadian population with and without PD. Socioeconomic status was delineated using two variables: the highest level of education; and the receipt of social assistance as an income source.

From a list of 27 chronic medical conditions, respondents were asked to identify conditions diagnosed by a health professional and which had been present for at least 6 months, or would be expected to last for at least 6 months. The identification of all chronic conditions was based upon a self-reported diagnosis, with the exception of depression. A summative score of the total number of chronic conditions was generated as a disability indicator.

15.2.4
Analysis

Differences in overall HUI3 and single attribute scores between respondents with and without PD were assessed using analysis of covariance (ANCOVA). All models were adjusted for age, gender, education, marital status, social assistance, and number of chronic medical conditions, other than PD. The number of respondents who failed to report their personal or household income was relatively large, which limited the usefulness of this variable as a covariate. Thus, the receipt of social assistance during the previous 12 months was included as an indicator of low income instead of income. Normalized sampling weights were applied to the analysis, and bootstrap variance estimates were used to adjust for clustering and stratification and to estimate 95% confidence intervals (CI) and *P*-values. All analyses were carried out using WESTVAR version 4.2, with bootstrap weights provided by Statistics Canada.

15.2.5
Results

The average age of respondents with PD was 68.9 years (95% CI: 66.6 to 71.2) compared to 44.8 years (95% CI: 44.8 to 44.9) in the general population (Table 15.1). The PD and general populations did not differ significantly with respect to marital status, social assistance, and gender, but some differences were noted

Table 15.1 Demographic characteristics of the Canadian population with and without Parkinson disease.

	Parkinson disease	General population
Age [mean (95% CI)] (years)	68.9 (66.6 to 71.2)*	44.8 (44.8 to 44.9)
Gender		
Female	44.1	51.0
Male	55.9	49.0
Level of education (%)		
Less than secondary	42.8*	22.4
Secondary graduation	18.2	20.5
Some post-secondary, college, trade school	24.4*	36.5
University degree	14.6	20.7
Marital status (%)		
Married	67.8	64.0
Not married	32.2	36.0
Social assistance as income source (%)		
Yes	9.7	5.3
No	90.4	94.7
Medical conditions [mean (95% CI)][a]	3.0 (2.5 to 3.4)*	1.5 (1.5 to 1.5)
HUI3 [mean (95% CI)]		
Overall	0.56 (0.48 to 0.63)*	0.87 (0.87 to 0.88)
Vision	0.93 (0.89 to 0.96)*	0.97 (0.97 to 0.97)
Hearing	0.95 (0.91 to 0.99)	0.99 (0.99 to 0.99)
Speech	0.98 (0.96 to 1.00)	1.00 (1.00 to 1.00)
Ambulation	0.84 (0.78 to 0.89)*	0.98 (0.98 to 0.98)
Dexterity	0.88 (0.81 to 0.96)*	1.00 (1.00 to 1.00)
Emotion	0.89 (0.85 to 0.93)*	0.97 (0.97 to 0.97)
Cognition	0.84 (0.80 to 0.89)*	0.96 (0.96 to 0.96)
Pain	0.76 (0.68 to 0.83)*	0.93 (0.93 to 0.93)

*$P < 0.05$.

a) Number of chronic conditions other than PD; CI, confidence interval.

according to the level of education. When compared to the general population, a higher proportion of respondents with PD had less than secondary education, whilst a smaller proportion of respondents with PD had some post-secondary education. The mean number of comorbid conditions for persons with PD was 3.0 (95% CI 2.5, 3.4).

The unadjusted overall HUI3 scores were significantly lower in the PD population compared to the general population (0.56, 95% CI: 0.48 to 0.63 versus 0.87, 95% CI: 0.87 to 0.88, $P < 0.05$). Clinically important and statistically significant differences in the unadjusted single attribute scores were observed for ambulation, dexterity, emotion, cognition, and pain (see Table 15.1).

After adjusting for the model covariates, the differences in overall HUI3 scores, ambulation, dexterity, emotion, cognition, and pain scores between respondents with and without PD persisted (see Table 15.2). The adjusted mean overall HUI3 scores were significantly lower for respondents with PD (0.61 versus 0.83, $P < 0.05$) (Figure 15.1), with the difference between groups being sevenfold larger than what would be considered clinically important (–0.22, 95% CI: –0.29 to –0.15, $P < 0.05$) (Table 15.2). Across the single attributes, the greatest burden was found for pain and cognition in both populations (Figure 15.1). As seen in Table 15.2, large differences in single attribute scores between respondents with and without PD were observed for ambulation (–0.11, 95% CI: –0.16 to –0.06, $P < 0.05$), dexterity (–0.11, 95% CI: –0.19 to –0.03, $P < 0.05$), cognition (–0.10, 95% CI: –0.18 to –0.02, $P < 0.05$), and pain (–0.09, 95% CI: –0.14 to –0.05, $P < 0.05$). Clinically important differences between respondents with and without PD were also observed for the emotion attribute (Table 15.2).

Table 15.2 Adjusted[a] mean difference in overall and single attribute HUI3 scores in Parkinson disease and the general population.

	Mean difference	95% CI
HUI3		
Overall	–0.22[*]	–0.29 to –0.15
Vision	–0.02	–0.05 to 0.02
Hearing	–0.02	–0.06 to 0.02
Speech	–0.02	–0.03 to 0.00
Ambulation	–0.11[*]	–0.16 to –0.06
Dexterity	–0.11[*]	–0.19 to –0.03
Emotion	–0.06[*]	–0.10 to –0.02
Cognition	–0.09[*]	–0.14 to –0.05
Pain	–0.10[*]	–0.18 to –0.02

a) Adjusted for age, gender, education, marital status, social assistance and number of chronic conditions other than PD.
*P <0.05.

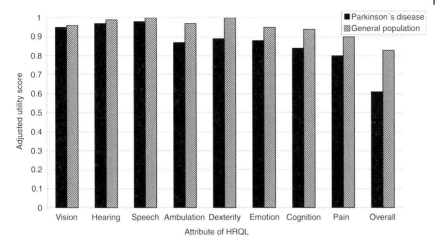

Figure 15.1 Overall and single attribute utility scores for respondents with and without Parkinson disease, adjusted for age, gender, education, marital status, social assistance, and number of chronic conditions other than PD.

15.3
Discussion

Within a representative sample of community-dwelling Canadians, persons with PD reported a substantially lower health status than the general population, when statistically adjusted for a number of covariates (including age) that could potentially impact the scores. The difference between persons with PD and the general population was sevenfold what is considered a clinically important difference. From this analysis, it was possible to quantify the burden of PD, affecting both physical and mental dimensions of HRQoL (ambulation, dexterity, emotion, cognition, and pain) relative to the general population. Such HRQoL instruments can capture relevant information about patients with PD that would otherwise not be captured by using standard clinical scales or disease-specific health measures [26]. For this reason, HRQoL data are essential for understanding the burden associated with disease, particularly when such information can be compared to the general population without the disease. Generic HRQoL measures allow such comparisons to be made between populations, and are pertinent to a wide range of health issues.

The average adjusted overall HUI3 score of all respondents with PD was 0.61, compared to 0.83 for respondents without the disease. In order to better understand the relative HRQoL burden of the two populations, the overall HUI3 scores could be grouped into categories which reflected the level of impairment: none/mild (0.89–1.00), moderate (0.70–0.88), and severe (<0.70). Thus, the community-dwelling population with PD experienced a severe HRQoL impairment on average, while those without PD experienced only a moderate impairment.

The overall HUI3 scores of PD can also be compared to other chronic conditions to further understand the burden of the disease. In a Canadian population-based study, the average overall HUI3 score in individuals with diabetes, heart disease, arthritis or stroke ranged from 0.74 to 0.89 [22]. For those patients with three of these conditions (in any combination), the overall HUI3 scores ranged from 0.62 to 0.66 [22]. Thus, the HRQoL of burden associated with PD was substantially higher than diabetes, heart disease, arthritis or stroke alone, but similar to having three of these chronic conditions in combination, again highlighting the magnitude of the burden associated with PD.

Multiattribute utility measures, such as the HUI3 and the EQ-5D, differ with respect to the attributes included in the instrument, the range of possible scores, and the scoring algorithms. Yet, despite these differences, the average unadjusted overall HUI3 score observed in the Canadian community-dwelling population with PD (mean = 0.56) was similar to the EQ-5D index scores from a population-based study of community-dwelling individuals with PD in the UK (mean = 0.54) [3], and from clinical settings [25, 27]. Thus, the burden experienced by the Canadian population is similar to what has been estimated in other population and clinical studies.

Both, motor (tremor, rigidity, bradykinesia, and postural instability) [8] and non-motor (anxiety, depression, sleep disturbance, pain, fatigue, and cognitive decline) [28] symptoms of PD affect multiple dimensions of the HRQoL [1, 4]. Although clinically well recognized, problems with ambulation, dexterity, emotion, cognition, and pain were quantified relative to the population without the disease. The importance of non-motor symptoms to the HRQoL in PD is increasingly being recognized [7, 28], with pain and loss of energy having been identified as two of the three most disabling symptoms in the disease [28]. Depression can be a stronger predictor of HRQoL in PD than even clinical features or postural instability [7]. Whilst it may not be immediately intuitive that difficulties with emotion and pain should be observed in the PD population, these findings are consistent with previous observations. The impairments observed on the emotion, cognition, and pain attributes demonstrated that attention to non-motor symptoms can also be important for improving or maintaining the HRQoL in PD.

While the present study has the strength of using population-based data and sound external validity, the results should be interpreted in light of a number of limitations. First, the ascertainment of PD was via self-reporting. Although questions regarding the presence of medical conditions specified that the condition had been diagnosed by a health professional, there remained the potential for individuals to either over-report or under-report PD. The estimated population prevalence of PD in the CCHS Cycle 1.1, however, was similar to other population-based estimates [1].

Second, despite over 98% of the Canadian community-dwelling population being represented in the survey, the generalizability of the results to the entire Canadian population with PD is limited by the fact that individuals who resided in institutions were not captured by the sampling frame. Accordingly, the results are only generalizable to the community-dwelling population with PD. It is expected, however, that individuals with PD who resided in institutions would have a poorer health status and greater impairment. A previous study of community-dwelling individuals found that relatively few were in the advanced stages of the disease [26]. Thus, the true burden of entire Canadian population with PD (both community- and institutional-dwelling combined) would likely be underestimated by these results.

15.4
Conclusion

In summary, PD has detrimental effects on both the physical and mental attributes of the HRQoL, creating a substantial HRQoL burden for persons with this neuro-degenerative disease.

The progressive nature of the disease, with its complex treatment, underscores the importance of the diverse impact of burden and the need to manage all aspects of the disease. The findings presented here provide only baseline population estimates of disease burden for PD in which the efficacy and efficiency of promising disease modifying therapy can be evaluated.

Acknowledgments

The authors would like to thank Statistics Canada for allowing access to the data through the Research Data Center at the University of Alberta and the University of Alberta for providing facilities to access the data. The research and analysis reported here are based on data from Statistics Canada. The opinions expressed do not represent the views of Statistics Canada.

References

1 Damiano, A.M., Snyder, C., Strausser, B., and Willian, M.K. (1999) A review of health-related Quality-of-life concepts and measures for Parkinson's disease. *Quality of life Research*, **8** (3), 235–243.

2 Global Parkinson's Disease Survey Steering Committee (2002) Factors impacting on quality of life in Parkinson's disease: results from an international survey. *Movement Disorders*, **17** (1), 60–67.

3 Schrag, A., Jahanshahi, M., and Quinn, N. (2000) How does Parkinson's disease affect quality of life? A comparison with quality of life in the general population. *Movement Disorders*, **15** (6), 1112–1118.

4 Karlsen, K.H., Larsen, J.P., Tandberg, E., and Maeland, J.G. (1999) Influence of clinical and demographic variables on quality of life in patients with Parkinson's disease. *Journal of Neurology, Neurosurgery, and Psychiatry*, **66** (4), 431–435.

5 Rubenstein, L.M., Chrischilles, E.A., and Voelker, M.D. (1997) The impact of Parkinson's disease on health status, health expenditures, and productivity. Estimates from the National Medical Expenditure Survey. *Pharmacoeconomics*, **12** (4), 486–498.

6 Hobson, P., Holden, A., and Meara, J. (1999) Measuring the impact of

Parkinson's disease with the Parkinson's Disease Quality of Life questionnaire. *Age and Ageing*, **28** (4), 341–346.

7 Schrag, A., Jahanshahi, M., and Quinn, N. (2000) What contributes to quality of life in patients with Parkinson's disease? *Journal of Neurology, Neurosurgery, and Psychiatry*, **69** (3), 308–312.

8 Jenkinson, C., Fitzpatrick, R., and Peto, V. (1999) Health-related quality-of-life measurement in patients with Parkinson's disease. *Pharmacoeconomics*, **15** (2), 157–165.

9 Riazi, A., Hobart, J.C., Lamping, D.L., Fitzpatrick, R., Freeman, J.A., Jenkinson, C., *et al.* (2003) Using the SF-36 measure to compare the health impact of multiple sclerosis and Parkinson's disease with normal population health profiles. *Journal of Neurology, Neurosurgery, and Psychiatry*, **74** (6), 710–714.

10 Dodel, R.C., Berger, K., and Oertel, W.H. (2001) Health-related quality of life and healthcare utilisation in patients with Parkinson's disease: impact of motor fluctuations and dyskinesias. *Pharmacoeconomics*, **19** (10), 1013–1038.

11 Chrischilles, E.A., Rubenstein, L.M., Voelker, M.D., Wallace, R.B., and Rodnitzky, R.L. (1998) The health burdens of Parkinson's disease. *Movement Disorders*, **13** (3), 406–413.

12 Cordato, D.J., Schwartz, R., Abbott, E., Saunders, R., and Morfis, L. (2006) A comparison of health-care costs involved in treating people with and without Parkinson's disease in Southern Sydney, New South Wales, Australia. *Journal of Clinical Neuroscience*, **13** (6), 655–658.

13 Noyes, K., Liu, H., Li, Y., Holloway, R., and Dick, A.W. (2006) Economic burden associated with Parkinson's disease on elderly Medicare beneficiaries. *Movement Disorders*, **21** (3), 362–372.

14 Dowding, C.H., Shenton, C.L., and Salek, S.S. (2006) A review of the health-related quality of life and economic impact of Parkinson's disease. *Drugs and Aging*, **23** (9), 693–721.

15 Beland, Y. (2002) Canadian community health survey-methodological overview. *Health Reports*, **13** (3), 9–14.

16 Statistics Canada (2004) CCHS Cycle 1.1, Public Use Microdata File Documentation.

17 Svenson, L.W., Platt, G.H., and Woodhead, S.E. (1993) Geographic variations in the prevalence rates of Parkinson's disease in Alberta. *Canadian Journal of Neurological Science*, **4**, 307–311.

18 Feeny, D., Furlong, W., Torrance, G.W., Goldsmith, C.H., Zhu, Z., Depauw, S., *et al.* (2002) Multiattribute and single-attribute utility functions for the health utilities index mark 3 system. *Medical Care*, **40** (2), 113–128.

19 Horsman, J., Furlong, W., Feeny, D., and Torrance, G. (2003) The Health Utilities Index (HUI(R)): concepts, measurement properties and applications. *Health Quality of Life Outcomes*, **1** (1), 54.

20 Maddigan, S.L., Feeny, D.H., and Johnson, J.A. (2003) A comparison of the Health Utilities Indices Mark 2 and Mark 3 in type 2 diabetes. *Medical Decision Making*, **23**, 489–501.

21 Maddigan, S.L., Feeny, D.H., and Johnson, J.A. (2004) Construct validity of the RAND-12 and Health Utilities Index Mark 2 and Mark 3 in type 2 diabetes. *Quality of Life Research*, **13**, 435–448.

22 Maddigan, S.L., Feeny, D.H., and Johnson, J.A. (2005) Health-related quality of life deficits associated with diabetes and comorbidities in a Canadian National Population Health Survey. *Quality of Life Research*, **14** (5), 1311–1320.

23 Grootendorst, P., Feeny, D., and Furlong, W. (2000) Health Utilities Index Mark 3: evidence of construct validity for stroke and arthritis in a population health survey. *Medical Care*, **38** (3), 290–299.

24 Jenkinson, C., Fitzpatrick, R., Peto, V., Greenhall, R., and Hyman, N. (1997) The Parkinson's Disease Questionnaire (PDQ-39): development and validation of a Parkinson's disease summary index score. *Age & Ageing*, **26** (5), 353–357.

25 Siderowf, A., Ravina, B., and Glick, H.A. (2002) Preference-based quality-of-life in patients with Parkinson's disease. *Neurology*, **59** (1), 103–108.

26 Rubenstein, L.M., Voelker, M.D., Chrischilles, E.A., Glenn, D.C., Wallace, R.B., and Rodnitzky, R.L. (1998) The usefulness of the Functional Status Questionnaire and Medical Outcomes Study Short Form in Parkinson's disease research. *Quality of Life Research*, **7** (4), 279–290.

27 Reuther, M., Spottke, E.A., Klotsche, J., Riedel, O., Peter, H., Berger, K., *et al.* (2007) Assessing health-related quality of life in patients with Parkinson's disease in a prospective longitudinal study. *Parkinsonism & Related Disorders*, **13** (2), 108–114.

28 Welsh, M. (2004) Parkinson's disease and quality of life: issues and challenges beyond motor symptoms. *Neurologic Clinics*, **22** (Suppl. 3), S141–S148.

A Patient's Story

Living with Parkinson's

Al Smith

My name is Al Smith, and I was diagnosed with Parkinson's disease in the fall of 1999. I was devastated and shocked, but it wasn't the disease itself that scared me the most – it was my lack of knowledge about it.

I had been a golf professional during the late 1960s and early 1970s, and in my spare time had enjoyed riding my motorcycle and playing with my grand-kids. I didn't know if I'd be able to continue doing the things I loved, or for how long.

What I came to realize is that Parkinson's is a disease, not a death sentence. It's a bump in a very long road.

Since my diagnosis I have participated in a number of different research programs. I've met many people from across North American in different stages of Parkinson's and I learned that, besides the disease, there is one thing we all share in common – a positive attitude. Our attitudes, in combination with medication, exercise and diet would allow us to take control of Parkinson's, not fall victim to it.

In September 2004, I had to take long-term disability which was financially stressful, but the lack of work stress has made a tremendous difference in my quality of life.

I consider myself incredibly fortunate to have the loving support of my wife Nancy, my son Paul (Krisa), daughter Melissa (Blair), grand-kids Madison, Darby, Morgan, Josh, Shelby, and more friends than I can mention. With their help I know I'll get through this bump in my road.

To the 100`000 other travelers on this journey – know your limits and have the courage to push them. I still play golf and ride my Gold Wing when I can. I play with my grandkids and I live life to the fullest.

To everyone who's been touched by someone living with Parkinson's – be patient with us, we are a little slower than we used to be. Please support fund-raising efforts, as research is the only way we are going to beat this disease and many others like it.

Good luck, and may God bless us all.

16
Policy Considerations for Alberta

Katharina Kovacs Burns, Egon Jonsson, Oksana Suchowersky, Wayne Martin, Bin Hu, and John Petryshen

In the general Summary and Policy Considerations section laid out at the beginning of this book, it was proposed that a special committee be established to review the findings presented in the book and other information about the situation for people with PD and other neurological diseases. That committee should develop a proposal for how to improve services for these people. Some of the issues raised there include the importance of building a structured surveillance system for PD, the concern about accurate diagnosis of PD, the availability and access to needed treatment and services, and the concern about the burden for caregivers. Specifically for Alberta, two directions for action are suggested from a policy perspective. Both are based on the findings presented in this book, and on the deliberations of the working group that produced this book and that has met repeatedly over a period of two years.

16.1
Coordinate Neurological Services – Establish Specialized Centers Within a New Framework

Good management of PD is part of solid management of neurological disorders, which in turn is part of chronic disease management. The development of the Alberta Health Services (AHS) provides an opportunity to better coordinate access to neurological expertise. Within a reorganization of neurological services there could be different specialized centers, of which one would be dedicated to PD.

   An important rationale for this is the need to refer persons with suspected PD to a specialist with expertise in the differential diagnosis of this condition. The diagnosis should be reviewed regularly and reconsidered if other clinical manifestations develop. Once diagnosed, the person should have access to clinical monitoring, medication adjustment, and a continuing point of contact to other service providers for support. This includes assessment within the local community, or

Parkinson Disease – A Health Policy Perspective. Edited by Wayne Martin, Oksana Suchowersky,
Katharina Kovacs Burns, and Egon Jonsson
Copyright © 2010 WILEY-VCH Verlag GmbH & Co. KGaA, Weinheim
ISBN: 978-3-527-32779-9

even in the home when appropriate, and a reliable source of information about clinical and social matters of concern to both the people with PD and their caregivers. Patients should also have access to physiotherapy, occupational therapy, speech therapy, social services, counseling, and palliative care as needed. This will ensure a continuum of care for persons with PD.

We recommend that a virtual Alberta Center for Parkinson Disease be developed with the available resources already present at the hospitals and the universities in Edmonton and Calgary. The Center should be given mandate and resources to gradually build up a functional network including researchers, specialists and caregivers throughout Alberta. It should establish a provincial registry of patients, their treatments and outcomes. It should become the focus of new innovations in the field. The Center should continuously perform what is known as Comparative Effectiveness Analyses, in which all potential options for treatment are reviewed and compared as to their safety, efficacy, effectiveness, and cost-effectiveness.

Some of the more specific responsibilities of the virtual Center could be to:

- provide persons with PD timely and easy access to specialist consultation via telephone/telehealth or traditional in-person consultation;
- establish and monitor existing provincial quality standards in PD, starting with existing information from previous regional and provincial efforts;
- develop a forum of best practices in the management of PD, and to determine or evaluate what is working as best practices in existing chronic disease management programs in Alberta, particularly those associated with Primary Care Networks;
- engage in health surveillance activities focused on identifying problem areas and monitoring progress towards the reduction of the burden of PD across the province;
- engage in patient navigation approaches to help persons with PD and their caregivers to access available services [1];
- educate the primary care workforce about evidence-based management of PD through the review of currently available interdisciplinary, evidence-informed clinical practice guidelines and chronic disease management program formats; and the development of new guidelines as needed; and
- create an inventory of existing PD research programs in Alberta and identify their potential research synergies with research in other neurological diseases. The Center could also coordinate these research activities.

16.2
Establish a Committee to Review the Management of People with Neurological Diseases

The committee should develop a comprehensive proposal for health policy that supports improved services and outcomes for people with PD and other neurological diseases in the province. In particular for PD, this would include:

1) Ensuring that resources are in place for adequate diagnostic work-up, appropriate medical treatments, and active community-based health and social support. Investments in early PD diagnosis and access to a variety of treatment programs and community services have been shown to delay the need for more intense and costly interventions, as well as to improve the quality of life (see Chapters 2 and 12). The Alberta Health Service, in its 2010 vision document, stressed its intention to focus on improvements in the access to different types and levels of care, including reducing waiting times for diagnostic services, a greater focus on prevention services, more efficient methods for providing primary health care, and creating a home care program (www.albertahealthservices.ca).

2) Reducing the obstacles of access to treatment and other services for patients, regardless of location. Alternative approaches to healthcare and service delivery that may be enhanced include the Alberta Telehealth for persons with PD (similar to what has been explored for mental health) [2], information portals, care pathways [3], mobile outreach units [4], and chronic disease management programs through the Primary Care Networks [5].

3) Reducing the economic burden for socially and economically vulnerable populations with PD and their caregivers, and recognizing the contributions and needs of caregivers of persons with PD.

4) Identifying clinically important research gaps as well as gaps in health services and policy research, and health-related quality of life determinants. It is suggested that a new approach is needed in the "research to policy cycle," whereby decision makers will need to be integrated into knowledge translation [6–8].

5) Reviewing and implementing clinical practice guidelines for PD. This ensures that the protocols for best treatment outcomes are evidence-based, and that the knowledge translation is applicable to all health and allied health professionals [7].

6) Involving health policy makers in knowledge translation related to PD.

7) Developing chronic disease management programs for PD.

8) Establishing mechanisms to continuously assess outcomes and quality improvements in services and PD management.

9) Exploring the possibility of providing research funding and incentives as part of recruitment packages to new and internationally known PD researchers to come to Alberta, either at one of the universities or through Alberta Health Services, to explore basic, clinical and best practices research in chronic disease management interventions for PD.

10) The committee should develop an evaluation framework to monitor and assess the progress or completion of strategies and their outcomes, particularly related to provincial quality standards in PD services.

The committee should also establish a process for regularly reporting to professional associations and policy makers the progress of proposed strategies and on the quality, accessibility, and effectiveness of services for PD patients across the province.

References

1 Alberta Health and Wellness (2008) New Patient Navigators Improve Access to Cardiac Care (news release from the Alberta Government, 23 July 2008). Available at: http://www.gov.ab.ca/acn/200807/2405950B149CC-ADD6-4C01-F1B723737E389748.html.

2 Institute of Health Economics (2007) *Evidence of Benefits from Telemental Health: A Systematic Review*, IHE, Edmonton.

3 Holloway, M. (2006) Traversing the network: a user-led Care Pathway approach to the management of Parkinson's disease in the community. *Health and Social Care in the Community*, **14** (1), 63–73.

4 Majumbar, S., Lewanczuk, R., Guirguis, L., Lee, T., Toth, E., and Johnson, J. (2003) Controlled trial of a multifaceted intervention for improving quality of care for rural patients with Type 2 diabetes. *Diabetes Care*, **26**, 3061–3066.

5 Every, B. (2007) Better for ourselves and better for our patients: chronic disease management in Primary Care Networks. *Healthcare Quarterly*, **10** (3), 70–74.

6 Interdisciplinary Chronic Disease Collaboration (2008) The research to health policy cycle: a tool for better management of chronic noncommunicable diseases. *Journal of Nephrology*, **21**, 621–631.

7 Hakkennes, S. and Dodd, K. (2008) Guideline implementation in allied health professions: a systematic review of the literature. *Quality Safe Health Care*, **17**, 296–300.

8 Institute of Health Economics (2008) *Effective Dissemination of Findings from Research – A Compilation of Essays*, IHE, Edmonton.

Appendices

Parkinson Disease – A Health Policy Perspective. Edited by Wayne Martin, Oksana Suchowersky,
Katharina Kovacs Burns, and Egon Jonsson
Copyright © 2010 WILEY-VCH Verlag GmbH & Co. KGaA, Weinheim
ISBN: 978-3-527-32779-9

Appendix A: Parkinson Disease FAQ Sheet

What is Parkinson Disease?

Parkinson disease is a progressive, neurologic disorder caused by damage to the part of the brain that produces dopamine (the substantia nigra). When 60–80% of the neurons in the substantia nigra are lost, symptoms affecting an individual's movement begin to surface.

Who Does Parkinson Disease Affect?

It is estimated that approximately 100`000 Canadians have Parkinson disease. The number of cases increases with age. Parkinson affects 1% of the population aged over 65 years, and this proportion increases to 2% in those aged 70 years and older. Although Parkinson disease can also occur in younger people, there may be some differences in the symptoms that people in this age group experience.

What are the Symptoms of Parkinson Disease?

Parkinson disease is clinically characterized by the following motor symptoms:

- Resting tremor (shaking back and forth when the limb is relaxed)
- Rigidity (stiffness, or resistance of the limb to passive movement)
- Postural instability (poor balance)
- Bradykinesia (slowness of movement)

Other motor symptoms include:

- Micrographia (smaller handwriting)
- Hypophonia (softening of the voice)
- Hypomimia (mask-like face with little expression)
- Shuffling gait
- Freezing of gait

Parkinson Disease – A Health Policy Perspective. Edited by Wayne Martin, Oksana Suchowersky,
Katharina Kovacs Burns, and Egon Jonsson
Copyright © 2010 WILEY-VCH Verlag GmbH & Co. KGaA, Weinheim
ISBN: 978-3-527-32779-9

- Dystonia (sustained contraction of muscles)
- Dysphagia (difficulty swallowing)

What Are the Non-Motor Symptoms of Parkinson Disease?

Many people with Parkinson disease experience a spectrum of other symptoms outside of the motor system. These may be related to the pathophysiology of the disease. Further research is being carried out to identify the specific causes of non-motor symptoms in Parkinson. Some non-motor symptoms include:

- Depression
- Weight loss
- Apathy
- Hallucinations
- Sleep disturbances
- Social dysfunction
- Memory loss
- Impairment in decision-making and executive function
- Fatigue
- Sweating disturbances
- Constipation
- Disturbed smell and taste

How is Parkinson Disease Diagnosed?

The diagnosis of Parkinson disease is made through assessment of the following:

- Clinical evaluation
- Patient history
- Neurologic examination
- Response to dopamine replacement therapy

Who Treats People with Parkinson Disease?

Typically, once a diagnosis of Parkinson disease is suspected, the patient's family physician will refer them to a neurologist who specializes in the care of Parkinson disease and other related disorders. Other allied health professionals, such as nurses, speech language pathologists, occupational therapists, and physiotherapists are also involved in helping the Parkinson patient manage his or her symptoms.

How is Parkinson Disease Treated?

There are many different treatments for the various symptoms and side effects of Parkinson disease, including:

- Medication
  - Six classes of medication are available to treat the primary symptoms of Parkinson.
  - Levodopa remains the most effective medicine to date for treating symptoms. It is always combined with another medication, such as carbidopa or benserazide to prevent the rapid breakdown of levodopa in the digestive system.
- Neurosurgery
  - Pallidotomies, which involve lesioning the globus pallidus (a part of the brain), have been used to improve dyskinesia.
  - Deep brain stimulation, which involves the implantation of a medical device called a brain pacemaker, has also been established as an effective treatment for cardinal motor symptoms.
- Other therapies
  - Physiotherapists and occupational therapists can help patients with Parkinson maintain their motor skills and adapt to physical challenges.
  - Speech language pathologists can help patients prevent and adapt to hypophonia.
- Alternative approaches (massage, chiropractic treatment, acupuncture, osteopathy, homeopathy, reflexology).
  - Some patients have found these therapies beneficial in helping to manage symptoms. However, there is not enough evidence in place to demonstrate their safety and efficacy.

What Other Support Services Are Available?

Various support groups and services are available through community non-profit Parkinson Disease Societies. Community organizations have a significant role to play in assisting people living with Parkinson's and their families or caregivers, with information on the disease, services in the community and through the healthcare system, and other social supports. Persons with Parkinson disease need the support of different medical, health, allied health, social and community professionals. The progressive nature of Parkinson disease calls for planned, proactive treatments and continuing supports.

There are two non-profit Parkinson Disease Societies in Alberta for people to contact:

- The Parkinson Society of Alberta in Edmonton.
- The Parkinson Society of Southern Alberta in Calgary.

Appendix B: Glossary of Terms

Action tremor: A tremor that occurs or increases during voluntary movement.

Adjunctive: Supplemental or secondary (but not essential) treatment.

Adverse event: Injury to the patient resulting from a medical intervention; a side effect.

Agonist: A chemical or drug that mimics the activity of a neurotransmitter such as dopamine.

Akathisia: A compelling need to be in constant motion (rocking, fidgeting, pacing) and feeling inner restlessness. This is often a side effect of neuroleptic (antipsychotic drugs).

Akinesia: Impaired initiation of movement, or the inability to move (i.e., "freezing").

Age/gender-standardized: A statistical technique used when the study population does not have the same age or gender distribution as the entire population. For example: When you age-standardize the prevalence of PD, you estimate the number of people in the actual population with PD by using the rate of PD in the study population for each age group, and then apply the rate to the actual population.

Ambulation: The act of traveling by foot; walking.

Amantadine (Tradename: Symmetrel): An antiparkinsonian medication which improves PD symptoms by stimulating the release of available dopamine in the brain. It may be used early in the disease, or added to levodopa.

Anticholinergics: Drugs that block acetylcholine, a neurotransmitter that has opposing effects to dopamine. By blocking acetylcholine's action, these drugs increase dopamine's ability to control movement.

Autonomic nervous system: The part of the nervous system that controls involuntary body functions, such as heart rate, blood pressure, intestinal movements, and temperature control.

Parkinson Disease – A Health Policy Perspective. Edited by Wayne Martin, Oksana Suchowersky,
Katharina Kovacs Burns, and Egon Jonsson
Copyright © 2010 WILEY-VCH Verlag GmbH & Co. KGaA, Weinheim
ISBN: 978-3-527-32779-9

Autonomic dysfunction (or autonomic disturbances or autonomic failure): Dysfunction or failure of the autonomic nervous system. Autonomic dysfunction may result in dizzy spells, urinary incontinence, constipation, sweating and flushing, sexual dysfunction, drooling, and other problems.

Aspiration: Accidental sucking in of food particles or fluids into the lungs.

Atypical neuroleptics (also known as atypical antipsychotics): Atypical neuroleptics tend to have fewer side effects than "typical neuroleptics." Neuroleptics block dopamine receptors, and are usually prescribed to treat psychiatric symptoms.

Basal ganglia: A group of nerve cells, located at the base of the brain, responsible for initiating and regulating movements. Basal ganglia function is abnormal in people with PD.

Bradykinesia: Abnormal slowness of movement; one of the main symptoms of PD.

Carbidopa: A drug that is combined with levodopa, in order to block the breakdown of levodopa in the intestinal tract and in the blood. It can also reduce the side effects of levodopa, such as nausea.

Case-control study: A study where a group of people with a disease are matched with a group of healthy people with similar age, gender, and other characteristics. The two groups are compared to see if a particular risk factor is more common in one group than the other. For example, eight out 40 people with PD might have been exposed to a particular chemical, whereas only two out of 40 healthy people were exposed. Thus, it appears there is a connection between the chemical and PD. These studies are generally considered to be weak because they can be easily biased, and should be followed-up with more rigorous methods.

Catechol-*O*-methyl transferase (COMT) inhibitors: A class of antiparkinsonian drugs that blocks the enzyme catchol-*O*-methyltransferase (COMT), which prevents the breakdown of levodopa in the intestinal tract. This allows more levodopa to cross into the blood, and then into the brain. Entacapone (Comtan) is the most widely used.

Cholinesterase inhibitors (also known as acetylcholinesterase inhibitors): A class of drugs used to treat mild to moderate dementia in PD. These drugs increase the brain levels of a neurotransmitter called acetylcholine, which helps neurons communicate with each other in relation to memory, learning, and thinking.

Cohort study: The people in a study are assembled into two groups according to exposure or lack of exposure, and then followed over time to determine outcome. For example, a group of smokers and a group of non-smokers are followed for five years to see how many in each group develop PD.

Colostomy: A surgical procedure that results in a portion of the large intestine being brought through the abdominal wall in order to carry stool out of the body.

Comorbidities: The coexistence of two or more diseases.

Construct validity: A test or instrument has construct validity if it actually measures what it is intended to measure. For example, does PDQ-39 actually measure the quality of life, or is it possible that someone could feel they have a high quality of life but score poorly on the PDQ-39?

95% Confidence intervals (CI): A way of stating the error associated with a number. Essentially, there is a 95 % probability that the "true" number (e.g., the effect of treatment in the whole population) lies within the range of numbers given as the confidence interval.

Cross-sectional study: A study in which disease and exposure are measured simultaneously (e.g., Parkinson disease and caffeine consumption). This type of study can discover relationships between diseases and exposures, but because the study represents only one moment in time it is impossible to identify cause and effect relationships. In other words, if it is discovered that people with PD have a lower than average caffeine consumption, it cannot be determined whether a high caffeine consumption has a protective effect against PD, or if people with PD simply drink fewer caffeinated drinks due to some aspect of the disease; for example, it might make a symptom worse or it may become too much of a bother to make coffee.

Daytime somnolence: Un-natural daytime sleepiness or drowsiness.

Deep-brain stimulation (DBS): A surgical method used in some patients with PD whose motor fluctuations are not being satisfactorily controlled with medication. Permanent electrodes are implanted in specific areas of the brain, and deliver electrical stimulation to block the abnormal nerve signals that cause tremor and PD symptoms. The electrodes are connected to a programmable power source inserted in the chest wall (similar to a cardiac pacemaker).

Dopamine: A chemical produced by the brain, which assists in the effective transmission of messages from one nerve cell to the next. Dopamine helps to control movement, balance and walking. A lack of dopamine is the primary cause of Parkinsonian motor symptoms.

Dopamine (or dopaminergic) agonists: Drugs that mimic the effects of dopamine and stimulate the dopamine receptors in nerve cells. They may be used by themselves, or in combination with levodopa.

Dopamine receptors: The area of the nerve cell in the striatum that receives the dopamine message from the substantia nigra.

Diplopia: Commonly known as "double vision." With diplopia, two images are perceived of a single object. The images may be displaced horizontally, vertically or diagonally (both vertically and horizontally) in relation to each other.

Dysarthria: Difficulty pronouncing words; muffled speech.

Dysautonomia: *see* **Autonomic dysfunction**

Dyskinesia: Abnormal involuntary movement that is frequently induced by medications taken by Parkinson patients.

Dysphagia: Difficulty swallowing. This common problem in PD increases the risk of inhaling food or liquids into the airways. In its later stages it can lead to a condition known as "aspiration pneumonia."

Dystonia: A type of dyskinesia that causes abnormal postures, twisting body motions. It may be a side effect of long-term drug treatment in PD, or due to the levodopa dose being too low.

Dysesthesia: A condition in which touch is distorted. Dysesthesia can cause an ordinary stimulus to be unpleasant or painful.

Dyspnea: Difficult or painful breathing; shortness of breath.

Epidemiology: The study of the patterns, causes, distribution and control of disease in groups of people.

Etiology: The cause, or the study of the causes, of a disease.

External validity: A study's results have external validity if they are true in the "outside world," and not just for the study population. For example, if 25% of PD patients in a study testing a new antiparkinsonian drug vastly improved on the drug, this should mean that 25% of ALL PD patients will also have a good reaction. This may not be the case if there is a confounding factor, for example if the study had too-few patients, the patients were not representative of most people with Parkinson (they may have been younger or better educated, or were institutionalized), or some other form of bias was introduced into the study.

Freezing of gait: Temporary, involuntary inability to take a step or initiate walking; the person essentially feels "stuck" to the ground. It is a common symptom of advanced PD, and can lead to falls and loss of mobility.

Globus pallidus: A structure of nerve cells in the corpus striatum (part of the basal ganglia) that is involved in movement. It is targeted during pallidotomy or deep-brain stimulation.

Hoehn & Yahr scale: A system used to categorize the severity of PD into five stages: stage 0 means no symptoms, while stage 5 means the most severe disease stage.

Hypokinesia: A clinical term for the slow or diminished movement associated with PD.

Hypophonia: An abnormally soft voice.

Idiopathic Parkinson disease: PD with unknown cause. Genetically related PD is included in this group. This differs from Parkinsonism caused by exposure to toxins or drugs.

Incidence: The number of newly diagnosed cases of a disease during a specific time period. The incidence is distinct from the prevalence, which refers to the number of cases alive on a certain date.

Levodopa (also know as L-dopa): The most commonly administered and most effective drug to treat PD. After administration, levodopa is converted into dopamine, which in turn raise the levels of dopamine in the brain. It produces an effective control of PD symptoms, although its long-term use may be associated with complications.

Lewy bodies: Abnormal protein clumps that accumulate in dead or dying dopamine-producing cells of the substantia nigra in PD. At autopsy, the presence of Lewy bodies is used to confirm a PD diagnosis.

Medically refractory: Resistant to treatment.

Micrographia: Small cramped handwriting that is a symptom of many PD patients.

Monoamine oxidase-B (MAO-B) inhibitors: A class of drugs that stop dopamine from being broken down in the brain. They can be used by themselves in patients with mild PD, or added to levodopa to help ease motor fluctuations.

Morbidity: The presence of a disease or illness. Also expresses the rate of incidence of a disease.

Mortality: A measure of deaths in a given population during a specified time period.

Motor fluctuations: When the PD patient's movement control switches between good and bad.

Neurotransmitter: A biochemical substance (such as dopamine, acetylcholine, or norepinephrine) that carries impulses from one nerve cell to another.

Nocturia: The need to wake up at night in order to urinate.

Non-motor symptoms: These are problems related to PD other than movement. They include cognitive impairment, autonomic dysfunction, sleep problems, and depression. They typically do not respond to dopamine replacement therapy.

Orthostatic hypotension: A drop in blood pressure usually due to rapid changes in body position, such as standing up.

On–off phenomenon: Fluctuations that occur in response to levodopa therapy, in which the person's mobility changes suddenly and unpredictably from a good response (on) to a poor response (off).

Palliative care: Care that focuses on reducing the symptoms of a disease rather than curing it.

Pallidotomy: The surgical destruction of a small group of cells in the internal globus pallidus, the major area from which information leaves the basal ganglia, in order to relieve dyskinesias and other symptoms of advanced PD. Deep-brain stimulation has mostly replaced this surgery in current practice.

Peripheral neuropathy: Condition that causes pain and numbness in the hands and feet.

Positron emission tomography (PET): An imaging method that allows the brain function to be visualized following the injection of a radioactive tracer.

Postural instability: Problems with keeping steady body positions during standing, sitting upright, or walking.

Prevalence: The number of people in a population who have a disease at a given time (frequency).

Prognosis: A forecast of the expected future course of a disease.

Putamen: Part of the basal ganglia.

P-value: A statistical term that measures the probability that the difference in outcome between two groups (e.g., the group receiving a drug and one receiving a placebo) happened by chance. The lower the P-value, the more likely it is that the difference was caused by the treatment.

Quality of Life: A person's sense of well being, self-perceived health status and ability to carry out activities of daily living.

Quality-Adjusted Life Years (QALY): A year of life adjusted for its quality or its value. A year in perfect health is equal to 1.0 QALY. The value of a year in ill health is discounted. For example, a year bedridden might have a value equal to 0.5 QALY.

Randomized Controlled Trial (RCT): An experimental study where people are randomly assigned to an intervention (e.g., given a drug) or a control group (e.g., not given drug or given a placebo). The groups are assessed at the end to compare which group has the better outcome. The study may also be "blinded" – that is, the participants and/or healthcare providers do not know who is in what group – in order to reduce the potential of bias.

Resting tremor: Shaking back and forth when the limb is relaxed.

Rigidity: Stiffness or resistance to passive movement of a limb. This is one of the four main clinical features of PD.

Risk factor: Something that increases a person's chances of developing a disease.

Schwab & England disability scale: Scale that rates the level of independence of a person with PD. A value of 100% relates to total independence, while 0% indicates a state of complete dependence.

Seborrhea: An increased discharge of the oily secretion sebum from the sebaceous glands of the skin.

Selegiline: A type of MAO-B inhibitor.

Substantia nigra: The area of the brain where dopamine is produced. In PD, the loss of nerve cells from this region leads to a dopamine deficit and subsequently to PD symptoms.

Subthalamic nucleus (STN): A nerve center near the substantia nigra. The STN may be targeted for deep-brain stimulation to reduce PD symptoms.

Striatum: An area of the brain that controls movement, walking, and balance. The largest component of the basal ganglia, it receives connections from the substantia nigra and contains the dopamine receptors.

Thalamotomy: A surgical procedure which now is much less frequently performed, in which cells in the thalamus (part of the brain) are destroyed in an effort to eradicate debilitating tremors.

Thermal paresthesias: An abnormal sensation of warmth or cold in different parts of the body, experienced by some PD patients.

Unified Parkinson Disease Rating Scale Motor Examination (UPDRS): A scoring system that is used to follow the progression of PD by monitoring a patient's physical and mental abilities, and their response to treatment.

Validity: Truth.

Wearing off: Waning of the effect of the last dose of levodopa, associated with a loss of mobility and movement.

A number of sources were used to compile this glossary.

National Parkinson Foundation Glossary of terms: http://www.parkinson.org/NETCOMMUNITY/Page.aspx?pid=231&srcid=482

Parkinsons-disease.info Glossary: http://www.parkinsons-disease.info/glossary/ MedicineNet.com Glossary of Terms: http://www.medicinenet.com/parkinsons_disease/glossary.htm

Michael J. Fox Foundation Glossary: http://www.michaeljfox.org/living_additionalResources_glossary.cfm

American Parkinson Disease Association Glossary: http://www.parkinsonsapda.org/glossary.html

NCI Dictionary of Cancer Terms (For general terms): http://www.cancer.gov/dictionary/

Index

Parkinson Disease – A Health Policy Perspective. Edited by Wayne Martin, Oksana Suchowersky,
Katharina Kovacs Burns, and Egon Jonsson
Copyright © 2010 WILEY-VCH Verlag GmbH & Co. KGaA, Weinheim
ISBN: 978-3-527-32779-9